MTP International Review of Science

Physiology
Series One

Consultant Editor
A. C. Guyton

Publisher's Note

The MTP International Review of Science is an important new venture in scientific publishing, which is presented by Butterworths in association with MTP Medical and Technical Publishing Co. Ltd. and University Park Press, Baltimore. The basic concept of the Review is to provide regular authoritative reviews of entire disciplines. Chemistry was taken first as the problems of literature survey are probably more acute in this subject than in any other. Physiology and Biochemistry followed naturally. As a matter of policy, the authorship of the MTP Review of Science is international and distinguished, the subject coverage is extensive, systematic and critical, and most important of all, it is intended that new issues of the Review will be published at regular intervals.

In the MTP Review of Chemistry (Series One), Inorganic, Physical and Organic Chemistry are comprehensively reviewed in 33 text volumes and 3 index volumes. Physiology (Series One) consists of 8 volumes and Biochemistry (Series One) 12 volumes, each volume individually indexed. Details follow. In general, the Chemistry (Series One) reviews cover the period 1967 to 1971, and Physiology and Biochemistry (Series One) reviews up to 1972. It is planned to start in 1974 the MTP International Review of Science (Series Two), consisting of a similar set of volumes covering developments in a two year period.

The MTP International Review of Science has been conceived within a carefully organised editorial framework. The overall plan was drawn up, and the volume editors appointed by seven consultant editors. In turn, each volume editor planned the coverage of his field and appointed authors to write on subjects which were within the area of their own research experience. No geographical restriction was imposed. Hence the 500 or so contributions to the MTP Review of Science come from many countries of the world and provide an authoritative account of progress.

Butterworth & Co. (Publishers) Ltd.

PHYSIOLOGY
SERIES ONE

Consultant Editors
A. C. Guyton,
*Department of Physiology and
Biophysics, University of Mississippi
Medical Center* and
D. Horrobin,
*Department of Medical Physiology,
University College of Nairobi*

Volume titles and Editors

1 CARDIOVASCULAR PHYSIOLOGY
Professor A. C. Guyton and Dr. C. E. Jones,
University of Mississippi Medical Center

2 RESPIRATORY PHYSIOLOGY
Professor J. G. Widdicombe, *St. George's
Hospital, London*

3 NEUROPHYSIOLOGY
Professor C. C. Hunt, *Washington
University School of Medicine, St. Louis*

4 GASTROINTESTINAL PHYSIOLOGY
Professor E. D. Jacobson and Dr. L. L.
Shanbour, *University of Texas Medical
School*

5 ENDOCRINE PHYSIOLOGY
Professor S. M. McCann, *University of
Texas*

6 KIDNEY AND URINARY TRACT
PHYSIOLOGY
Professor K. Thurau, *University of Munich*

7 ENVIRONMENTAL PHYSIOLOGY
Professor D. Robertshaw, *University
of Nairobi*

8 REPRODUCTIVE PHYSIOLOGY
Professor R. O. Greep, *Harvard Medical
School*

BIOCHEMISTRY
SERIES ONE

Consultant Editors
H. L. Kornberg, F.R.S.
*Department of Biochemistry
University of Leicester* and
D. C. Phillips, F.R.S., *Department of
Zoology, University of Oxford*

Volume titles and Editors

1 CHEMISTRY OF MACRO-
MOLECULES
Professor H. Gutfreund, *University of
Bristol*

2 BIOCHEMISTRY OF CELL WALLS
AND MEMBRANES
Dr. C. F. Fox, *University of California*

3 ENERGY TRANSDUCING
MECHANISMS
Professor E. Racker, *Cornell University,
New York*

4 BIOCHEMISTRY OF LIPIDS
Professor T. W. Goodwin, F.R.S.,
University of Liverpool

5 BIOCHEMISTRY OF CARBO-
HYDRATES
Professor W. J. Whelan, *University
of Miami*

6 BIOCHEMISTRY OF NUCLEIC
ACIDS
Professor K. Burton, F.R.S., *University of
Newcastle upon Tyne*

7 SYNTHESIS OF AMINO ACIDS
AND PROTEINS
Professor H. R. V. Arnstein, *King's
College, University of London*

8 BIOCHEMISTRY OF HORMONES
Professor H. V. Rickenberg, *National
Jewish Hospital & Research Center,
Colorado*

9 BIOCHEMISTRY OF CELL DIFFER-
ENTIATION
Dr. J. Paul, *The Beatson Institute
for Cancer Research, Glasgow*

10 DEFENCE AND RECOGNITION
Professor R. R. Porter, F.R.S., *University
of Oxford*

11 PLANT BIOCHEMISTRY
Professor D. H. Northcote, F.R.S.,
University of Cambridge

12 PHYSIOLOGICAL AND PHARMACO-
LOGICAL BIOCHEMISTRY
Dr. H. F. K. Blaschko, F.R.S., *University
of Oxford*

INORGANIC CHEMISTRY SERIES ONE

Consultant Editor
H. J. Emeléus, F.R.S.
Department of Chemistry
University of Cambridge

Volume titles and Editors

1 **MAIN GROUP ELEMENTS—HYDROGEN AND GROUPS I-IV**
Professor M. F. Lappert,
University of Sussex

2 **MAIN GROUP ELEMENTS—GROUPS V AND VI**
Professor C. C. Addison,
F.R.S. and Dr. D. B.
Sowerby, *University of Nottingham*

3 **MAIN GROUP ELEMENTS—GROUP VII AND NOBLE GASES**
Professor Viktor Gutmann,
Technical University of Vienna

4 **ORGANOMETALLIC DERIVATIVES OF THE MAIN GROUP ELEMENTS**
Dr. B. J. Aylett, *Westfield College, University of London*

5 **TRANSITION METALS— PART 1**
Professor D. W. A. Sharp,
University of Glasgow

6 **TRANSITION METALS— PART 2**
Dr. M. J. Mays, *University of Cambridge*

7 **LANTHANIDES AND ACTINIDES**
Professor K. W. Bagnall,
University of Manchester

8 **RADIOCHEMISTRY**
Dr. A. G. Maddock,
University of Cambridge

9 **REACTION MECHANISMS IN INORGANIC CHEMISTRY**
Professor M. L. Tobe,
University College,
University of London

10 **SOLID STATE CHEMISTRY**
Dr. L. E. J. Roberts, *Atomic Energy Research Establishment, Harwell*

INDEX VOLUME

PHYSICAL CHEMISTRY SERIES ONE

Consultant Editor
A. D. Buckingham
Department of Chemistry
University of Cambridge

Volume titles and Editors

1 **THEORETICAL CHEMISTRY**
Professor W. Byers Brown,
University of Manchester

2 **MOLECULAR STRUCTURE AND PROPERTIES**
Professor G. Allen,
University of Manchester

3 **SPECTROSCOPY**
Dr. D. A. Ramsay, F.R.S.C.,
National Research Council of Canada

4 **MAGNETIC RESONANCE**
Professor C. A. McDowell,
F.R.S.C., *University of British Columbia*

5 **MASS SPECTROMETRY**
Professor A. Maccoll,
University College,
University of London

6 **ELECTROCHEMISTRY**
Professor J. O'M Bockris,
University of Pennsylvania

7 **SURFACE CHEMISTRY AND COLLOIDS**
Professor M. Kerker,
Clarkson College of Technology, New York

8 **MACROMOLECULAR SCIENCE**
Professor C. E. H. Bawn,
F.R.S., *University of Liverpool*

9 **CHEMICAL KINETICS**
Professor J. C. Polanyi, F.R.S.,
University of Toronto

10 **THERMOCHEMISTRY AND THERMO- DYNAMICS**
Dr. H. A. Skinner, *University of Manchester*

11 **CHEMICAL CRYSTALLOGRAPHY**
Professor J. Monteath
Robertson, F.R.S., *University of Glasgow*

12 **ANALYTICAL CHEMISTRY —PART 1**
Professor T. S. West,
Imperial College, University of London

13 **ANALYTICAL CHEMISTRY —PART 2**
Professor T. S. West,
Imperial College, University of London

INDEX VOLUME

ORGANIC CHEMISTRY SERIES ONE

Consultant Editor
D. H. Hey, F.R.S.,
Department of Chemistry
King's College, University of London

Volume titles and Editors

1 **STRUCTURE DETERMINATION IN ORGANIC CHEMISTRY**
Professor W. D. Ollis, F.R.S.,
University of Sheffield

2 **ALIPHATIC COMPOUNDS**
Professor N. B. Chapman,
Hull University

3 **AROMATIC COMPOUNDS**
Professor H. Zollinger, *Swiss Federal Institute of Technology*

4 **HETEROCYCLIC COMPOUNDS**
Dr. K. Schofield, *University of Exeter*

5 **ALICYCLIC COMPOUNDS**
Professor W. Parker,
University of Stirling

6 **AMINO ACIDS, PEPTIDES AND RELATED COMPOUNDS**
Professor D. H. Hey, F.R.S.,
and Dr. D. I. John, *King's College, University of London*

7 **CARBOHYDRATES**
Professor G. O. Aspinall,
Trent University, Ontario

8 **STEROIDS**
Dr. W. F. Johns, *G. D. Searle & Co., Chicago*

9 **ALKALOIDS**
Professor K. Wiesner, F.R.S.,
University of New Brunswick

10 **FREE RADICAL REACTIONS**
Professor W. A. Waters,
F.R.S., *University of Oxford*

INDEX VOLUME

MTP International Review of Science

Physiology
Series One

Volume 5
Endocrine Physiology

Edited by **S. M. McCann**
University of Texas

Butterworths · London
University Park Press · Baltimore

THE BUTTERWORTH GROUP

ENGLAND
Butterworth & Co (Publishers) Ltd
London: 88 Kingsway, WC2B 6AB

AUSTRALIA
Butterworths Pty Ltd
Sydney: 586 Pacific Highway 2067
Melbourne: 343 Little Collins Street, 3000
Brisbane: 240 Queen Street, 4000

NEW ZEALAND
Butterworths of New Zealand Ltd
Wellington: 26–28 Waring Taylor Street, 1

SOUTH AFRICA
Butterworth & Co (South Africa) (Pty) Ltd
Durban: 152–154 Gale Street

ISBN 0 408 70485 3

UNIVERSITY PARK PRESS

U.S.A. and CANADA
University Park Press
Chamber of Commerce Building
Baltimore, Maryland, 21202

Library of Congress Cataloging in Publication Data

McCann, Samuel McDonald, 1925–
  Endocrine physiology.

  (Physiology, series one, v. 5) (MTP international
  review of science)
  1. Endocrinology. I. Title. II. Series.
III. Series: MTP international review of science.
[DNLM: 1. Endocrine glands—Physiology. 2.
Hormones—Physiology. W1PH951D v. 5 1974/
WK102 E56 1974]
QP1.P62 vol. 5 [QP187]   599'.01'08s   [599'.01'42]
ISBN 0–8391–1054–5   74–2264

First Published 1974 and © 1974
MTP MEDICAL AND TECHNICAL PUBLISHING CO LTD
St Leonard's House
St Leonardgate
Lancaster, Lancs
and
BUTTERWORTH & CO (PUBLISHERS) LTD

Typeset and printed in Great Britain by
REDWOOD BURN LIMITED
Trowbridge & Esher
and bound by R. J. Acford Ltd, Chichester, Sussex

Consultant Editor's Note

The International Review of Physiology, a review with a new format, is hopefully also new in concept. But before discussing the new concept, those of us who are joined in making this review a success must admit that we asked ourselves at the outset: Why should we promote a new review of physiology? Not that there is a paucity of reviews already, and not that the present reviews fail to fill important roles, because they do. Therefore, what could be the role of an additional review?

The International Review of Physiology has the same goals as all other reviews for accuracy, timeliness, and completeness, but it has new policies that we hope and believe will engender still other important qualities that are often elusive in reviews, the qualities of critical evaluation and instructiveness. The first decision toward achieving these goals was to design the new format, one that will allow publication of approximately 2500 pages per edition, divided into eight different sub-speciality volumes, each organised by experts in their respective fields. It is clear that this extensiveness of coverage will allow consideration of each subject in far greater depth than has been possible in the past. To make this review as timely as possible, a new edition of all eight volumes will be published every two years giving a cycle time that will keep the articles current. And in addition to the short cycle time, the publishers have arranged to produce each volume within only a few months after the articles themselves have been completed, thus further enhancing the immediate value of each author's contribution.

Yet, perhaps the greatest hope that this new review will achieve its goals of critical evaluation and instructiveness lies in its editorial policies. A simple but firm request has been made to each author that he utilise his expertise and his judgement to sift from the mass of biennial publications those new facts and concepts that are important to the progress of physiology; that he make a conscientious effort not to write a review consisting of annotated lists of references; and that the important material he does choose be presented in thoughtful and logical exposition, complete enough to convey full understanding and also woven into context with previously established physiological principles. Hopefully, these processes will bring to the reader each two years a treatise that he will use not merely as a reference in his own personal field but also as an exercise in refreshing and modernising his whole body of physiological knowledge.

Mississippi   A. C. Guyton

Preface

The purpose of this volume on endocrine physiology is to present comprehensive reviews of nearly all aspects of the subject. Sufficient background information will be presented so as to make the review understandable to the reader new to the subject and yet the latest research will be discussed so that the reviews will be useful to the specialist in the field as well.

Endocrinology has developed along with the rest of the biological sciences making use of advances in physics, chemistry and mathematics. There have been notable breakthroughs in recent years. Perhaps the most noteworthy is the development of radioimmunoassay which has made possible the accurate measurement of minute amounts of hormones in body fluids. Although a separate chapter is not devoted to this methodology, much new information has been discovered or quantitated using this new technique.

Since the endocrine system represents a means by which the nervous system can control internal processes, the book begins with the consideration of a gland completely under neural control, namely the neurohypophysis. It then moves on to a consideration of the hypothalamic releasing and inhibiting hormones. Although it has been realised for some time that the anterior lobe of the pituitary was under neural control, the discovery, purification, isolation and synthesis of hypothalamic peptides which specifically stimulate and inhibit anterior pituitary hormone release has been one of the most exciting chapters of recent endocrinology. We then pass on to consideration of pituitary-target gland relationships with chapters on the pituitary-thyroid, pituitary-adrenal systems. The pituitary secretes growth hormone which has as a target general body tissues, and this hormone is the topic of a separate chapter. We continue with the consideration of hormones which effect metabolism by discussing the pancreas as a regulator of metabolism. Because of lack of space we will concentrate on the hormone from the a-cells, glucagon, and its interrelationship with the well known hormone from the β-cells, insulin. There is also an endocrine control over mineral metabolism, and we will first consider the hormonal control of salt and water excretion and then pass on to the parathyroid and thyroid as controllers of mineral metabolism. Very recently the pineal gland has come into its own as a regulator of endocrine function and a separate chapter is therefore devoted to the rapid and recent advances in pineal physiology. Lastly, recent events have brought a revolution in our concept of the mechanism of hormonal action. The most dramatic advance has been the realisation that cyclic-AMP is a second messenger which mediates many hormonal effects in diverse tissues. Consequently, we have allocated a separate chapter to the cyclic-AMP story.

It is hoped that at frequent intervals the subject of endocrinology can be brought up to date with additional reviews of this type.

Dallas   S. M. McCann

Contents

1
The Neurohypophysis

L. SHARE and C. E. GROSVENOR
The University of Tennessee Medical Units

1.1 INTRODUCTION

Although the evidence points to the conclusion that, in general, the supraoptic and paraventricular nuclei are involved in the production and release of
vasopressin and oxytocin respectively[1,2], there is a long-standing controversy
as to whether the neurohypophysis can release oxytocin independently of
vasopressin and vice versa. The minute by minute control of osmotic pressure
of the blood requires the release of small amounts of vasopressin over rather
long periods of time; the release of oxytocin, on the other hand, is abundant
and intermittent. Whereas volume and osmoreceptors monitor the plasma
continuously and in turn translate any changes into either the need for
release or shut-off of release of vasopressin, oxytocin release, as far as is
known, is not regulated by alterations in any plasma constituent. The release
of oxytocin apparently occurs only in response to neurogenic stimuli, e.g.
suckling, cervical stretch.

Various stimuli evoke simultaneous, though not necessarily synchronous,
release of both hormones. For example, an antidiuretic response is frequently
but not always recorded after suckling or after electrical stimulation of the
mammary nerve endings[1,2]. The proportions of the two hormones which are
released, however, vary with the stimulus, with oxytocin usually secreted in
the greater amount. The vasopressin-oxytocin ratio in the blood has been
recorded after suckling as 1:100 in the rabbit[3] and 1:30 in the dog[4]. After
stimulation of the supraoptico-hypophysial tract the vasopressin:oxytocin
ratio has been recorded as 1:5[5] and following intracarotid injections of hypertonic saline in the dog the ratio has been recorded as 1:20[6]. Some authors
have reported a selective fall in the oxytocin content in the neurohypophysis
of lactating animals[7,8] while other authors have detected no change[9,10]. In
contrast, oxytocin and vasopressin are liberated in large but fairly equal
amounts during labour[11], and during severe acute haemorrhage in rats and
cats large amounts of vasopressin are liberated without equivalent amounts
of oxytocin[12-14].

The functions of vasopressin and oxytocin appear so different in kind, in
spite of the intimate anatomical association and chemical similarity of the
two hormones, that we have chosen, in much of the discussion which follows,
to treat them as two quite separate entities.

1.2 BIOSYNTHESIS

It was early postulated, by Scharrer and by Bargmann[15] that vasopressin
(ADH) and oxytocin are synthesised in the supraoptic and paraventricular
nuclei of the hypothalamus, packaged into membrane bounded neurosecretory granules, and transported down the axons of the hypothalamo-neurohypophysial tract to the neurohypophysis for storage and release. Evidence
important for the confirmation of this hypothesis, and indeed most of our
current information concerning the biosynthesis of ADH, is found in the well
designed, meticulous experiments of Sachs and his associates (for review, see
Reference 16). First, when ^{35}S-labelled cysteine was infused into anaesthetised
dogs, the specific activity of ADH isolated from the hypothalamus was
several times that of the hormone obtained from the posterior pituitary, and
when the stalk was sectioned, no labelled ADH appeared in the neural
lobe[16]. Second, the isolated hypothalamus–median eminence complex of the
guinea-pig can synthesise ADH *de novo* when incubated under appropriate
conditions[17]. The isolated posterior pituitary, incubated under the same conditions, is unable to synthesise ADH.
     Sachs has proposed[18] that ADH is synthesised on ribosomes in a biologically
inactive form, as part of a precursor molecule, and that biologically active
ADH appears during the formation and maturation of the neurosecretory
granules, possibly in the Golgi region of the cell body. This hypothesis is
based upon: the intracellular distribution of labelled ADH following the
infusion of labelled amino acids[19], the inhibition of ADH biosynthesis by
puromycin[18], evidence for a lag period in the biosynthesis of ADH, and the
fact that puromycin can inhibit only the initial synthetic events[18]. ADH
biosynthesis is to some extent under physiological control. Thus, a chronic
stimulus for increased ADH release, such as dehydration, resulted in an
increased rate of ADH synthesis[17]. An acute stimulus such as haemorrhage,
however, was without effect[16]. Recently, Sachs *et al.*[20] have been able to maintain fragments of guinea-pig hypothalamus in organ culture. Incorporation
of labelled amino acids into ADH could be demonstrated for periods of
up to 12 days. This incorporation could be blocked by inhibitors of protein
synthesis.
     Although there have been no similar studies of the biosynthesis of oxytocin,
it is presumed that the biosynthesis of this hormone follows a pathway similar
to that for ADH.

1.3 NEUROPHYSIN

The neurohypophysial hormones within the neurosecretory granules are
found in association with a family of small proteins, the neurophysins[21], with
molecular weights of approximately 10,000[22,23]. Three neurophysins have
been found in each of the following: the ox[24], the pig[25], the rat[26] and sheep[27].
In man two neurophysins have been identified to date[22]. Evidence derived
from differential centrifugation of homogenates of posterior lobes[28], release
patterns of neurophysin, ADH and oxytocin[29,30], and the study of the rat with
hereditary diabetes insipidus[31] suggests that oxytocin may be largely associated with neurophysin I and ADH with neurophysin II. Based upon the

properties of neurophysin, it is generally presumed that the neurohypophysial hormones are bound to neurophysin within the posterior pituitary. Although ADH and oxytocin are released from the neurohypophysis together with neurophysin *in vivo*[28a,29,30,32,33] and *in vitro*[32-36], it is unlikely that these hormones are bound to neurophysin in the blood, since the pH optimum for this binding is 5.2–5.8, and the binding is decreased with dilution[37].

Neurophysin apparently functions to retain ADH and oxytocin within the axon endings of the posterior pituitary until the arrival of a stimulus for release. Neurophysin secreted into the blood, however, has no known function.

1.4 MECHANISMS OF RELEASE

The neurosecretory cells have electrophysiological properties common to other neurones[38]. Oxytocin and ADH are released from the posterior pituitary when the membranes of the axon terminals are depolarised due to the arrival of an action potential[39,41].

The coupling of stimulus to secretion requires calcium[39,40]. There are currently two general theories for the mechanism by which this coupling is achieved. In one, advanced by Ginsburg and Ireland[42] and by Thorn[43], Ca^{2+}, which diffuses into the axon ending when its membrane depolarises, dissociates hormone from neurophysin in the axoplasm. The free hormone then diffuses across the cell membrane into the blood. Consistent with this concept are the observations that a portion of the neurophysin-bound hormone is in the axoplasm, outside of the neurosecretory granules[42], and that there is a readily releasable pool, presumably the extragranular moiety, of ADH within the posterior pituitary[43,44].

The second theory, proposed by Douglas and Poisner[39], is more in keeping with current information. In this view, ADH and oxytocin are released by exocytosis. This is supported by the observations that neurophysin is released with ADH and oxytocin[29-36] and the identification of exocytotic figures in electron micrographs of the posterior pituitary[44,45].

1.5 CONTROL OF ADH RELEASE

1.5.1 Plasma osmolality

The first definitively characterised stimulus for the release of ADH was an increase in the osmotic pressure of the plasma. Verney, in his classic studies[47], showed that a 2% increase in the osmolality of carotid artery blood inhibited a water diuresis in the conscious dog, and that this response was most likely due to the release of ADH from the posterior pituitary. Subsequently, Jewell and Verney[48] located the receptors which sense changes in plasma osmolality, the osmoreceptors, in or near the supraoptic nuclei of the hypothalamus. Since that time, there have been any number of confirmatory reports, showing that an increase in the plasma osmotic pressure, due either to dehydration (e.g. References 49, 50) or to the administration of hypertonic salt solution (e.g. References 51, 52), stimulates ADH release. In addition,

Eggena and Thorn[53] have reported that the isolated complex of the hypothalamus and posterior pituitary reponds to an increased osmolality of the incubation medium with an increased release of ADH.

The hypothalamic osmoreceptors have not been precisely identified. Electrophysiological studies suggest that the neurosecretory cells themselves may function as osmoreceptors. Neurosecretory cells in the supraoptic and paraventricular nuclei, identified by antidromic stimulation of the posterior pituitary, respond to an injection of hypertonic saline into a common carotid artery with a change in electrical activity[54, 55]. However, Bridges and Thorn[56] have suggested that at least two synapses, one cholinergic and one monoaminergic, lie between the osmoreceptor and the neurosecretory cell body, since antiadrenergic and ganglionic blocking agents inhibited the release of ADH in response to an osmotic stimulus. These findings must be interpreted with caution; the pharmacological agents which were used may have themselves caused the release of substantial quantities of ADH, which may have been responsible for the impaired response to a subsequent osmotic stimulus.

The attempts to quantify the relationship between plasma osmolality and the plasma concentration of ADH are not wholly satisfactory. Changes in the osmotic pressure of the plasma of the order of 1.5–3% result in appropriate changes in the release of ADH[47, 57-59]. Moore[60], Robertson et al.[61], Beardwell[62] and Shimizu et al.[52] found a highly significant positive correlation between ADH concentration and plasma osmolality. A problem with all of these studies is that it is difficult to vary plasma osmolality without concomitantly changing blood volume, and the latter itself has an important effect on ADH release.

The central osmoreceptors can apparently be stimulated by an increase in the osmotic pressure of the cerebrospinal fluid. Andersson et al.[63] have extended earlier observations that small injections of hypertonic saline into the third ventricle of the brain inhibited a water diuresis in the conscious hydrated goat. That this response was due to the release of ADH is supported by the observation that the response could no longer be elicited after diabetes insipidus was produced by lesioning the median eminence. On the other hand, Mouw and Vander[64] reported that perfusion of the ventriculo-cisternal system with a hypo-osmolar solution had no consistent effect on the plasma ADH concentration. Since this is based on measurements in only three dogs, it cannot be considered conclusive.

The injection of hypertonic solutions of sucrose[65] and fructose[66] into the third ventricle of the conscious hydrated goat does not inhibit a water diuresis although these agents are effective when injected into the common carotid artery[47, 66, 67]. This raises the possibility that receptors which respond to an increased osmolality of the cerebrospinal fluid may be different from those which sense changes in the osmolality of the cerebral blood.

Verney[47] proposed that the osmoreceptor cells are activated as a consequence of a reduction in their volume. An important consideration in advancing this suggestion was the failure of hypertonic solutions of urea, injected into a common carotid artery, to inhibit a water diuresis. Andersson and his colleagues[68-70] have suggested that this concept of osmoreceptor function may be oversimplified, in view of evidence that urea crosses the blood-brain barrier only very slowly and the failure of hypertonic sucrose to stimulate ADH release when injected into the cerebral ventricles[65]. However, the possibility that the blood-brain barrier is incomplete in the region of the hypothalamic osmoreceptors and that urea freely diffuses across the cell membranes of these osmoreceptors should be considered.

Haberich et al.[72,73] have proposed the existence in the liver of osmoreceptors with afferents in the vagus[73]. No definitive conclusions can be drawn about the mechanism of action of this osmosensitive reflex, since no measurements were made of the plasma ADH concentration, glomerular filtration rate, or free water clearance.

Further support for an hepatic osmoreceptor mechanism was provided by Niijima[74]. When isolated guinea-pig livers were perfused with hypertonic Ringer solution, he recorded an increased firing rate from the hepatic branch of the vagus. However, the minimal effective increase in the osmotic pressure of the perfusate was 17 mosmol kg^{-1}. On the other hand, Schneider et al.[75] were unable to confirm in the dog the work of Haberich and his associates in the rat, but this may be due to species difference. In any event, it seems premature to speculate about the possible physiological role of hepatic osmoreceptors until this problem has been subjected to additional study.

1.5.2   Blood volume

It is firmly established that a reduction in blood volume is an effective, potent stimulus for the release of ADH[76-80]. Conversely, an acute expansion of blood volume results in a reduction in the plasma ADH concentration[50,58]. The receptors for this neuroendocrine reflex are the left atrial stretch receptors and the arterial baroreceptors.

Based largely upon the demonstration that distension of the left atrium resulted in an increased urine volume, Henry et al.[81] postulated that the left atrial stretch receptors play an important role in controlling water excretion by the kidney. It was subsequently shown that stimulation of these receptors, which are innervated by the vagus, does indeed result in an inhibition of ADH release[82-84] and that they function within a physiological range of left atrial pressures[84].

An apparent challenge to this view is the report by Goetz et al.[85] that a reduction in atrial transmural pressure by pericardial tamponade in the conscious dog failed to produce the expected reduction in the plasma ADH concentration. However, anatomical location of the atrial receptors concerned in the control of ADH release is such that they may not have been affected by the tamponade. Alternatively, these receptors may not have been tonically active under the circumstances of these experiments.

The question of whether receptors in chambers of the heart other than the left atrium may participate in the control of ADH release has not as yet been satisfactorily answered. Henry et al.[81] failed to find effects on urine flow of procedures designed to increase pressure in the right side of the heart and pulmonary vascular tree. Since the plasma concentration of ADH was not measured, the results of these experiments cannot be considered definitive. Brennan et al.[86] have claimed that distension of the right atrium in the anaesthetised dog did not affect the plasma ADH concentration. However, in those experiments in which it was measured, left atrial pressure fell when the right atrium was distended by balloon inflation, possibly demonstrating opposing effects of stimulation of right atrial receptors.

In addition to the atrial receptors, the other major group of 'volume receptors' are the arterial baroreceptors. Of these, attention has been directed primarily to the carotid sinus receptors because of technical difficulties in studying receptors in the aortic arch. When stimulation of the carotid sinus baroreceptors is reduced[87,88], there is an increase in the plasma ADH concentration. Although it is presumed that aortic arch baroreceptors function in a similar fashion in the control of ADH secretion, the only evidence for this is that section of the aortic nerves in the vagotomised rabbit results in an increase in the plasma concentration of ADH[89]. Why vagotomy was necessary for the demonstration of this response is not apparent.

It appears that the left atrial receptors may be primarily involved in the release of ADH in response to small to moderate changes in blood volume. First, in the conscious dog or the dog anaesthetised with an anaesthetic mixture which preserves cardiovascular reflexes (e.g. morphine sedation followed by a mixture of chloralose and urethane), left atrial pressure varies directly with changes in blood volume over a broad range, whereas mean arterial pressure holds constant[79,80,90,91]. Although there may be small changes in arterial pulse pressure under these circumstances, available evidence suggests that only large changes in pulse pressure can affect ADH release[88]. Second, Zehr et al.[92] have found that in dogs with chronic mitral stenosis, the ADH response to haemorrhage was considerably blunted, although the haemodynamic responses were normal. Presumably, the morphological changes in the left atrial myocardium in this condition interfered with the ability of the atrial receptors to sense changes in blood volume. Third, manoeuvres which result in changes in intrathoracic blood volume effect changes in the plasma ADH concentration[93-96]. Thus, the arterial receptors may function as a redundant auxiliary system, coming into play when arterial pressure falls, e.g. following severe haemorrhage or overexpansion of the vascular compartment.

The volume receptor system controlling ADH secretion appears to be as sensitive as the osmoreceptor system. A reduction in blood volume of as little as 2.6% can increase the plasma ADH concentration[91]. However, sodium depletion, with its attendant reduction in extracellular fluid volume does not increase the plasma ADH concentration[97-98].

The volume receptor and osmoreceptor systems interact in an additive fashion[58-59]. The conclusion by Johnson et al.[58] that, with small changes in blood volume and plasma osmolality neither system appears to be dominant, appears reasonable.

1.5.3 Renin–angiotensin system

Considerable current interest and controversy are centred upon the role of the renin–angiotensin system in the control of ADH release. There are several reports that angiotensin II, presumably acting at some locus in the central nervous system, stimulates the release of ADH. The injection of angiotensin

II into the cerebral ventricles resulted in an increased blood pressure[99] and an inhibition of a water diuresis[70]. Since plasma ADH concentrations were not measured in these two studies, their conclusions can be accepted only with reservation. A more direct approach to this problem is found in the report by Bonjour and Malvin[100] that the intravenous infusion of pressor doses of renin or angiotensin II increased the plasma ADH concentration in the conscious dog. However, the response was small, and a dose–response relationship was not reproducibly obtained. Subsequently, Mouw et al.[101] reported that plasma ADH levels were elevated in the anaesthetised dog when angiotensin was infused into a common carotid artery, but not intravenously, at a rate of 10 ng kg^{-1} min^{-1}. This was based on only three experiments, two of which were completely satisfactory. It was additionally found that perfusion of the ventriculo-cisternal system with solutions containing angiotensin elevated the plasma ADH concentration. There was no dose–response relationship; instead, the magnitude of the response was proportional to the control levels of ADH.

There is considerable evidence which challenges the concept that circulating angiotensin II directly stimulates ADH release. Andersson and Eriksson[69] found that in conscious goats the intravenous infusion of angiotensin II (3 ng kg^{-1} min^{-1}) failed to inhibit a water diuresis. Similarly, Claybaugh et al.[102] were unable to demonstrate in anaesthetised dogs any effect on the plasma ADH concentration when angiotensin was infused intravenously or via a common carotid artery over a broad dose range. Furthermore, exclusion of the kidneys from the circulation failed to impair the ADH response to haemorrhage[103]. Finally, when dogs were bled at a slow constant rate, the plasma ADH concentration rose before a change in plasma renin activity occurred, and, as the haemorrhage continued, circulating levels of ADH and renin did not change in a parallel fashion[91]. There are other situations in which there is no correlation between changes in plasma levels of ADH and renin (e.g. References 97, 104).

Although angiotensin in the systemic circulation may not directly stimulate the release of ADH, it may potentiate the secretion of ADH in response to other stimuli. Andersson and his associates[68-70] found that angiotensin and hypertonic saline injected into the third ventricle of the brain of the conscious goat interacted synergistically to inhibit a water diuresis. Similarly, the infusion of angiotensin into a common carotid artery in the anaesthetised dog enhanced the release of ADH in response to an osmotic stimulus[52]. The route and method of administration of angiotensin may be important in determining its action. In anaesthetised cats[105], microelectrophoretic application of angiotensin II to neurosecretory cells in the supraoptic nucleus (identified antidromically) increased their rate of firing, whereas the injection of large doses of angiotensin had no effect on the firing rate of these neurones.

Tagawa et al.[239] have made the intriguing observation that infusion of Pitressin at rates which resulted in physiological increases in plasma ADH levels resulted in an inhibition of renin secretion in conscious, sodium-deprived dogs. Thus, there may be a negative feed-back relationship between ADH and the renin–angiotensin system, which serves to dampen fluctuations in the plasma concentrations of these humoral agents under basal conditions. It is obvious, however, that appropriate stimuli, e.g. changes in blood volume or composition can override this relationship, resulting in increased secretion of ADH, or renin, or both ADH and renin.

Certainly the regulation of body water and electrolyte metabolism requires integrated control of ADH and the renin–angiotensin–aldosterone system. However, the level at which this integration takes place and the manner in which it occurs remain to be determined.

1.5.4 Adrenal cortex

Because of the impaired ability of the kidney to excrete a water load in adrenal insufficiency, there has been for many years considerable interest in the possibility that the adrenocortical hormones play a role in either the control of the release of ADH (e.g. Reference 106) or its action on the nephron (e.g Reference 107). Much of this dispute centres upon the question of whether or not plasma levels of ADH are elevated in adrenal insufficiency. A resolution of at least this controversy may be found in the work of Share and Travis[108]. Their data suggest that whether or not the plasma ADH concentration rises during the early stages of adrenal insufficiency may depend in large part upon the degree to which blood volume and pressure fall. Green et al.[109] supported the view that the impaired renal handling of water is not entirely due to an elevated plasma ADH concentration. Adrenalectomy impaired the ability of rats with hereditary diabetes insipidus to excrete a water load and dilute the urine. Treatment with both glucocorticoids and mineralocorticoids was required to correct this disorder.

Under certain conditions glucocorticoids can inhibit ADH secretion. Aubry et al.[110] found that treatment of normal human subjects with cortisol resulted in an elevation of the plasma osmolality at which a water diuresis is inhibited. Travis and Share[104] reported that in conscious, adrenally insufficient dogs, the intravenous injection of 100 mg cortisol prevented an acute, marked increase in the plasma ADH concentration in response to a poorly defined stimulus, apparently associated with the experimental situation. Finally, addition of prednisolone to the incubation medium inhibited the release of ADH in response to an elevated potassium concentration in the medium[111].

1.5.5 Prostaglandins

A possible action of the prostaglandins on the control of ADH release has received little attention. Most investigators have found that the prostaglandins of the E and A series increase the renal excretion of sodium and water, and have attributed this effect to a direct action of the prostaglandins upon the kidney (e.g. Reference 112). Vilhardt and Hedqvist[113], however, have observed that although PGE_2 was without effect on the release of ADH from isolated rat neural lobes, it inhibited a water diuresis in the intact rat when injected into the carotid circulation. On this basis they have suggested that PGE_2 acts on some element in the central nervous system to stimulate ADH release. Further investigation in this area seems warranted.

1.5.6   Role of the central nervous system

Recently, there has been little interest in mapping the pathways within the central nervous system responsible for the neural control of ADH release. However, Bisset et al.[114], in an extension of earlier work, have provided additional evidence that ADH is released following electrical stimulation of the supraoptic and paraventricular nuclei and median eminence in the anaesthetised cat.

Study of the neurosecretory cells themselves and their responses to neurotransmitters has been facilitated by the use of antidromic activation following electrical stimulation of the posterior lobe to identify the neurosecretory cells. Koizumi and Yamashita[38], using this technique, have concluded that the neurosecretory cells in the supraoptic and paraventricular nuclei are functionally similar to other neurones, but have some unique features which may in part be the result of the accumulation of neurosecretory material within the cells.

It is generally held that release of ADH from the axon endings in the posterior pituitary is directly dependent upon an increased electrical activity of the ADH-containing neurosecretory cells. However, attempts to correlate changes in the electrical activity of hypothalamic neurosecretory cells with stimuli known to release ADH have been less than satisfying. It has frequently been observed that a stimulus expected to either increase or decrease ADH release increased the activity of some responding cells and decreased the activity of others[54, 55, 115, 116, 117]. Dyball[55] found that electrical activity of neurosecretory cells with a slow spontaneous discharge rate was more apt to be increased by intracarotid hypertonic saline and vice versa, and that peak ADH release appeared to occur after changes in the electrical activity of the cells had subsided. Thus, Dyball[55] suggested that there may not be a simple direct relationship between electrical activity of the neurosecretory cells and quantity of ADH released. This view merits careful consideration.

Evidence continues to accumulate that a hypothalamic cholinergic synapse is a component in the reflex control of ADH release. The intraventricular injection of acetylcholine or carbachol inhibited a water diuresis in the goat[118] and rat[119]. The addition of acetylcholine to the incubation medium induced an increased release of ADH from the isolated rat hypothalamo–posterior pituitary complex[53]. In the rat, atropine prevented the inhibition of a water diuresis by hypertonic saline[56]. The direct application of acetylcholine by iontophoresis has been reported to stimulate[120] and to stimulate and inhibit[121] antidromically identified hypothalamic neurosecretory cells. In the latter work, the stimulatory activity of acetylcholine was reported to be nicotinic and the inhibitory activity muscarinic, but Bhargava et al.[122] concluded that the stimulatory effect of acetylcholine is muscarinic.

The monoamines play a role in the control of ADH release, but the nature of their role is controversial. The intraventricular infusion of epinephrine and norepinephrine inhibited a water diuresis in the conscious goat[118], and antiadrenergic drugs blocked the osmotic inhibition of a water diuresis in the rat[56]. On the basis of the effects of the intraventricular injection of adrenergic agonists and antagonists on the plasma ADH concentration in the dog, Bhargava et al.[122] concluded that central α-adrenoceptors are concerned with stimulating and central β-adrenoceptors with inhibiting ADH release. Apparently not consonant with this view is the report by Barker *et al.*[121] that the iontophoretic application of dopamine, norepinephrine and serotonin to supra-optic neurosecretory cells inhibited their electrical activity.

On the basis of the failure of acetylcholine to affect the release of ADH by the posterior pituitary *in vitro* (e.g. Reference 39), it has been concluded that acetylcholine does not act directly upon the axon endings in the posterior lobe to modify ADH release. This view may be incorrect. Gosbee and Lederis[123] found that direct application of acetylcholine to the posterior pituitary *in vivo* inhibited a water diuresis in the hydrated, ethanol-anaesthetised rat, presumably due to an increased release of ADH. The authors present the possibility of a cholinergic link in the stimulus–secretion coupling in the neurohypophysis.

1.6 METABOLISM OF ADH

The concentration of ADH in plasma is obviously a function of both the rate of secretion of the hormone and the rate of its removal from the circulating blood. It is particularly important to be cognisant of this, since because of the extreme difficulty in measuring directly the rate of secretion of ADH, changes in its plasma concentration are commonly taken as an index of changes in secretion rate. In as much as the metabolism of ADH has been well reviewed by Lauson[124, 125], no attempt will be made to deal with this subject definitively. Rather, recent developments will be highlighted.

The following are well established[124, 125]. (1) The organs which are primarily, if not solely, responsible for the irreversible clearance of ADH from the circulating blood are the liver and kidneys. (2) Circulating ADH is confined to the plasma fraction of blood. (3) The half-life of ADH is relatively short, with estimates ranging from 0.69 min in the rat to 8 min in dog and man. On the other hand, the questions of the volume of distribution of ADH and its binding to plasma protein remain controversial. Thus, with respect to the latter, for example, Vorherr *et al.*[126] found little or no binding of ADH to plasma protein in humans, whereas Fabian *et al.*[127] reported 30% binding. However, Lauson[125] has concluded with good reason that the binding of neurohypophysial hormones to plasma protein, regardless of its extent, probably plays only a minor role in the kinetics of the removal of the hormones from plasma.

The complexity of the problems facing studies in this area is highlighted by the report by Pliska *et al.*[128]. These investigators infused ADH intravenously into anaesthetised, hydrated dogs at a very high rate (135 to 900 mU h^{-1} kg^{-1}) for 1.5–2 h. When the infusion was stopped, the plasma ADH concentration fell rapidly for the first 7–10 min with a half-life of 1.5–5.7 min. During the next 15 to 20 min, the plasma ADH concentration rose transiently to 45 to 100% of the steady-state level. The authors suggested that the second peak in the plasma ADH concentration was the result of the release of ADH from some tissue, possibly the neurohypophysis, which had accumulated the ADH during the infusion phase of the experiment.

Miller and Moses[129] have reported that, in normal human subjects, the urinary excretion of ADH averaged 28.9 mU 24 h^{-1}. Following oral water loading there was no detectable ADH in the urine, whereas a period of dehydration resulted in an increased urinary excretion of ADH. These workers have proposed that measurement of the urinary excretion of ADH might serve as an 'effective method for assessing neurohypophysial function in man'.

1.7 ACTIONS OF ADH

The primary physiological action of ADH is apparently to increase the reabsorption of water by the kidney by increasing the permeability of the collecting duct and, in some species at least, of the distal convoluted tubule[130]. It is generally accepted that this is accomplished by increasing the area of pores through which the osmotic flow of water can occur. This can be achieved by either an enlargement of pre-existing pores or the opening up of additional pores. Evidence favouring the latter has been presented for the collecting duct[131] and the epithelial cells of the toad bladder[132].

It has been suggested[133] that ADH exerts its action upon the renal tubule and other epithelial structures by accelerating the formation of cyclic-3',5'-AMP from ATP, and that it is the cyclic-3',5'-AMP which is the intra-cellular mediator of the action of ADH. Although there is much evidence to support this hypothesis[134], the finding by Graziani and Livne[135] that ADH in low concentrations markedly increased the permeability to water of an artificial lipid membrane suggests that ADH may exert its hydro-osmotic effect on living tissue, at least in part, independently of cyclic-3',5'-AMP.

An additional physiological action of ADH upon the kidney may be to modify the intrarenal distribution of blood flow. In the conscious dog in the transient phase of diabetes insipidus (resulting from section of the hypothal-amohypophysial tract), Fisher et al.[136] observed an increased total renal and outer cortical blood flow, and a decreased inner cortical and outer medullary blood flow. These workers proposed that postglomerular renal resistance is under ADH control.

A possible role for ADH in the release of ACTH has been the subject of controversy for many years. Recently, Yates et al.[137] reported that ADH under physiological circumstances potentiates the action of CRF on the anterior pituitary. These workers point out that ADH also can directly stimulate the release of ACTH and CRF. However, the physiological role of ADH in the control of the release of ACTH cannot yet be fully assessed.

A variety of other physiological actions have been attributed to ADH, including inhibition of gastrointestinal secretions (e.g. Reference 138), inhibition of absorption of water and salt from the small intestine[139], enhanced sodium transport by the ciliary epithelium of the eye[140], and prolonged maintenance of a conditioned avoidance response[141, 142].

Maximum concentration of the urine occurs at a plasma ADH concentra-tion of approximately 4 mU ml^{-1} [60], yet a reduction in blood volume can result in plasma ADH levels considerably in excess of this value. In as much as ADH is a potent pressor agent, it is tempting to speculate that it may play a role in regulation of blood pressure. Thus, with severe haemorrhage, plasma levels of ADH are probably sufficiently high for the hormone to exert a direct pressor action. In addition, Bartelstone and Nasmyth[143] reported that low, sub-pressor doses of ADH potentiate the pressor action of catecholamines, and Frieden and Keller[144] have observed that the ability of the dog to maintain arterial pressure in the face of haemorrhage was impaired by surgically induced diabetes insipidus. It is, however, still premature to evaluate the physiological importance of ADH as a pressor agent.

1.8 PHYSIOLOGICAL CONTROL OF THE RELEASE OF OXYTOCIN

1.8.1 Effect of genital stimulation in the female

Milk ejection often occurs in the cow and goat after mechanical stimulation of the vulva and vagina[145]; in fact, manual stimulation of this area has been exploited by the tribal Hottentots as a means of inducing milk ejection in their domesticated animals. In the experiments in cows, Debackere and Peeters[146] inflated a balloon in the vagina to pressures of 50–200 mmHg. This caused milk ejection and antidiuresis. Cervical distension also caused milk ejection in some animals although comparable distension of the rectum was without effect. In other experiments, Debackere et al.[147, 148] anastomosed the jugular veins in sheep so that the jugular outflow in each animal passed into the venous system and thus returned to the heart of the other animal. Stimulation of the vagina in one ewe resulted in an increase in the intramammary pressure not in the udder of the stimulated ewe but in the other ewe. The intramammary pressure responses of the udder could be matched with the intravenous injection of 20–50 mU of oxytocin. Their conclusion was that vaginal distension caused a discharge of hormones from the head and that the release occurred almost immediately after vaginal distension. Van Demark and Hays[149] found that of the several sites of stimulation of the reproductive tract of cows the greatest effects on oxytocin release were seen following stimulation of the cervix, especially the external os of the cervix. In sheep, vaginal distension ordinarily causes a threefold increase in plasma-oxytocin concentration, but this response disappears in advanced pregnancy[150]. Furthermore, normally responsive sheep do not respond to vaginal distension following a week of treatment with progesterone. On the other hand, the response is markedly potentiated after a week of treatment with oestradiol[151]. Apparently the release of oxytocin in response to vaginal distension is seasonally related; vaginal distension causes a greater release of oxytocin during the first part of the year than during the latter part of the year[152].

Increased uterine activity and milk ejection has been observed following coitus in the females of several species including man and this has been attributed to the release of oxytocin[145]. Recently, Fox and Knaggs[153] observed that an increase occurred in the plasma oxytocin levels after female orgasm. An antidiuresis has been demonstrated in female rats[154] and in men[155] after coitus suggesting that vasopressin as well, is released. The interpretation of the release of oxytocin at coitus is obscure. Although it is quite possible that a reflex release of oxytocin is initiated by the local stimulation of the genitalia, this certainly is not the only source of impulses impinging upon the hypothalmus during coitus since courtship phenomenon without any physical contact between male and female apparently can release oxytocin[156,157].

The spurting of milk from the teats at parturition has been commonly observed in various domesticated animals including cows, mares, and sows. Gunther[158] reported that milk was expressed from the breast synchronously with labour pains in a woman still lactating from a previous pregnancy. The effect was simulated by injection of a posterior pituitary extract. Similar observations have been made in women in which elevations in the intramammary pressure have been used to mark the release of oxytocin[159]. Cross[160] observed milk ejection in rabbits occurred precisely at the time of delivery of their litters and observed also that the milk ejection effect at parturition was somewhat greater than that produced by physiological doses of oxytocin (50 mU). Fuchs[161] recorded intrauterine pressure continuously throughout the last 48 h of pregnancy and throughout labour in fully conscious rabbits. Only minor changes in spontaneous activity were recorded until just a few minutes before parturition. Contractions of considerable frequency and intensity then appeared which were followed closely by the delivery of the entire litter. The intrauterine pressure responses closely resembled those following a single intravenous injection of 250–300 mU of oxytocin.

More recently, oxytocin has been assayed in the jugular blood of parturient sheep, goats, horses and cows[162-165]. In the domestic species an increase in blood oxytocin was detected only during the expulsive stage of labour and much lower amounts, if any, were detected during the stage of cervical dilation suggesting that the maximum rate of secretion of oxytocin occurred during the passage of the foetus through the vagina and cervix, particularly at the time the head emerges from the vulva. The oxytocin levels quickly subsided after parturition. Coch et al.[166] measured milk-ejecting activity in both internal jugular and peripheral vein blood of women at the time of labour and found that the concentration in the jugular blood was 69 times greater than that found in the peripheral blood. From this they concluded that the active substance, probably oxytocin or a mixture of oxytocin and vasopressin, was secreted at some site in the head, probably the neurohypophysis.

1.8.2   Effect of genital stimulation in the male

Although there is no recognised physiological function for oxytocin in male animals, the store of oxytocin in the neurohypophysis is not less in males than in females. It is clear also that stimulation of the neurohypophysis in males releases oxytocin as well as vasopressin. The association between the neurohypophysis and the male reproductive tract is best illustrated from experiments[148] in which the circulation of a ram and a lactating ewe were connected by attaching the distal end of a severed jugular vein of each animal to the central stump in the other so that the ram received the jugular blood of the female and vice versa. Stimulation of the seminal vesicles and the ampullae of the male resulted in a milk-ejection response in the ewe which was clearly similar to that produced by an intravenous injection of oxytocin. These results suggest that the release of oxytocin may occur in the male during coitus, though in man Fox and Knaggs[153] failed to note a rise in plasma oxytocin during coitus or following orgasm. There is, however, evidence for a release of vasopressin during coitus in men[155,167].

1.8.3 Sensory nerve endings in the genital tract

There is a paucity of information concerning the localisation of and identification of the receptors in the male or female reproductive tracts which transmit information to the neurohypophysis. Bower[168] detected an action potential discharge in the afferent nerves leading from the rabbit uterus when the intrauterine pressure was increased by about 40 mmHg. This was interpreted as demonstrating the presence of uterine baroceptors. Recently, potential changes have been demonstrated in the hypothalamus and in regions of the cerebral cortex following discrete electrical stimulation of the uterus[169]. Electroencephalographic changes have been recorded from the hypothalamus in association with vaginal stimulation or coitus in cats[170]. Barraclough and Cross[171] found that an increased firing rate occurred in certain of the hypothalamic neurones when the os cervix was subjected to pressure stimulation.

1.8.4 Effect of suckling

The ejection of milk is mediated via a neurohumoral reflex. Oxytocin is released from the neurohypophysis by suckling or milking stimuli and is carried by the circulation to the mammary gland, where a few seconds after it has been released it causes the contraction of the alveolar myoepithelium which expels the alveolar milk, under pressure, into the larger ducts or cisterns where it is available for withdrawal[1,2,172]. The stimulation provided by the acts of suckling or milking is of a very complex nature and probably involves the simultaneous activation of various types of mammary receptors such as touch, heat, etc. Local anaesthesia of the teats of conscious rabbits prevents milk ejection in response to suckling presumably because of blockade of afferent impulses from the teat receptors[173]. The frequency characteristics that mammary stimulation must fulfil in order to induce milk ejection have been studied in the goat by Grachev[174] who found that milk ejection was not produced at frequencies of milking below 12 per min whereas rates of stimulation between 84 and 142 stimuli per minute were found to be maximally effective.

Some evidence exists[175,176] that the amount of oxytocin released by suckling is roughly directly proportional to the number of pups suckling. The discharge of the hormone appears to be intermittent though suckling or milking may be rather continuous[153,175,177-180]. Perhaps a refractoriness of the oxytocin release mechanism occurs following suckling which is similar to that observed with regards to prolactin release[181]. In addition to the release of oxytocin in response to suckling, there is in some species a release first as a result of premilking stimuli, e.g. the presence of the milker. This may represent a conditioned response in the Pavlovian sense to auditory, olfactory and visual stimuli. In fact, there are several reports which indicate that the suckling-induced release of oxytocin may be conditioned[182-187].

Although the suckling-induced release of oxytocin is essential for the ejection of milk in many mammals, in the sheep and goat the occurrence of the reflex is not vital for the removal of milk, although the reflex may occur under normal circumstances. Moreover, it is possible that in these, and in other species as well, milk removal might be assisted by local contraction of myoepithelial cells in response to direct mechanical stimulation of the udder[188].

1.8.5 Sensory nerve endings in the mammary gland

There is little detailed information concerning the structure and arrangement of sensory receptors in the teat and within the mammary gland. Whereas there is good evidence for a profuse innervation of the teat, there is no unanimity of opinion regarding the type of receptor found there. The walls of the teats contain numerous free nerve endings, though in addition, superficial and deep nerve plexuses with numerous encapsulated ends, including Merkels, Golgi-Mazzoni, and Pacini corpuscles, are thought to be present in some species (see References 2,189–191). The richly innervated areola apparently does not contain any corpuscular formations.

The properties of teat receptors have been examined in the rabbit by Findlay[192] using electrophysiological afferent nerve recording techniques. He demonstrated that the teat contains mechanoreceptors which are responsive to suction and to pressure, some of which were slowly adapting, though most of which appeared to be of the rapidly adapting type.

The existence of receptors sensitive to changes in intramammary pressure has been established though the function, if any, of such receptors is unknown. Subjective sensations occurring in human lactation associated with the milk-ejection reflex have been described by Isbister[193], and Forbes et al.[194] noted that similar sensations usually accompanied the injection of posterior pituitary extract. Grachev[195] separated the goat udder from the body of the animal with the exception of the nerves and perfused its blood vessels with oxygenated Tyrode solution at 38°C. Artificial distension of the udder with air, milk or water brought about a rise in systemic blood pressure and respiration rate which he believed to be due to the activation of pressure receptors within the gland.

In later studies, Grachev[196] noted that higher intramammary pressures resulting from the introduction of fluid or air into the udder elicited signs of acute discomfort in the goat. Cobo et al.[197] found that in humans, suckling by the baby and duct dilation of the mammary gland each produced a clear milk-ejection response. The characteristic waves of mammary contraction seen with suckling and duct dilation could be simulated by intermittent injections of oxytocin.

The analysis of the afferent connections between the mammary gland and the neurohypophysis in different species with respect to the pathway of the milk-ejection reflex has been the subject of several recent reviews[1,2,191,198-200] and will not be discussed here. At present, it is considered that paraventricular (PV) and supraoptic (SO) neurones of the hypothalamus constitute the last relay, i.e. final common pathway, of the milk-ejection reflex (see References 28, 54) and stimulation of these neurones precipitates hormone release.

Lincoln et al.[177,201] observed that in the anaesthetised rat, suckling caused a dramatic acceleration in the activity of the neurosecretory cells immediately prior to oxytocin release. Although the pups then respond by vigorous suckling and obtain the milk, there was no increase in the activity of the neurosecretory cells.

1.8.6 Inhibition of oxytocin release

The milk-ejection reflex appears to be easily inhibited by various somatic and psychological stressors. Ely and Petersen[202] reported that a reduction of milk yield occurred in cows when paper bags filled with air were exploded or when a cat was placed on the back of the cow during milking. Similar inhibition was obtained in cows by Whittlestone[203] when faradic shocks were applied shortly before milking. Newton and Newton[204] have reported that embarassment, fear or discomfort while nursing partially inhibited milk ejection in women. A reduction in milk ejection also occurs in rabbits[205] and guinea-pigs[206] when the mothers are forcibly restrained in a supine position during suckling. Severe stresses, e.g. a leg break or an open wound under ether anaesthesia[207] or milder stresses such as the odour of the oil of peppermint, intermittent low intensity sounds or intermittent bright light[208] have been shown to drastically reduce milk ejection in rats.

The mechanisms underlying emotional inhibition of milk ejection were first studied by Cross[209] who concluded that one of the main factors in the emotional disturbance of the milk-ejection reflex is a partial inhibition of oxytocin release from the neurohypophysis. Aulsebrook and Holland[210] found in the rabbit that the release of oxytocin elicited by stimulation of the forebrain could be suppressed by simultaneous excitation of some regions of the brain stem, e.g. mesencephalic tegmentum, central grey, pretectal regions, etc. The participation of the cerebral cortex in the emotional inhibition of oxytocin release also has been demonstrated by Taleisnik and Deis[207] who found that cortical spreading depression prevented the inhibition of the milk-ejection reflex produced by painful stimuli. Chaudhury et al.[206] showed that blockage of the milk-ejection reflex induced by stress in guinea-pigs could be reduced by injecting tranquillising drugs into the mothers before suckling, but that adrenergic blocking drugs were without effect. Koizumi et al.[211] found that electrical or chemical excitation of the anterior lobe of the cerebellum and the mesencephalic reticular formation inhibited the discharge rate of many of the neurosecretory neurones in the supraoptic and paraventricular nuclei.

1.9 ACTIONS OF OXYTOCIN

Of the several actions of oxytocin described for the mammalian organism the two most important physiological actions are those upon the lactating mammary gland and uterus. This is not surprising when considering that the major sources of sensory input regulating oxytocin secretion, as described in the previous section, emanate from the female reproduction tract and mammary gland.

1.9.1 Action on mammary gland

The milk in the alveoli and in the small ducts of the mammary gland must be ejected, in contrast to that contained in the sinuses, cisterns or other dilations of the large ducts which can be withdrawn passively, i.e. drained through a teat cannula. The amount of milk which can be withdrawn passively may comprise a large percentage of the total milk in cows and goats whose glands have large cisterns, but constitutes only a small percentage in such species as the rat, rabbit and mouse, whose glands lack a cistern or other dilation of the major ducts (see References 1, 2, 189, 190).

The contractile tissues of the mammary gland have been shown by Richardson[212] to be of two types: myoepithelium which covers the stromal surface of the epithelium of the alveoli, ducts and cistern of the entire gland, and smooth muscle which is found in the teat and forms scattered interlobular bundles closely associated with the blood vessels. On the alveoli the myoepithelial cells are arranged in a stellate form so that their contraction in response to oxytocin compresses the alveoli and raises the pressure within the gland. On the small ducts the cells are disposed longitudinally and the effects of their contraction in response to oxytocin is to widen and shorten the ducts[213]. The mammary myoepithelial cells of a variety of species have been shown also to contract in response to direct mechanical stimulation and thus constitute a subsidiary system for the expulsion of milk (see Reference 188).

1.9.2 Mode of action of oxytocin on the mammary gland

It was first shown in 1960 by Mendez-Bauer et al.[215] that an isolated strip of mammary gland suspended in Tyrode solution would contract in response to oxytocin. Moore and Zarrow[216] showed that when sodium was replaced by potassium in the Tyrode solution the response of the strip of isolated rabbit mammary gland to oxytocin, although not abolished, decreased exponentially with time; the decrease then was reversed when the strip was replaced in normal Tyrode solution. However, an increase in the potassium concentration has no effect on the response of rat mammary strips[217]. Omission of calcium from Tyrode solution results both in rats and in rabbits in the mammary strip eventually becoming inexcitable to oxytocin; the excitability can be restored and even increased up to a point by adding calcium to the bath. Larger increases in calcium, though, produce an irreversible loss of responsiveness of the mammary strip to oxytocin[217]. The exact function of calcium remains uncertain but evidence indicates that multiple sites of action for calcium are present on the myoepithelial cells[217-219]. As far as this reviewer is aware, there have been no experiments in which the action of oxytocin on the membrane potential and action potential of the myoepithelial cells of the lactating mammary gland have been recorded.

1.9.3 Peripheral inhibition of milk ejection

The injection of adrenaline has been shown to inhibit the milk ejection normally evoked by endogenous or exogenous oxytocin in a variety of species as well as in the perfused isolated bovine udder preparation (see References 1, 2, 214).

The mechanism by which adrenaline prevents the milk-ejection response to oxytocin has not been clearly defined. Presumably mammary arteriolar vaso-constriction plays a large part in inhibiting the mammary gland responses to oxytocin by preventing access of oxytocin to the myoepithelium. Adrenaline also acts directly to inhibit the effect of oxytocin on the mammary myo-epithelial cells[220-222] and more recently activation of the sympathetic system has been found to increase the resistance to flow of milk within the mammary ducts[223, 224].

Presumably these effects of adrenaline and noradrenaline are mediated through alpha-adrenergic receptors which have been described in the mammary gland blood vessels and through beta receptors which have been described in the myoepithelial cells[220, 225].

Grosvenor et al.[224] found that either administration of KCl to the cerebral cortices or section of the spinal cord of anaesthetised lactating rats greatly increased the slope and amplitude of the intramammary pressure response to intravenously injected oxytocin. In the case of spinal cord section, only the glands caudal to the section were affected. The effect of KCl persisted in rats which were pre-treated either with phenoxybenzamine or with pentolinium. These data would seem to implicate a central mechanism in the regulation of ductal resistance within the mammary gland.

1.9.4 Action on the uterus

The uterus under certain conditions contracts in response to oxytocin. The contraction is not due to direct stimulation of the myometrium by the hormone, a point which was made clear by the experiments of Csapo[226] in which potentially contractile isolated uterine actomyosin-ATP systems failed to contract in the presence of oxytocin. It is generally thought instead that the mechanism of action of oxytocin, at least in part, is through affecting the electro-physiological status of the myometrial membrane (see Reference 227).

It has been known for many years that the status of the ovaries of animals can influence the contractile effect of oxytocin upon the uterus. Chan et al.[228] found that oxytocin contracts the uterus more potently in oestrous and metoestrous than during the dioestrous or proestrous states of the oestrous cycle. Munsick and Jeronimus[229] found that diethylstilboesterol materially altered the potencies of oxytocin and some of its analogues in the rat uterus preparation. However, the changes in sensitivity of the human uterus to oxytocin during the menstrual cycle, pregnancy and during the puerperium are not clear. The confusing, often conflicting reports have been reviewed[230, 231].

The changes in responsivity of the uterus during the menstrual or oestrous cycle and during pregnancy undoubtedly are related to some extent to the effect of oestrogen or progestagens which are known to have a profound influence on the resting potential of uterine smooth muscle membranes (see Reference 227). In general, oxytocin causes a depolarisation of the oestrogen-dominated uterus. In pregnancy or in castrated rats treated with oestrogen plus progesterone, the resting membrane potential is elevated and oxytocin is ineffectual in depolarising the membrane or in producing a contractile response. These observations have led many to postulate that the pregnant uterus is refractory to oxytocin because of a progesterone 'block'[232]. It appears that calcium plays an important part in the membrane phenomena and in the mechanism by which oxytocin affects the membrane. Likewise, calcium apparently plays some role in determining the difference in response between oestrogen- and progesterone-dominated uteri. It has been suggested that oxytocin acts by liberating calcium from the membrane and that the demonstrable difference in oxytocin response between oestrogen and progesterone–dominated uterine muscle may be accounted for by supposing that progesterone causes a far tighter binding of calcium than does oestrogen[227].

1.10   METABOLISM OF OXYTOCIN

It appears likely that there is very little inactivation of circulating oxytocin by factors in the blood[233] with the possible exception of the case in those primates in which circulating oxytocinase is present during pregnancy.

The rapid inactivation of oxytocin *in vitro* has been demonstrated with homogenates of various tissues[233], and at least in the non-lactating rat, the kidneys and the splanchnic area are principally involved in removing oxytocin from the circulation[12]. Lactating rats clear oxytocin more rapidly[12] which indicates that these animals in addition to the kidney and liver possess a subsidiary site for oxytocin inactivation—probably the actively secreting mammary gland. The liver in the lactating rat, however, is larger than it is during the non-lactating state. The lactating mammary gland also may excrete oxytocin since small amounts of oxytocin have been found in the milk of goats and cows after injections of large quantities of oxytocin[234].

In pregnant women and also in some anthropoid apes there is an enzyme, oxytocinase, which circulates in the plasma during pregnancy and which splits the pentapeptide ring of oxytocin between cystine and tyrosine, thus acting as a cystine aminopeptidase[233]. Since the structural requirements for the substrate of this enzyme are fulfilled also by vasopressin, it is not surprising that human pregnancy serum also inactivates the antidiuretic properties of vasopressin. Small but significant amounts of oxytocinase are present in the plasma of pregnant women as early as 8 weeks after conception[235]. The oxytocinase activity in the plasma increases throughout the course of pregnancy[236], then after parturition, decreases slowly and reaches a non-pregnant level in about 3 weeks post-partum. Dicker and Tyler[237] reported that a sharp decline in plasma oxytocinase activity occurred during the first stage of labour and suggested that this might be a factor in determining the onset of labour. Later investigations, however, have failed to substantiate this observation[238].

References

1. Bisset, G. W. (1968). The milk-ejection reflex and the actions of oxytocin, vasopressin and synthetic analogues on the mammary gland. *Handbook Exp. Pharmacol.*, Vol. 23, 475 (B. Berde, editor) (New York: Springer-Verlag)
2. Denamur, R. (1965). The hypothalamo-neurohypophysial system and the milk-ejection reflex. *Dairy Sci. Abstr.*, **27**, 193

3. Cross, B. A. (1951). Suckling antidiuresis in rabbits. *J. Physiol. (London)*, **114**, 447
4. Pickford, M. (1960). Factors affecting milk release in the dog and the quantity of oxytocin liberated by suckling. *J. Physiol. (London)*, **152**, 515
5. Harris, G. W. (1948). The excretion of an antidiuretic substance by the kidney after electrical stimulation of the neurohypophysis in the unanaesthetized rabbit. *J. Physiol. (London)*, **107**, 436
6. Abrahams, V. C. and Pickford, M. (1954). Simultaneous observations on the rate of urine flow and spontaneous uterine movement in the dog and their relationship to posterior lobe activity. *J. Physiol. (London)*., **126**, 329
7. Dicker, S. E. and Tyler, C. (1953). Vasopressin and oxytonix activities of the pituitary glands of rats, guinea pigs, and cats and of human foetuses. *J. Physiol. (London)*, **121**, 206
8. Acher, R. and Fromageot, C. (1957). The relationship of oxytocin and vasopressin to active proteins of posterior pituitary origin. *The Neurohypophysis* (H. Heller, editor) (London: Butterworths)
9. Whittlestone, W. G., Basset, E. G. and Turner, C. W. (1952). Source of secretion of milk 'let-down' hormone in domestic animals. *Proc. Soc. Exp. Biol. Med.*, **80**, 191
10. Barer, R., Heller, H. and Lederis, K. (1963). The isolation, identification and properties of the hormonal granules of the neurohypophysis. *Proc. Roy. Soc. B*, **153**, 388
11. Fuchs, A. R. and Saito, S. (1971). Pituitary oxytocin and vasopressin content of pregnant rats before, during and after parturition. *Endocrinology*, **88**, 547
12. Ginsburg, M. and Smith, M. W. (1959). The fate of oxytocin in male and female rats. *Brit. J. Pharmacol. Chemother.*, **14**, 237
13. Beleslin, D., Bisset, G. W., Haldar, J. and Polak, R. L. (1967). The release of vasopressin without oxytocin in response to haemorrhage. *Proc. Roy. Soc. B*, **166**, 443
14. Clark, B. J. and Rocha, E., Silva, M., Jr. (1967). An afferent pathway for the selective release of vasopressin in response to carotid occlusion and hemorrhage in the cat. *J. Physiol. (London)*, **191**, 529
15. Bargmann, W. and Scharrer, E. (1951). The site of origin of the hormones of the posterior pituitary. *Amer. Sci.*, **39**, 255
16. Sachs, H. (1970). Biosynthesis of the neurohypophysial hormones. *International Encyclopedia of Pharmacology and Therapeutics*, Section 41, Vol. 2, 155 (H. Heller and B. T. Pickering, editors) (Oxford: Pergamon)
17. Takabatake, Y. and Sachs, H. (1964). Vasopressin biosynthesis. III. *In vitro* studies. *Endocrinology*, **75**, 934
18. Sachs, H. and Takabatake, Y. (1964). Evidence for a precursor in vasopressin biosynthesis. *Endocrinology*, **75**, 943
19. Sachs, H. (1963). Vasopressin biosynthesis-II incorporation of [^{35}S] cysteine into vasopressin and protein associated with cell fractions. *J. Neurochem.*, **10**, 299
20. Sachs, H., Goodman, R., Osinchak, J. and McKelvy, J. (1971). Supraoptic neurosecretory neurons of the guinea pig in organ culture. Biosynthesis of vasopressin and neurophysin. *Proc. Nat. Acad. Sci. USA*, **68**, 2782
21. Ginsburg, M. and Ireland, M. (1966). The role of neurophysin in the transport and release of neurohypophysial hormones. *J. Endocrinol.*, **35**, 289
22. Cheng, K. W. and Friesen, H. G. (1972). The isolation and characterization of human neurophysin. *J. Clin. Endocrinol.*, **34**, 165
23. Cheng, K. W. and Friesen, H. G. (1971). Isolation and characterization of a third component of porcine neurophysin. *J. Biol. Chem.*, **246**, 7656
24. Rauch, R., Hollenberg, M. D. and Hope, D. B. (1969). Isolation of a third bovine neurophysin. *Biochem. J.*, **115**, 473
25. Uttenthal, L. O. and Hope, D. B. (1970). The isolation of three neurophysins from porcine posterior pituitary lobes. *Biochem. J.*, **116**, 899
26. Watkins, W. B. (1972). Neurophysins of the rat. *J. Endocrinol.*, **53**, 331
27. Watkins, W. B. (1972). Neurophysins of the sheep. *Biochem. J.*, **126**, 759
28. Dean, C. R., Hope, D. B. and Kazic, T. (1968). Evidence for the storage of oxytocin with neurophysin-I and of vasopressin with neurophysin II in separate neurosecretory granules. *Brit. J. Pharmacol.*, **24**, 192P
28a. Fawcett, C. P., Powell, A. E. and Sachs, H. (1968). Biosynthesis and release of neurophysin. *Endocrinology*, **83**, 1299

29. Robinson, A. G., Zimmerman, E. A. and Frantz, A. G. (1971). Physiologic investigation of posterior pituitary binding proteins neurophysin I and neurophysin II. *Metabolism*, **20**, 1148
30. McNeilly, A. S., Legros, J. J. and Frosling, M. L. (1972). Release of oxytocin, vasopressin and neurophysin in the goat. *J. Endocrinol.*, **52**, 209
31. Burford, G. D., Jones, C. W. and Pickering, B. T. (1971). Tentative identification of a vasopressin-neurophysin and an oxytocin-neurophysin in the rat. *Biochem. J.*, **124**, 809
32. Cheng, K. W. and Friesen, H. G. (1970). Physiological factors regulating secretion of neurophysin. *Metabolsim*, **19**, 876
33. Cheng, K. W., Martin, J. B. and Friesen, H. G. (1972). Studies of neurophysin release. *Endocrinology*, **91**, 177
34. Legros, J. J., Stewart, U., Nordmann, J. J., Dreifus, J. J. and Franchimont, P. (1971). Libération de vasopressine, d'ocytocine et de neurophysine appréciée par méthode radio-immunologique lors de la stimulation *in vitro* de neuro-hypophyses de rat. *C.R. Soc. Biologie*, **165**, 2443
35. Nordmann, J. J., Dreifuss, J. J. and Legros, J. J. (1971). A correlation of release of polypeptide hormone and of immunoreactive neurophysin from isolated rat neurohypophyses. *Experientia*, **27**, 1344
36. Uttenthal, L. O., Livett, B. G. and Hope, D. B. (1971). Release of neurophysin together with vasopressin by a Ca^{2+} dependent mechanism. *Phil. Trans. Roy. Soc. Lond. B*, **261**, 379
37. Ginsburg, M. and Ireland, M. (1964). Binding of vasopressin and oxytocin to protein in extracts of bovine and rabbit neurohypophyses. *J. Endocrin.*, **30**, 131
38. Koizumi, K. and Yamashita, H. (1972). Studies of antidromically identified neurosecretory cells of the hypothalamus by intracellular and extracellular recordings. *J. Physiol. (London)*, **221**, 683
39. Douglas, W. W. and Poisner, A. N. (1964). Stimulus-secretion coupling in a neurosecretory organ: The role of calcium in the release of vasopressin from the neurohypophysis. *J. Physiol. (London)*, **172**, 1
40. Douglas, W. W. (1963). A possible mechanism of neurosecretion: release of vasopressin by depolarization and its dependence on calcium. *Nature (London)*, **197**, 81
41. Daniel, A. R. and Lederis, K. (1967). Release of neurohypophysial hormones *in vitro*. *J. Physiol. (London)*, **190**, 171
42. Ginsburg, M. and Ireland, M. (1966). The role of neurophysin in the transport and release of neurohypophysial hormones. *J. Endocrinol.*, **35**, 289
43. Thorn, N. A. (1966). *In vitro* studies of the release mechanism for vasopressin in rats. *Acta Endocrinol.*, **53**, 644
44. Sachs, H., Share, L., Osinchak, J. and Carpi, A. (1967). Capacity of the neurohypophysis to release vasopressin. *Endocrinology*, **81**, 755
45. Nagasawa, J., Douglas, W. W. and Schulz, R. A. (1970). Ultrastructural evidence of secretion by exocytosis and of 'synaptic vesicle' formation in posterior pituitary glands. *Nature (London)*, **227**, 407
46. Douglas, W. W., Nagasawa, J. and Schulz, R. (1971). Electron microscopic studies on the mechanism of secretion of posterior pituitary hormones and significance of microvesicles ('synaptic vesicles'): evidence of secretion by exocytosis and formation of microvesicles as a by-product of this process. *Mem. Soc. Endocrin.*, **19**, 353
47. Verney, E. B. (1947). The antidiuretic hormone and the factors which determine its release. *Proc. Roy. Soc. Med B*, **135**, 25
48. Jewell, P. A. and Verney, E. B. (1957). An experimental attempt to determine the site of the neurohypophysial osmoreceptors in the dog. *Phil. Trans. Roy. Soc. London B*, **240**, 197
49. Yoshida, S., Motohashi, K., Ibayashi, H. and Okinaka, S. (1963). Method for the assay of antidiuretic hormone in plasma with a note on the antidiuretic titer of human plasma. *J. Lab. Clin. Med.*, **62**, 279
50. Zehr, J. E., Johnson, J. A. and Moore, W. W. (1969). Left atrial pressure, plasma osmolality, and ADH levels in the unanaesthetized ewe. *Amer. J. Physiol.*, **217**, 1672
51. Saito, T., Yoshida, S. and Nakao, K. (1969). Release of antidiuretic hormone from neurohypophysis in response to hemorrhage and infusion of hypertonic saline in dogs. *Endocrinology*, **85**, 72
52. Shimizu, K., Share, L. and Claybaugh, J. R. (1973). Potentiation by angiotensin II

of the vasopressin response to an increasing plasma osmolality. *Endocrinology*, in the press
53. Eggena, P. and Thorn, N. A. (1970). Vasopressin release from the rat supraoptico-neurohypophysial system *in vitro* in response to hypertonicity and acetylcholine. *Acta Endocrinol.*, **65**, 442
54. Dyball, R. E. J. and Koizumi, K. (1969). Electrical activity in the supraoptic and paraventricular nuclei associated with neurohypophysial hormone release. *J. Physiol.* (*London*), **201**, 711
55. Dyball, R. E. J. (1971). Oxytocin and ADH secretion in relation to electrical activity in antidromically identified supraoptic and paraventricular units. *J. Physiol.* (*London*), **214**, 245
56. Bridges, T. E. and Thorn, N. A. (1970). The effect of autonomic blocking agents on vasopressin release *in vivo* induced by osmoreceptor stimulation. *J. Endocrinol.*, **48**, 265
57. Arndt, J. O. and Gauer, O. H. (1965). Diuresis induced by water infusion into the carotid loop of unanaesthetised dogs. *Pflügers Arch.*, **282**, 301
58. Johnson, J. A., Zehr, J. E. and Moore, W. W. (1970). Effects of separate and concurrent osmotic and volume stimuli on plasma ADH in sheep. *Amer. J. Physiol.*, **218**, 1273
59. Moses, A. M. and Miller, M. (1971). Osmotic threshold for vasopressin release as determined by saline infusion and by dehydration. *Neuroendocrinology*, **7**, 219
60. Moore, W. W. (1971). Antidiuretic hormone levels in normal subjects. *Fed. Proc.*, **30**, 1387
61. Robertson, G. L., Klein, L. A., Roth, J. and Gorden, P. (1970). Immunoassay of plasma vasopressin in man. *Proc. Nat. Acad. Sci. USA*, **66**, 1298
62. Beardwell, C. G. (1971). Radioimmunoassay of arginine vasopressin in human plasma. *J. Clin. Endocrin. Metabolism.*, **33**, 254
63. Andersson, B., Dallman, M. F. and Olsson, K. (1969). Observations on central control of drinking and of the release of antidiuretic hormone (ADH). *Life Sci.*, **8**, 425
64. Mouw, D. R. and Vander, A. J. (1971). Evidence for hormonal mediation of the renal response to low-sodium stimulation of the brain. *Proc. Soc. Exp. Biol. Med.*, **137**, 179
65. Olsson, K. (1969). Studies on central regulation of secretion of anti-diuretic hormone (ADH) in the goat. *Acta Physiol. Scand.*, **77**, 465
66. Eriksson, L., Fernandez, O. and Olsson, K. (1971). Differences in the antidiuretic response to intracarotid infusions of various hypertonic solutions in the conscious goat. *Acta Physiol. Scand.*, **83**, 554
67. Olsson, K. and McDonald, I. R. (1970). Lack of antidiuretic response to osmotic stimuli in the early stages of a water diuresis in sheep. *J. Endocrinol.*, **48**, 301
68 Andersson, B. and Westbye, O. (1970). Synergistic action of sodium and angiotensin on brain mechanisms controlling fluid balance. *Life Sci.*, **9**, 601
69 Andersson, B. and Eriksson, L. (1971). Conjoint action of sodium and angiotensin on brain mechanisms controlling water and salt balance. *Acta Physiol. Scand.*, **81**, 18
70. Andersson, B., Eriksson, L. and Oltner, R. (1970). Further evidence for angiotensin-sodium interaction in central control of fluid balance. *Life Sci.*, **9**, 1091
71. Haberlich, F. J., Aziz, O. and Nowacki, P. E. (1965). Über einen osmoreceptorisch tätigen mechanismus in der leber. *Pflügers Arch.*, **285**, 73
71. Haberich, F. J., Aziz, O. and Nowacki, P. E. (1965). Über einen osmoreceptorisch osmoreceptoren in der leber. *Pflügers Arch.*, **313**, 289
73. Dennhardt, R., Ohm, W. W. and Haberich, F. J. (1971). Die ausschaltung der leberäste des N. vagus an der wachen ratte und ihr einflub auf die hepatogene diurese-indirekter beweis für die afferente leitung der leber-osmo-receptoren über den N. vagus. *Pflügers Arch.*, **328**, 51
74. Niijima, A. (1969). Afferent discharges from osmoreceptors in the liver of the guinea pig. *Science*, **166**, 1519
75. Schneider, E. G., Davis, J. O., Robb, C. A., Baumber, J. S., Johnson, J. A. and Wright, F. S. (1970). Lack of evidence for a hepatic osmoreceptor mechanism in conscious dogs. *Amer. J. Physiol.*, **218**, 42
76. Ginsburg, M. and Heller, H. (1953). Antidiuretic activity in blood obtained from various parts of the cardiovascular system. *J. Endocrinol.*, **9**, 274
77. Weinstein, H., Berne, R. M. and Sachs, H. (1960). Vasopressin in blood: effect of hemorrhage. *Endocrinology*, **66**, 712

78. Share, L. (1962). Vascular volume and blood level of antidiuretic hormone. *Amer. J. Physiol.*, **202,** 791
79. Henry, J. P., Gupta, P. D., Meehan, J. P., Sinclair, R. and Share, L. (1968). The role of afferents from the low-pressure system in the release of antidiuretic hormone during non-hypotensive hemorrhage. *Can. J. Physiol. Pharmacol.*, **46,** 287
80. Share, L. (1968). Control of plasma ADH titer in hemorrhage: role of atrial and arterial receptors. *Amer. J. Physiol.*, **215,** 1384
81. Henry, J. P., Gauer, O. H. and Reeves, J. L. (1956). Evidence of the atrial location of receptors influencing urine flow. *Circulation Res.*, **4,** 85
82. Baïsset, A. and Montastruc, P. (1957). Polyuric par distension auriculaire chez le chien; rôle de l'hormone antidiurétique. *J. Physiol. Paris*, **49,** 33
83. Share, L. (1965). Effects of carotid occlusion and left atrial distension on plasma vasopressin titer. *Amer. J. Physiol.*, **208,** 219
84. Johnson, J. A., Moore, W. W. and Segar, W. E. (1969). Small changes in left atrial pressure and plasma antidiuretic hormone titers in dogs. *Amer. J. Physiol.*, **217,** 210
85. Goetz, L. K., Bond, G. C., Hermreck, A. S. and Trank, J. W. (1970). Plasma ADH levels following a decrease in mean atrial transmural pressure in dogs. *Amer. J. Physiol.*, **219,** 1424
86. Brennan, L. A., Jr., Malvin, R. L., Jochim, K. E. and Roberts, D. E. (1971). Influence of right and left atrial receptors on plasma concentrations of ADH and renin. *Amer. J. Physiol.*, **221,** 273
87. Share, L. and Levy, M. N. (1962). Cardiovascular receptors and blood titer of antidiuretic hormone. *Amer. J. Physiol.*, **203,** 425
88. Share, L. and Levy, M. N. (1966). Carotid sinus pulse pressure, a determinant of plasma antidiuretic hormone concentration. *Amer. J. Physiol.*, **211,** 721
89. Bond, G. C. and Trank, J. W. (1972). Plasma antidiuretic hormone concentration after bilaterial aortic nerve section. *Amer. J. Physiol.*, **222,** 595
90. Gupta, P. D., Henry, J. P., Sinclair, R. and von Baumgarten, R. (1966). Responses of atrial and aortic baroreceptors to nonhypotensive hemorrhage and to transfusion. *Amer. J. Physiol.* **211,** 1429
91. Claybaugh, J. R. and Share, L. (1973). Vasopressin, renin and cardiovascular responses to continuous slow hemorrhage. *Amer. J. Physiol.*, **224,** 519
92. Zehr, J. A., Hawe, A., Tsakiris, A. G., Rastelli, G. C., McGoon, D. C. and Segar, W. E. (1971). ADH levels following nonhypotensive hemorrhage in dogs with chronic mitral stenosis. *Amer. J. Physiol.*, **221,** 312
93. Rogge, J. D., Moore, W. W., Segar, W. E. and Fasola, A. F. (1967). Effect of $+G_z$ and $+G_x$ acceleration on peripheral venous ADH levels in humans. *J. Appl. Physiol.*, **23,** 870
94. Segar, W. E. and Moore, W. W. (1968). The regulation of antidiuretic hormone release in man. I. Effects of change in position and ambient temperature on blood ADH levels. *J. Clin. Invest.*, **47,** 2143
95. Bengele, H. H., Moore, W. W. and Wunder, C. C. (1969). Decreased antidiuretic activity measured in the blood of chronically centrifuged rats. *Aerospace Med.*, **40,** 518
96. Auger, R. G., Zehr, J. E., Siekert, R. G. and Segar, W. E. (1970). Position effect on antidiuretic hormone. *Arch. Neurol.*, **23,** 513
97. Share, L., Claybaugh, J. R., Hatch, F. E., Johnson, J. G., Lee, S., Muirhead, E. E. and Shaw, P. (1972). Effects of change in posture and of sodium depletion on plasma levels of vasopressin and renin in normal human subjects. *J. Clin. Endocrin. Metab.*, **35,** 171
98. Brennan, L. A., Bonjour, J.-P. and Malvin, R. L. (1971). ADH levels during salt depletion in dogs. *Europ. J. Clin. Invest.*, **2,** 43
99. Severs, W. B., Summy-Long, J., Taylor, J. S. and Connor, J. D. (1970). A central effect of angiotensin: release of pituitary pressor material. *J. Pharmacol. Exp. Therap.*, **174,** 27
100. Bonjour, J.-P. and Malvin, R. L. (1970). Stimulation of ADH release by the renin-angiotensin system. *Amer. J. Physiol.*, **218,** 1555
101. Mouw, D., Bonjour, J.-P., Malvin, R. L. and Vander, A. (1971). Central action of angiotensin in stimulating ADH release. *Amer. J. Physiol.*, **220,** 239
102. Claybaugh, J. R., Share, L. and Shimizu, K. (1972). The inability of infusions of

angiotensin to elevate the plasma vasopressin concentration in the anesthetized dog. *Endocrinology*, **90**, 1647

103. Claybaugh, J. R. and Share, L. (1972). Role of the renin-angiotensin system in the vasopressin response to hemorrhage. *Endocrinology*, **90**, 453

104. Travis, R. H. and Share, L. (1971). Vasopressin-renin-cortisol inter-relations. *Endocrinology*, **89**, 246

105. Nicholl, R. A. and Barker, J. L. (1971). Excitation of supraoptic neuro-secretory cells by angiotensin II. *Nature New Biol.*, **233**, 172

106. Ahmed, A. B. J., George, B. C., Gonzalez-Auvert, C. and Dingman, J. F. (1967). Increased plasma arginine vasopressin in clinical adrenocortical insufficiency and its inhibition by glucosteroids. *J. Clin. Invest.*, **46**, 111

107. Kleeman, C. R., Czaczkes, J. W. and Cutler, R. (1964). Mechanisms of impaired water excretion in adrenal and pituitary insufficiency. IV. Antidiuretic hormone in primary and secondary adrenal insufficiency. *J. Clin. Invest.*, **43**, 1641

108. Share, L. and Travis, R. H. (1970). Plasma vasopressin concentration in the adrenally insufficient dog. *Endocrinology*, **86**, 196

109. Green, H. H., Harrington, A. R. and Valtin, H. (1970). On the role of antidiuretic hormone in the inhibition of acute water diuresis in adrenal insufficiency and the effects of gluco- and mineralocorticoids in reversing the inhibition. *J. Clin. Invest.*, **49**, 1724

110. Aubry, R. H., Nankin, H. R., Moses, A. M. and Streeten, D. H. P. (1965). Measurement of the osmotic threshold for vasopressin release in human subjects and its modification by cortisol. *J. Clin. Endocrinol.*, **25**, 1481

111. Vilhardt, H. (1970). Influence of corticosteroids and chlorpromazine on the release of vasopressin from isolated neural lobes of rats. *Acta Endocrinol.*, **65**, 490

112. Shimizu, K., Kurosawa, T., Maeda, T. and Yoshitoshi, Y. (1969). Free water excretion and washout of renal medullary urea by prostaglandin E_1. *Jap. Heart J.*, **10**, 437

113. Vilhardt, H. and Hedqvist, P. (1970). A possible role of prostaglandin E_2 in the regulation of vasopressin secretion in rats. *Life Sci.*, **9**, 825

114. Bisset, G. W., Clark, B. J. and Errington, M. L. (1971). The hypothalamic neuro-secretory pathways for the release of oxytocin and vasopressin in the cat. *J. Physiol. (London)*, **217**, 111

115. Menninger, R. P. and Frazier, D. T. (1972). Effects of blood volume and atrial stretch on hypothalamic single-unit activity. *Amer. J. Physiol.*, **223**, 288

116. Barker, J. L., Crayton, J. W. and Nicoll, R. A. (1971). Supraoptic neurosecretory cells: autonomic modulation. *Science*, **171**, 206

117. Hayward, J. N. and Vincent, J. D. (1970). Osmosensitive single neurones in the hypothalamus of anaesthetized monkeys. *J. Physiol. (London)*, **210**, 947

118. Olsson, K. (1970). Effects on water diuresis of infusions of transmitter substances into the 3rd ventricle. *Acta Physiol. Scand.*, **79**, 133

119. Kühn, E. R. and McCann, S. M. (1971). Release of oxytocin and vasopressin in lactating rats after injection of carbachol into the third ventricle. *Neuroendocrinology*, **8**, 48

120. Dreifuss, J. J. and Kelly, J. S. (1972). The activity of identified supraoptic neurones and their response to acetylcholine applied by iontophoresis. *J. Physiol. (London)*, **220**, 105

121. Barker, J. L., Crayton, J. W. and Nicoll, R. A. (1971). Noradrenaline and acetylcholine responses of supraoptic neurosecretory cells. *J. Physiol. (London)*, **218**, 19

122. Bhargava, K. P., Kulshrestha, V. K. and Srivastava, Y. P. (1972). Central cholinergic and adrenergic mechanisms in the release of antidiuretic hormone. *Brit. J. Pharmacol.*, **44**, 617

123. Gosbee, J. L. and Lederis, K. (1972). *In vivo* release of antidiuretic hormone by direct application of acetylcholine or carbachol to the rat neurohypophysis. *Can. J. Physiol. Pharmacol.*, **50**, 618

124. Lauson, H. D. (1967). Metabolism of antiduretic hormones. *Amer. J. Med.*, **42**, 713

125. Lauson, H. D. (1970). Fate of the neurohypophysial hormones. *International Encyclopaedia of Pharmacology and Therapeutics*, Section 41, Vol. 2, 377 (H. Heller and B. T. Pickering, editors) (Oxford: Pergamon)

126. Vorherr, H., Kleeman, C. R. and Hoghoughi, M. (1968). Factors influencing the

sensitivity of rats under ethanol anesthesia to antidiuretic hormone (ADH). *Endocrinology*, **82**, 218

127. Fabian, M., Forsling, M. L., Jones, J. J. and Pryor, J. S. (1969). The clearance and antidiuretic potency of neurohypophysial hormones in man, and their plasma binding and stability. *J. Physiol. (London)*, **204**, 653

128. Pliska, V., Heller, J. and Tata, P. S. (1970). Anomalous changes in the plasma antidiuretic activity of hydrated dogs after the cessation of intravenous infusion of arginine vasopressin. *Experientia*, **26**, 1108

129. Miller, M. and Moses, A. M. (1972). Radioimmunoassay of urinary antidiuretic hormone in man: response to water load and dehydration in normal subjects. *J. Clin. Endocrinol.*, **34**, 537

130. Berliner, R. W. and Bennett, C. M. (1967). Concentration of urine in the mammalian kidney. *Amer. J. Med.*, **42**, 777

131. Grantham, J. J. and Burg, M. B. (1966). Effect of vasopressin and cyclic AMP on permeability of isolated collecting tubules. *Amer. J. Physiol.*, **211**, 255

132. Hays, R. M., Franki, N. and Soberman, R. (1971). Activation energy for water diffusion across the toad bladder: evidence against the pore enlargement hypothesis. *J. Clin. Invest.*, **50**, 1016

133. Orloff, H. and Handler, J. S. (1962). The similarity of effects of vasopressin, adenosine-3',5'-phosphate (cyclic AMP) and theophylline on the toad bladder. *J. Clin. Invest.*, **41**, 702

134. Orloff, J. and Handler, J. S. (1967). The role of adenosine 3',5'-phosphate in the action of antidiuretic hormone. *Amer. J. Med.*, **42**, 757

135. Graziani, Y. and Livne, A. (1971). Vasopressin and water permeability of artificial lipid membranes. *Biochem. Biophys. Res. Commun.*, **45**, 321

136. Fisher, R. D., Grünfeld, J. P. and Barger, A. C. (1970). Intrarenal distribution of blood flow in diabetes insipidus: role of ADH. *Amer. J. Physiol.*, **219**, 1348

137. Yates, F. E., Russell, S. M., Dallman, M. F., Hedge, G. A., McCann, S. M. and Dhariwal, A. P. S. (1971). Potentiation by vasopressin of corticotropin release induced by corticotropin-releasing factor. *Endocrinology*, **88**, 3

138. Schapiro, H. and Britt, L. F. (1972). The action of vasopressin on the gastrointestinal tract. *Amer. J. Dig. Dis.*, **17**, 649

139. Dennhardt, R. and Haberich, F. J. (1972). Wirkung von ADH und den netto-wasser- und elektrolyttransport am dünndarm wacher ratten. *Pflügers Arch.*, **334**, 74

140. Cole, D. F. and Nagusubramanian, S. (1972). The effect of natural and synthetic vasopressins and other substances on active transport in ciliary epithelium of the rabbit. *Exp. Eye Res.*, **13**, 45

141. DeWied, D. (1971). Long term effect of vasopressin on the maintenance of a conditioned avoidance response in rats. *Nature (London)*, **232**, 58

142. DeWied, D., Greven, H. M., Lande, S. and Witter, A. (1972). Dissociation of the behavioural and endocrine effects of lysine vasopressin by tryptic digestion. *Brit. J. Pharmacol.*, **45**, 118

143. Bartelstone, H. and Nasmyth, P. A. (1965). Vasopressin potentiation of catecholamine actions in dog, rat, cat, and rat aortic strip. *Amer. J. Physiol.*, **208**, 754

144. Frieden, J. and Keller, A. (1954). Decreased resistance to hemorrhage in neurohypophysectomized dogs. *Circulation Res.*, **2**, 214

145. Fitzpatrick, R. J. (1966). The posterior pituitary gland and the female reproductive tract. *The Pituitary Gland*, Vol. 3, 453. (G. W. Harris and B. T. Donovan, editors) (Berkeley: University of California Press)

146. Debackere, M. and Peeters, G. (1960). The influence of vaginal distention on milk ejection and diuresis in the lactating cow. *Archiv. Int. Pharmacodyn.*, **123**, 462

147. Debackere, M. and Peeters, G. (1960). Le mechanism de l'ejection du lait par distension vaginale chez le mouton. *Archiv. Int. Pharmacodyn.*, **126**, 486

148. Debackere, M., Peeters, G. and Tuyttens, N. (1961). Reflex release of an oxytocic hormone by stimulation of genital organs in male and female sheep studied by a cross circulation technique. *J. Endocrinol.*, **22**, 321

149. Van Demark, N. L. and Hays, R. L. (1953). Effect of stimulation of the reproductive organs of the cow on the release of an oxytocin-like substance. *Endocrinology*, **52**, 634

150. Roberts, J. S. and Share, L. (1968). Oxytocin in plasma of pregnant, lactating and cycling ewes during vaginal stimulation. *Endocrinology*, **83**, 272

151. Roberts, J. S. and Share, L. (1969). Effects of progesterone and estrogen on blood levels of oxytocin during vaginal distention. *Endocrinology*, **84**, 1076
152. Roberts, J. S. (1971). Seasonal variations in the reflexive release of oxytocin and in the effect of estradiol on the reflex in goats. *Endocrinology*, **89**, 1029
153. Fox, C. A. and Knaggs, G. S. (1969). Milk-ejection activity (oxytocin) in peripheral venous blood in man during lactation and in association with coitus. *J. Endocrinol.*, **45**, 145
154. Eränko, O., Friberg, O. and Karvonen, M. J. (1953). The effect of the act of copulation on water diuresis in the rat. *Acta Endocrinol.*, **12**, 197
155. Friberg, O. (1953). The antidiuretic effect of coitus in human subjects. *Acta Endocrinol.*, **12**, 193
156. Van Demark, N. L. and Hays, R. L. (1952). Uterine motility responses to mating. *Amer. J. Physiol.*, **170**, 518
157. Harris, G. W. (1955). *Neural Control of the Pituitary Gland* (London: Edward Arnold)
158. Gunther, M. (1948). The posterior pituitary and labour. *Brit. Med. J.*, i, 567
159. Sica-Blanco, Y., Mendez-Bauer, C., Sala, N., Cabot, H. M. and Caldeyro-Barcia, R. (1959). Neuro metudo para el Estudio de la functionalidad mammaria en la mujer. *Arch. Ginecol. Obstet. (Montevideo)*, **17**, 63
160. Cross, B. A. (1955). The hypothalamus and the mechanism of sympathetico-adrenal inhibition of milk-ejection. *J. Endocrinol.*, **12**, 15
161. Fuchs, A. R. (1964). Oxytocin and the onset of labour in rabbits. *J. Endocrinol.*, **30**, 217
162. Fitzpatrick, R. J. and Walmsley, C. F. (1962). The concentration of oxytocin in bovine blood during parturition. *J. Physiol. (London)*, **163**, 13
163. Fitzpatrick, R. J. and Walmsley, C. F. (1965). The release of oxytocin during parturition. *Advances in Oxytocin*, 51 (J. Pinkerton, editor) (Oxford: Pergamon Press)
164. Folley, S. J. and Knaggs, G. S. (1964). Observations on oxytocin release in ruminants *J. Reprod. Fertil.*, **8**, 265
165. Folley, S. J. and Knaggs, G. S. (1965). Levels of oxytocin in the jugular vein blood of goats during parturition. *J. Endocrinol.*, **33**, 301
166. Coch, J. A., Brovetto, J., Cabot, H. M., Fielitz, C. A. and Caldeyro-Barcia, R. (1965). Oxytocin-equivalent activity in the plasma of women in labour and during the puerperium. *Amer. J. Obstet. Gynec.*, **91**, 10
167. Fitzpatrick, R. J. (1966). The neurohypophysis and the male reproductive tract *The Pituitary Gland*, Vol. 3, 505 (G. W. Harris and B. T. Donovan, editors) (Berkeley: University of California Press)
168. Bower, E. A. (1969). Action potentials from uterine sensory nerves. *J. Physiol. (London)*, **148**, 2P
169. Abrahams, V. C., Langworth, E. P. and Theobald, G. W. (1964). Potentials evoked in the hypothalamus and cerebral cortex by electrical stimulation of the uterus. *Nature (London)*, **203**, 654
170. Porter, R. W., Cavanaugh, E. B., Critchlow, B. V. and Sawyer, C. H. (1957). Localized changes in electrical activity of the hypothalamus in estrous cats following vaginal stimulation. *Amer. J. Physiol.*, **189**, 145
171. Barraclough, C. A. and Cross, B. A. (1963). Unit activity in the hypothalamus of the cyclic female rat: Effect of genital stimuli and progesterone. *J. Endocrinol.*, **26**, 339
172. Benson, G. K. and Fitzpatrick, R. J. (1966). The neurohypophysis and the mammary gland. *The Pituitary Gland*, Vol. 3, 414 (G. W. Harris and B. T. Donovan, editors) (Berkeley: University of California Press)
173. Findlay, A. L. R. (1968). The effect of teat anaesthesia on the milk-ejection reflex in the rabbit. *J. Endocrinol.*, **40**, 127
174. Grachev, I. I. (1953). The cerebral cortex and lactation. *Zh. Obshch. Biolog.*, **14**, 333
175. Fuchs, A. R. and Wagner, G. (1963). Quantitative aspects of release of oxytocin by suckling in unanesthetised rabbits. *Acta Endocrinol.*, **44**, 581
176. Mena, F. and Grosvenor, C. E. (1968). Effect of number of pups suckling upon suckling-induced fall in pituitary prolactin concentration and milk ejection in the rat. *Endocrinology*, **82**, 623
177. Lincoln, D.W., Hill, A. and Wakerley, J. B. (1973). The milk-ejection reflex of the rat: an intermittent function not abolished by surgical levels of anaesthesia. *J. Endocrinol.*, **57**, in the press.

178. Folley, S. J. and Knaggs, G. W. (1966). Milk-ejection activity (oxytocin) in the external jugular vein blood of the cow, goat and sow in relation to the stimulus of milking or suckling. *J. Endocrinol.*, **34**, 197

179. Sandholm, L. E. (1968). Variations in the milk ejection reflex in women during early stages of lactation. *Acta Obstet. Gynecol. Scand.*, **47**, 132

180. Fitzpatrick, R. J. (1961). The estimation of small amounts of oxytocin in blood. *Oxytocin*, 358 (R. Caldeyro-Barcia and H. Heller, editors) (London: Pergamon Press)

181. Grosvenor, C. E. and Mena, F. (1971). Evidence for a refractory period in the neuro-endocrine mechanism for the release of prolactin. *Endocrinol.*, **88**, 355

182. Newton, M. (1961). Human lactation. Milk: *The Mammary Gland and its Secretions*, Vol. 1, 281 (S. K. Kon and A. T. Cowie, editors) (New York: Academic Press)

183. Baryshnikov, I. A. and Kokorina, E. P. (1959). Higher nervous activity of cattle. *Proc. XV Int. Dairy Cong.*, **1**, 46

184. Cleverly, J. D. (1968). The detection of oxytocin release in response to conditioned stimuli associated with machine milking in the cow. *J. Endocrinol.*, **40**, 11

185. Deis, R. P. (1968). The effect of an exteroceptive stimulus on milk-ejection in lactating rats. *J. Physiol. (London)*, **197**, 37

186. Momongan, V. G. and Schmidt, G. H. (1970). Oxytocin levels in the plasma of Holstein-Friesian cows during milking with and without a premilking stimulus. *J. Dairy Sci.*, **53**, 747

187. McNeilly, A. S. (1972). The blood levels of oxytocin during suckling and hand-milking in the goat with some observations on the pattern of hormone release. *J. Endocrinol.*, **52**, 177

188. Findlay, A. L. R. and Grosvenor, C. E. (1969). The role of the mammary gland innervation in the control of the motor apparatus of the mammary gland. A review. *Dairy Sci. Abstr.*, **31**, 109

189. Cross, B. A. (1961). Neural control of lactation. Milk: *The Mammary Gland and its Secretions*, Vol. 1, 121 (S. K. Kon and A. T. Cowie, editors) (New York: Academic Press)

190. Linzell, J. L. (1959). Physiology of the mammary glands. *Physiol. Rev.*, **39**, 534

191. Grosvenor, C. E. and Mena, F. (1972). Neural and hormonal control of milk secretion and milk ejection. *Lactation* (B. L. Larson and V. R. Smith, editors) (New York: Academic Press)

192. Findlay, A. L. R. (1966). Sensory discharges from lactating mammary glands. *Nature (London)*, **211**, 1183

193. Isbister, C. (1954). A clinical study of the draught reflex in human lactation. *Arch. Dis. Childhood*, **29**, 66

194. Forbes, A., Forbes, A. P. and Neyland, M. (1955). Action potentials in the human mammary gland. *J. Appl. Physiol.*, **7**, 675

195. Grachev, I. I. (1949). Reflexes from the mammary gland. *Zh. Obshch. Biol.*, **10**, 401

196. Grachev, I. I. (1964). *Reflex Regulation of Lactation* (Leningrad: Izdatel stvo Leningradskogo Universitita)

197. Cobo, E., Bernal, M., Gaitan, E. and Quintero, C. A. (1967). Neurohypophyseal hormone release in the human. II. Experimental study during lactation. *Amer. J. Obstet. Gynec.*, **97**, 519

198. Beyer, C. and Mena, F. (1969). Neural factors in lactation. *Physiology and Pathology of Adaptive Mechanisms*, 310 (E. Bajus, editor) (New York: Pergamon Press)

199. Tindal, J. S. and Knaggs, G. S. (1970). Environmental stimuli and the mammary gland. *Mem. Soc. Endocrinol.*, **18**, 239

200. Cross, B. A. (1966). Neural control of oxytocin secretion. *Neuroendocrinology*, Vol. 1, 217 (L. Martini and F. Ganong, editors) (New York: Academic Press)

201. Wakerly, J. B. and Lincoln, D. W. (1973). The milk-ejection reflex of the rat: a 20- to 40-fold acceleration in the firing of paraventricular neurones during oxytocin release. *J. Endocrinol.*, **57**, in the press

202 Ely, F. and Peterson, W. E. (1941). Factors involved in the ejection of milk. *J. Dairy Sci.*, **24**, 211

203. Whittlestone, W. G. (1951). Studies on milk-ejection in the dairy cow. *N.Z.J. Sci. Tech.*, **A 32**, 1

204. Newton, M. and Newton, N. R. (1948). The let-down reflex in human lactation. *J. Pediat.*, **33**, 698

205. Cross, B. A. (1955). Neurohormonal mechanisms in emotional inhibition of milk-ejection. *J. Endocrinol.*, **12**, 29

206. Chaudhury, R. R., Chaudhury, M. R. and Lu, F. C. (1961). Stress-induced block of milk-ejection. *Brit. J. Pharmacol. Chemotherap.*, **17**, 305

207. Taleisnik, S. and Deis, R. P. (1964). Influence of cerebral cortex in inhibition of oxytocin release induced by stressful stimuli. *Amer. J. Physiol.*, **207**, 1394

208. Grosvenor, C. E. and Mena, F. (1967). Effect of auditory, olfactory and optic stimuli on milk ejection and suckling-induced release of prolactin in lactating rats. *Endocrinology*, **80**, 840

209. Cross, B. A. (1958). On the mechanism of labour in the rabbit. *J. Endocrinol.*, **16**, 261

210. Aulsebrook, L. H. and Holland, R. C. (1969). Central inhibition of oxytocin release. *Amer. J. Physiol.*, **216**, 830

211. Koizumi, K., Ishikawa, T. and Brooks, McC. (1964). Control of activity of neurons in the supraoptic nucleus. *J. Neurophysiol.*, **27**, 878

212. Richardson, K. C. (1949). Contractile tissues in the mammary glands with special reference to myoepithelium in the goat. *Proc. R. Soc. B*, **136**, 30

213. Linzell, J. L. (1955). Some observations on the contractile tissue of the mammary glands. *J. Physiol. (London)*, **130**, 257

214. Folley, S. J. and Knaggs, G. W. (1970). Physiological and pharmacological effects: mammary action. *Pharmacology of the Endocrine System and Related Drugs: The Neurohypophysis*, Vol. 1, 295 (H. Heller and B. T. Pickering, editors) (New York: Pergamon Press)

215. Mendez-Bauer, C., Cabot, H. M. and Caldeyro-Barcia, R. (1960). A new test for the biological assay of oxytocin. *Science*, **132**, 299

216. Moore, R. D. and Zarrow, M. X. (1965). Contraction of the rabbit mammary strip *in vitro* in response to oxytocin. *Acta Endocrinol.*, **48**, 186

217. Polacek, I., Krejci, I. and Rudinger, J. (1967). The action of oxytocin and synthetic analogues on the isolated mammary-gland myoepithelium of the lactating rat; effect of some ions. *J. Endocrinol.*, **38**, 13

218. Lawson, D. M. and Schmidt, G. H. (1972). Role of cations in the milk-ejecting action of oxytocin in rat mammary tissue. *Amer. J. Physiol.*, **222**, 444

219. Lawson, D. M. and Schmidt, G. H. (1972). Effects of lanthanum on ^{45}Ca movements of oxytocin-induced milk ejection in mammary tissue. *Proc. Soc. Exp. Biol. Med.*, **140**, 481

220. Bisset, G. W., Clark, B. J. and Lewis, G. P. (1967). The mechanism of the inhibitory action of adrenaline on the mammary gland. *Brit. J. Pharmacol. Chemotherap.*, **31**, 550

221. Chan, W. Y. (1965). Mechanism of epinephrine inhibition of the milk-ejecting response to oxytocin. *J. Pharmacol. Exp. Therap.*, **147**, 48

222. Houvenaghel, A. (1969). Biological determinants of plasma oxytocin. *Mém. Acad. r. Méd. Belg.*, **7**, 47

223. Grosvenor, C. E. and Findlay, A. L. R. (1968). Effect of denervation of fluid flow into rat mammary gland. *Amer. J. Physiol.*, **217**, 820

224. Grosvenor, C. E., DeNuccio, D. M., King, S. F., Maiweg, H. and Mena, F. (1972). Central and peripheral neural influences on the oxytocin-induced pressure response of the mammary gland of the anesthetized lactating rat. *J. Endocrinol.*, **55**, 299

225. Vorherr, H. (1971). Catecholamine antagonism to oxytocin-induced milk-ejection. *Acta Endocrinol. Copenhagen*, **67**, 1

226. Csapo, A. (1959). Function and regulation of the myoepithelium. *Ann. New York Acad. Sci.*, **75**, 790

227. Munsick, R. A. (1968). The effect of neurohypophysial hormones and similar peptides on the uterus and other extravascular smooth muscle tissue. *Handb. Exp. Pharmacol.*, Vol. 23, 443 (B. Berde, editor) (New York: Springer-Verlag)

228. Chan, W. Y., O'Connell, M. and Pomeroy, S. R. (1963). Effects of the estrous cycle on the sensitivity of rat uterus to oxytocin and desamino-oxytocin. *Endocrinology*, **72**, 279

229. Munsick, R. A. and Jeronimus, S. C. (1965). Effects of diethylstilbestrol and magnesium on the rat oxytocin potencies of some neurohypophysial hormones and analogues. *Endocrinology*, **76**, 90

230. Embrey, M. P. (1959). A criterion of oxytocin activity. *J. Obstet. Gynaec. Brit. Cwlth.*, **66**, 871

231. Calderyo-Barcia, R. and Sereno, J. A. (1961). The response of the human uterus to oxytocin throughout pregnancy. *Oxytocin*, 177 (R. Caldeyro-Barcia and H. Heller, editors) (New York: Pergamon Press)

232. Csapo, A. E. (1961). The effects of oxytocin substances on the excitability of the uterus. *Oxytocin*, 100 (R. Caldeyro-Barcia and H. Heller, editors) (New York: Pergamon Press)

233. Ginsburg, M. (1968). Production, release, transportation and elimination of the neuro-hypophysial hormones. *Handbook of Experimental Pharmacology*, Vol. 23, 286 (B. Berde, editor) (Berlin: Springer-Verlag)

234. Noddle, B. (1962). Metabolism of oxytocin in the mammary glands. *Proc. Int. Union Physiol. XXII Int. Congr. Leiden*, Abstr. Comm. No. 523

235. Page, E. W. (1946). The value of plasma pitocinase determination in obstetrics. *Amer. J. Obstet. Gynec.*, **52**, 1014

236. Werle, E. A., Hevelke, A. and Buthman, K. (1941). Zur Kenntnis des oxytocin-abbauenden Prinzips des Blutes. *Biochem. Z*, **309**, 270

237. Dicker, S. E. and Tyler, C. (1956). Inactivation of oxytocin and vasopressin by blood of pregnant women. *J. Obstet. Gynaec. Brit. Emp.*, **63**, 690

238. Dicker, S. E. and Whyley, G. A. (1959). Inactivation of oxytocin by plasma of pregnant women. *J. Obstet. Gynaec. Brit. Emp.*, **66**, 605

239. Tagawa, H., Vander, A. J., Bonjour, J.-P. and Malvin, R. L. (1971). Inhibition of renin secretion by vasopressin in unanesthetized sodium-deprived dogs. *Amer. J. Physiol.*, **220**, 949

2
Hypothalamic Hypophysial Releasing and Inhibiting Hormones

S. M. McCANN*, C. P. FAWCETT and L. KRULICH
University of Texas Southwestern Medical School, Dallas

* Research from the author's laboratory was supported by grants from NIH (AM10073
and AD05151), from the Ford Foundation, Texas Population Crisis and the R. A. Welch
Foundation.

2.1   INTRODUCTION

During the past 15 years there has been a complete revolution in our thinking about the control of adenohypophysial function. Whereas the pituitary gland was thought to be the master gland and the conductor of the endocrine symphony orchestra, it is now clear that it must be reduced to the role of concert master, the conductor residing in the hypothalamus. The ability of a variety of environmental stimuli to influence the secretion of the pituitary had long led to the recognition that there must be some degree of neural control over the gland. For example, seasonal factors play an important role in regulating reproductive cycles and a variety of stresses have been known since the early 1950s to stimulate release of adrenocorticotrophin (ACTH). The classical example of neural control of gonadotrophin secretion was provided by copulation-induced ovulation which occurs in the rabbit, ferret and a few other species. Until recently the view persisted that the pituitary, interacting with target gland secretions, was largely self-regulating and that CNS influences were only important in certain situations. It is now clear that the gland is under moment to moment control by the central nervous system via the hypothalamus. Furthermore, this control is neurohumoral in nature and mediated by a new family of releasing and inhibiting polypeptide neurohormones. At least two active substances, thyrotropin-releasing factor (TRF) and luteinising hormone-releasing factor (LRF), have been synthesised. These new hormones are stored largely in the median eminence and infundibular stem and are transported down the stalk by a specialised hypophysial portal system of veins to modulate the secretion of each and every adenohypophysial hormone.

In this review we will begin by summarising briefly the historical developments in the field and indicate the unique anatomical considerations which make possible the neurohumoral control of the gland. Then we will outline the evidence for the existence of the various hypothalamic factors, of which ten have now been postulated. Some of these have now reached the status where they certainly must be called hormones, whereas the existence of others is still somewhat in doubt. We will then try to consider the common features of the action of these new hormones on the gland, discuss their hypothalamic localisation and describe their interaction with target gland hormones both at the hypothalamic and pituitary level. We will consider some of the synaptic transmitters which may be involved in the release of these new hormones and lastly consider the present status of their chemistry.

2.2   HISTORICAL SUMMARY

The earliest evidence for hypothalamic control over the functions of the adenohypophysis came from classical techniques of lesions and electrical stimulations. As early as 1921, Bailey and Bremer[1] reported atrophy of the testis following lesions restricted to the hypothalamus of the dog. In the early 1930s, P. E. Smith[2] reported the tuberal syndrome in the rat in which lesions in the basal hypothalamus produced atrophy of various endocrine target glands and disruption of oestrous cycles. In the late thirties and early forties, a series of papers from Dey in Ranson's laboratory indicated that lesions in the median eminence region disrupted gonadal function and that lesions over the optic chiasm could induce constant vaginal oestrus in guinea-pigs[3]. It is now clear that median eminence lesions result in impairment in the secretion of all anterior pituitary hormones with the exception of prolactin, the secretion of which is enhanced[4]. In most cases these conclusions are now based on radioimmunoassay (RIA) of the various hormones in blood. This is coupled with a decrease in stored hormone content in the anterior lobe which indicates that there is deficiency not only in release but also in the synthesis of hormone[5].

As early as the mid-1930s, it was shown that electrical stimulation in the preoptic region or anterior hypothalamus would evoke ovulation[6]. Utilising radioimmunoassay, it has been possible to show that LH-release is enhanced by electrical or electrochemical stimulation of a broad band of tissue extending from the medial preoptic region through the anterior hypothalamus and into the median eminence arcuate region, whereas FSH-release is evoked from a slightly more caudal area extending from anterior hypothalamus into median eminence[7, 8]. ACTH release has been reported to occur from stimulation of a variety of hypothalamic sites including anterior hypothalamus and median eminence[9]. The evidence for ACTH release has been an increase in corticoid output by the adrenals rather than actual measurement of blood ACTH levels. TSH is also released by anterior hypothalamic stimulation[10], but growth hormone is released by stimulation of the lateral portions of the ventromedial nucleus[11]. Thus, these stimulation studies not only show that the hypothalamus can evoke secretion of anterior pituitary hormones but also give some evidence for localisation of function within this part of the brain. Conversely, lesion studies have shown that it is possible to interrupt selectively secretion of one or another pituitary hormone[12, 13].

These stimulation and lesion experiments clearly indicate a role for the hypothalamus in controlling pituitary function but cast no light on the mechanism by which this control is exerted. As early as 1933, Hinsey and Markee[14] suggested that the anterior pituitary might be controlled humorally via neurohypophysial hormones, a prophetic suggestion which is very close to the truth. At the time they made their suggestion, the hypophysial portal system of veins had not been discovered. This unique system was discovered in 1933 by Popa and Fielding[15], and the direction of flow was finally established to be from hypothalamus to pituitary by the anatomical studies of Wislocki and King[16] and by the direct observation of the direction of flow in the vessels by Houssay et al.[17] and, much later, by Green and Harris[18]. Since it was accepted that there was little if any innervation of the anterior lobe via the hypothalamus, the possibility of neurohumoral control by the hypophysial portal system of vessels was suggested by several investigators in the mid-1930s. Apparently Friedgood was the first to make this suggestion in 1936 in an oral address at the Harvard Tercentenary Exposition: however, his remarks were not published until very recently[19]. Hinsey[20] and Haterius[6] were the first to publish this hypothesis in 1937. Harris had found the anterior lobe to be electrically excitable and actually favoured a direct secretomotor innervation of the gland[21]. Later studies[22] showed that the gland was not directly excitable and these early results of Harris must be attributed to current spread to the hypothalamus.

Harris deserves the primary credit for developing the concept of neuro-humoral control of the pituitary gland. The results of stalk section had been quite variable with reports ranging from no effect to partial or complete disruption of pituitary function. Harris resolved this problem by showing that the hypophysial portal vessels were capable of rapid regeneration and that stalk section produced permanent disruption of pituitary function if this regeneration was prevented by placing a paper plate or other obstacle between the cut ends of the stalk[23]. With Jacobsohn, he showed that pituitaries grafted to a distant site had little ability to restore pituitary function but that similar grafts placed under the median eminence which were revascularised by the portal vessels were capable of fully restoring the functions of the gland[24].

These observations provided strong indirect evidence for the neuro-humoral hypothesis, but it remained for a group of young investigators stimulated by the work of Harris to provide direct evidence for the hypothesis by injecting extracts of hypothalamic tissue and stimulating the secretion of pituitary hormones. In retrospect, it is easy to see why this step was a formidable one. It is now clear that only minute amounts of the hypothalamic releasing and inhibiting hormones are stored in the median eminence, perhaps because they have preferential access to the gland via the portal vessels. Therefore, a prerequisite to obtain activity with hypothalamic extracts was a sensitive means for evaluating pituitary function.

The first such sensitive test of pituitary function was the estimation of ACTH secretion by adrenal ascorbic acid depletion[25]. It was also necessary to block the ubiquitous stress-induced release of ACTH. This could be accomplished either by pharmacological blockade utilising drugs to suppress CNS control, such as Nembutal plus morphine anaesthesia[26], or large doses of adrenal corticoids[27] or by means of hypothalamic lesions to eliminate CNS control[28]. Since the hypothalamus is a veritable storehouse of pharmaco-logically active agents, it was then necessary to determine if any of these played a role in stimulating ACTH secretion. Epinephrine, norepinephrine, histamine and serotonin were shown not to be effective in animals in which the stress response was blocked; however, the neurohypophysial hormone, vasopressin, could evoke ACTH release[28]. Controversy then ensued as to whether or not vasopressin was the only corticotrophin-releasing factor or whether there was, in addition, a specific corticotrophin-releasing factor (CRF). This controversy was magnified by utilisation of neural lobe extracts for most of the early studies of CRF[29, 30]. These contain mostly vasopressin and little if any CRF[31-33]. The controversy was settled with the use of hypo-thalamic extracts which could readily be shown to contain CRF distinct from vasopressin[31, 34]. There simply was too little vasopressin present to account for the biological activity. Hypothalamic CRF was purified[35-38] and, in the meantime, it had been shown that the ACTH-releasing activity of blood collected from the cut pituitary stalk could not be accounted for by vasopressin[39]. By the late 1950s the existence of a specific CRF had been established and this was followed by an intensified and successful search for the other factors (or activities).

2.3 ANATOMICAL CONSIDERATIONS

The unique features of the anatomy of the region from a functional standpoint are the absence of a secretomotor innervation to the anterior lobe and the presence of the hypophysial portal system of veins. There are two groups of these veins, the long portal vessels which originate from recurrent capillary loops in the median eminence and pass down the pituitary stalk to end in the sinusoids of the anterior lobe and the short portal vessels which take origin from capillaries in the neural lobe and pass across the intermediate lobe to join the anterior lobe sinusoidal network[40]. Flow in these vessels is predominantly in a direction from neural tissues to the anterior lobe; however, Török[41] has claimed to see some flow in the reverse direction under abnormal conditions. There appears to be no arterial supply to the anterior lobe in any species in which the question has been carefully examined. Thus, all blood which passes through the anterior lobe has previously passed through either the median eminence, infundibular stem or infundibular process where it would pick up neurosecretory products. Individual portal vessels appear to receive blood from rather restricted regions in the median eminence and to perfuse relatively restricted areas in the adenohypophysis[42]. This suggests some anatomical specificity, so that releasing factors released into particular portal vessels might act on particular types of pituitary cells lying in the bed perfused by that portal vessel. However, in vivo studies have not supported this concept probably because it is almost impossible to mimic the perfusion pressure which is normally operative[43].

Autoregulation appears to be operative in the portal circulation since lowering the blood pressure results in vasodilation and maintenance of adenohypophysial blood flow[44]. Vasoactive agents such as vasopressin and norepinephrine, constrict the bed as in other microcirculations[45].

Since this is a true portal circulation, one would expect relatively low pressures in the portal veins and a very low pressure in the pituitary sinusoids, but no measurements have been made. In order for Starling's hypothesis to operate, one would assume also a very high permeability of the pituitary sinusoids such that there would be a balance between colloid osmotic forces on the one hand and perfusion pressure on the other even at the very low sinusoidal pressures. No actual measurements of capillary permeability in the pituitary sinusoids have been made; however, electron microscope studies indicate that these sinusoids have the characteristics of the highly permeable vascular beds found in most glands[46]. This would be a requirement of this bed which must be permeable to relatively large protein and glycoprotein pituitary hormones on the one hand and the polypeptide-releasing factors on the other.

Since the rate of perfusion of the gland is very high, it is possible that flow is seldom a limiting factor in determining secretion of pituitary hormones; however, more data is really needed to settle this issue conclusively. Although hypothalamic lesions in the median eminence would be expected to interrupt the flow in the long portal vessels at least partially, it is clear that the defect in ACTH secretion following such lesions is not due to restricted blood flow in the gland since corticoid output was severely depressed in such animals in the presence of a normal blood flow and infusion of CRF was followed by a rapid release of ACTH[47].

2.4   CRITERIA FOR A RELEASING FACTOR

There are several criteria which must be fulfilled before a releasing or in-hibiting factor can be considered to be established as a hormone[48]. These can be listed as follows:

(a) The activity should be extractable from the hypothalamic region, in particular from the median eminence.

(b) The extract should be capable of producing an alteration in the secre-tion of the particular target pituitary hormone by a direct action on the gland as demonstrated by its ability to affect the *in vitro* release of hormone. Evidence for an action directly on the gland *in vivo* can be obtained if the extract is active in animals with median eminence lesions to interrupt neural control, or after injection into the interstices of the gland, or after direct infusion in a cannulated hypophysial portal vessel.

(c) There should be evidence for altered release of the factor in situations which alter the release of the pituitary hormone. The most direct evidence for this would be to monitor rates of release of the factor into hypophysial portal blood and the response to situations which produce parallel alterations in the release of the pituitary hormone in question. Alternatively, alterations in peripheral blood levels of the releasing factor in response to similar stimuli would constitute good evidence for the actual secretion of the factor, particu-larly if destruction of the median eminence led to disappearance of the circulating releasing factor. Lastly, indirect evidence of release of releasing factor can be obtained by monitoring changes in hypothalamic content of the factor. Acute changes can perhaps be interpreted in terms of release; however, chronic changes only indicate that an alteration has taken place but tell us nothing as to whether this is an increase or decrease in release of the factor, a change in its *in situ* destruction, or a combination of these changes.

Many assay systems have been developed to monitor releasing factor activity. *In vivo* assays have been utilised and in this instance it is necessary to eliminate possible indirect effects on the pituitary by use of hypothalamic lesions or pharmacological blockade as outlined above in the assay of CRF[48, 49]. *In vitro* techniques make use of pituitaries incubated *in vitro* in static situa-sions[50] or in a perfusion apparatus[51]. Recently, techniques of incubation of isolated cells either acutely[52] or in tissue culture[53] have been introduced which may offer advantages in terms of reproducibility and sensitivity. The various assay systems in use have been reviewed *in extenso* elsewhere[48-50].

2.5 THE RELEASING AND INHIBITING HORMONES

It is clear that a whole family of releasing and inhibiting hormones exist and at least one such hormone has been postulated to control the release of each anterior pituitary hormone. On the basis of the criteria outlined above, a number of these have reached the status of hormones.

There is no doubt that a corticotrophin-releasing factor (CRF) exists. Hypothalamic extracts increase the release of ACTH both *in vitro*[32] and *in vivo*[31-39], the extracts are active when injected into the interstices of the pituitary[54] or after hypothalamic lesions[31, 32] and there have been several reports of CRF activity in blood which has even been stated to increase following adrenalectomy and to be reduced by adrenal steroids[55]. Alterations in stored CRF have also been reported[56]. CRF has been found in a higher concentration in blood from the cut hypophysial stalk of the dog than in peripheral circulation[39]. In all probability this hormone is secreted and controls the minute to minute output of ACTH by the pituitary gland[47].

With the acceptance of a CRF, attention turned to other possible releasing factors and shortly thereafter an LH-releasing factor (LRF) was discovered in crude hypothalamic extracts[57]. This hormone is now firmly established on the basis of its activity directly on the gland both *in vitro*[58] and *in vivo*[59]. It is actually secreted into the circulation on the basis of measurements of both peripheral blood[60] and portal blood[61] LRF content. LRF content in the hypothalamus fluctuates in various physiological states. For example, it decreases following treatment of ovariectomised rats with small doses of oestrogen[62].

An FSH-releasing activity of crude hypothalamic extracts was also described[63, 64] and this activity is now well established. In earlier work utilising bioassay, a separation of the FSH-releasing from the LH-releasing activity in partially purified hypothalamic extracts was achieved by several groups[65-68]. Later work utilising radioimmunoassay failed to demonstrate clear separation of the two activities; however, further work suggests that an FSH-releasing factor (FRF) indeed exists (see Section 2.12). Alterations in stored FRF have been reported in hypothalamus[69, 70], and an increase in FRF in portal blood has also been observed following intraventricular injections of dopamine in the rat[71]. Increased levels of peripheral circulating FRF have been observed in hypophysectomised rats exposed to constant light[72].

Although the early claims of Shibusawa[73] and Schreiber[74] have been questioned, there is no doubt on the basis of the work of Guillemin's group[75] and that of Schally and associates[76] that a thyrotrophin-releasing factor (TRF) exists. This activity has yet to be demonstrated in blood, perhaps because of an enzymatic system present in blood for destruction of the hormone[77]; however, instances of alterations in stored TRF in the hypothalamus have been reported[78]. TRF is active when perfused directly into a cannulated hypophysial portal vessel[79].

It is almost certain that the hypothalamic control over prolactin release is mediated primarily by a prolactin-inhibiting factor (PIF). This follows from the fact that hypothalamic lesions result in enhanced prolactin release[80] and that crude hypothalamic extracts can inhibit prolactin release *in vitro*[81, 82].

Under certain circumstances an inhibitory activity of such extracts has also been demonstrated *in vivo* both on peripheral injection[83] and on injection directly into cannulated portal vessels[84]; however, it has sometimes been difficult to demonstrate this activity[85]. Work on the purification of PIF is sufficient to say that the activity can be separated from most other hypothalamic-releasing factors[86], but it is still not very far advanced (see Section 2.12).

A prolactin-releasing factor has also been postulated[87] and appears to be the primary regulator of prolactin release in birds[88]. Even in the rat, hypothalamic extracts can stimulate prolactin release *in vitro* under certain conditions, and recently a stimulation has been observed after very large doses of hypothalamic extracts in oestrogen-primed male rats *in vivo*[85]. A prolactin-releasing factor can be considered likely to exist, but it is not yet established.

On the basis of the results from transplantation of the pituitary to a distant site[89] or production of median eminence lesions[90], it appears that melanocyte-stimulating hormone (MSH) is predominately under inhibitory hypothalamic control. Consequently, it is not surprising that an MSH release-inhibiting factor (MIF) has been described on the basis of its effect on the release of MSH from pituitaries incubated *in vitro*[91]. In addition, an MSH-releasing factor (MRF) has been reported based on the ability of hypothalamic extracts to deplete pituitary MSH[92]. Because of the unsatisfactory state of MSH assay, these hypothalamic factors are still on rather insecure ground although peptides with both of these activities have already been described, as indicated below (see Section 2.12).

Although growth hormone (GH) was the first pituitary hormone to be discovered, the regulation of its secretion remained completely obscure for four decades following its discovery. The only evidence for a hypothalamic control of GH secretion was impairment of growth in animals with hypothalamic lesions or with pituitaries transplanted to an area distant from the hypothalamus and increased sensitivity to insulin in animals with lesions. More direct evidence for hypothalamic control was provided by Reichlin[93] who observed a considerable decrease of pituitary GH content following massive lesions of the ventral hypothalamus, an observation later confirmed by Krulich *et al.*[94]. After the specific RIA for human GH became available, making direct determination of plasma GH possible, it was soon apparent that the secretion of GH in humans is influenced by a wide variety of stimuli which by their very nature implied a nervous regulation[95].

The first effort to prove the existence of growth hormone-releasing factor (GRF) in hypothalamic extracts was made by Franz *et al.*[96], who found that extracts from porcine hypothalami increased GH release from pituitaries incubated *in vitro* and increased the width of the tibial epiphysial cartilage if injected *in vivo*. It was even claimed that overall growth was stimulated. GH content in the media in the *in vitro* experiment was determined by the tibia test. The conclusion reached by Franz *et al.* that hypothalamic extracts contain a GRF has been amply confirmed by other workers, in particular Deuben and Meites[97] who found increased formation of GH in pituitary tissue cultures incubated with rat hypothalamic extract. Many others have also observed the activity of hypothalamic extracts to increase the release of GH *in vitro* as measured by the tibia test. In addition, intravenous or intracarotid injection of hypothalamic extract was reported to decrease the pituitary GH content as measured by the tibia test[98, 99]. This was reported many times and dose-response relationships were obtained with both the *in vitro* and *in vivo* tests[100].

Alterations in GRF activity in rat hypothalamus were shown to occur in various situations[101]. For example, the content increased with age and decreased with insulin hypoglycaemia, starvation or exposure to cold. In these cases the activity was measured by the pituitary depletion test.

Krulich and McCann[102] even found that injection of plasma from hypophysectomised, hypoglycaemic rats depleted the pituitary GH in normal animals, and Müller *et al.*[103] found GRF activity in plasma of animals exposed to cold. Plasma GRF appears to increase with time in hypophysectomised animals[104]. GRF has even been reported in plasma of some acromegalics as measured by its effect on release of GH from pituitaries incubated *in vitro*[105]. Using radioimmunoassay, Wilbur and Porter[106] and later Worthington[107] observed increased amounts of GH in portal as compared to systemic plasma and Worthington also reported an increase in GH content of pituitaries incubated in the presence of portal plasma.

The work on GRF has been hampered by a discrepancy between the results with bioassay by the tibia test and with immunoassay of the hormone. It has not been possible to observe a depletion of pituitary GH determined by radioimmunoassay following injection of hypothalamic extracts[108]. On the other hand, there is agreement between bio and immunoassay that hypothalamic extracts can increase the release of pituitary GH from glands incubated *in vitro*. Even measuring the hormone by radioimmunoassay, it has been possible to show an increase in plasma GH following injection of partially purified factor into the interstices of the pituitary[109] and an increase in plasma levels following systemic injection of crude and purified extracts in sheep[110]. Only crude but not purified extracts have been active in monkeys[111]. Several hypotheses have been advanced to explain the discrepancy between radioimmunoassay and bioassay in measuring pituitary GH content in the rat, but so far the problem remains unresolved.

In contrast, to the controversies which have developed regarding GRF, the history of growth-hormone-inhibiting factor (GIF) is short and so far without controversy. Krulich *et al.*[112] observed that certain fractions from Sephadex-purified sheep hypothalamic extracts strongly inhibited GH release from rat pituitaries incubated *in vitro*. The inhibitory activity was ascribed to a specific GIF. The activity was further purified and separated from other hypothalamic factors[113]. At the same time evidence was obtained that GIF inhibited not only GH release but also synthesis of GH and counteracted the effects of GRF[114]. All of this work utilised the tibia test for bioassay of GH *in vitro*. The existence of GIF was reconfirmed using a different purification technique and RIA of GH[115]. Recently, Stachura *et al.*[116] using an elegant technique of sequential differential labelling of GH in pituitaries *in vitro* and RIA for GH confirmed the existence of GIF utilising a Sephadex-purified preparation and also noted that GIF inhibited both release and synthesis of GH. Very recently, the structure of GIF has been elucidated (see Section 2.12). In this work it was shown that GIF could diminish the rise in GH measured by RIA normally observed in rats anaesthetised with Nembutal[117].

2.6 CHARACTERISTICS OF RELEASING FACTOR ACTION

On the basis of results obtained by bio and radioimmunoassay, a general pattern of response to releasing factors can now be described. Following the injection of crude, purified or synthetic releasing factors there is a dramatic increase in release of the particular pituitary hormone stimulated which occurs within a minute or two of the intravenous injection of the releasing factor[118, 119]. Following a single intravenous pulse, the response rises to a peak at *ca.* 10 min in the rat and plasma levels then decay according to the half-time of the pituitary hormone in question. In the case of LRF, repeated pulses of releasing factor result in quite similar responses to each pulse[119]. Following infusion of extracts, a maximum level is reached after *ca.* 1 h and there is no decline in release for several hours, suggesting that pituitary exhaustion does not supervene with continued stimulation[120]. As in many other endocrine structures, it appears that the release takes place from a readily releasable pool of recently-synthesised hormone[121]. Although depletion of stored hormone has been observed in many bioassay studies[122], this has not been confirmed so far by immunoassay of hormone content. In fact, the fraction of hormone released is quite small in the case of FSH and LH so that one could hardly expect a depletion[123]. In *in vitro* studies it has been possible to demonstrate a net increase in assayable hormone in the system following exposure to releasing factors which indicates that these substances can stimulate additional synthesis of hormone either as another primary action or secondary to the releasing action[124, 125].

Another characteristic of the releasing factors is their specificity of action. Early studies suggested that this was absolute and that there was no effect on the release of other pituitary hormones. For example, this was shown to be the case for LRF, GRF and GIF and TRF[126, 127]. Recent work suggests that this may have to be modified somewhat. For example, TRF has a very potent effect in releasing prolactin in humans[128, 129]. Although its ability to effect release of prolactin is quite limited in normal rats[130], a releasing action has been observed in cell cultures of rat pituitary tumours[131].

2.7 MECHANISM OF ACTION OF RELEASING FACTORS

As is the case for many other hormones, the initial action of the releasing factors apparently is to combine with high affinity receptors on the surface of the cell. This has been demonstrated clearly now utilising synthetic TRF[132, 133]. Analogues of the synthetic hormone compete for the receptor site and the affinity to the receptor bears a direct relationship to the biological activity of the analogue[134].

Beyond this point theories of the mechanism of action diverge and there are two prominent theories at the present time. The first of these is an extension of the stimulus–secretion coupling hypothesis of Douglas and Poisner[135], which has been used to explain the secretory activity of the adrenal medulla, neurohypophysis and salivary glands. According to this theory, the releasing factors would alter the permeability of the cell membrane. This would lead to depolarisation of the membrane and uptake of calcium from the extracellular fluid. Calcium would in some manner activate the releasing mechanism which is generally agreed to be by a process of emiocytosis of secretory granules[136, 137]. In support of this theory is the ability of high potassium in the medium of pituitaries incubated *in vitro* to activate the release of all pituitary hormones[138, 139]. Potassium is postulated to depolarise the cell membrane leading to uptake of calcium and hormone release. Prolactin is a partial exception in that it is only slightly stimulated by potassium as might be predicted since it is under inhibitory hypothalamic control[140]. One could visualise that in this situation the permeability of the membrane is already almost maximally altered in the absence of high potassium. Alterations in membrane potential have also been reported both *in vitro*[141] and *in vivo*[142] but they do not seem to fit a simple depolarisation of the membrane.

Low sodium in the medium can also activate release[139, 143]. Ouabain stimulated release of GH, possible because it interferes with the sodium potassium-activated ATPase in the membrane[143].

There is no doubt about the requirement for calcium *in vitro* since removal of the ion from the medium can inhibit release, and in situations where this is not sufficient, the addition of a chelating agent can profoundly block resting and stimulated release by the glands[118, 138, 143]. The rate of release of hormone in some situations *in vitro* is directly proportional to the medium calcium[144]. An increase in intracellular calcium has even been observed following addition of high potassium media or growth hormone-releasing factor[145]. As in many other situations in which calcium is an activator, magnesium appears to inhibit release of pituitary hormones when added in high concentrations *in vitro*[139].

Strong evidence supports another mechanism of action via the second messenger, cyclic AMP. Addition of crude hypothalamic extracts to pituitaries incubated *in vitro* results in a very rapid increase in adenyl-cyclase activity and a dramatic increase in cyclic AMP levels[118, 146, 147]. There is no alteration in phosphodiesterase levels, so the increase in cyclic AMP presumably follows the activation of adenyl cyclase. The elevation in cyclic AMP levels occurs prior to any significant effect on release of hormone. Thus, it occurs quickly enough to account for the releasing action. There was great specificity of the effects of crude hypothalamic extracts on adenyl cyclase and cyclic AMP since these same extracts had no effect on the levels of the enzyme or the nucleotide in posterior pituitary, adrenal medulla or thyroid[118, 146, 147]. Cerebral cortical extracts prepared similarly had no effect on pituitary cyclase and cyclic AMP levels. Synthetic TRF[148] and LRF[149] have also been reported to increase the cyclic AMP in the gland, although the increase following synthetic LRF was delayed which is difficult to reconcile with the hypothesis. If cyclic AMP were the physiological mediator of releasing factor action, then one should be able to obtain release of hormones with cyclic AMP or its derivative, dibutyryl cyclic AMP. Indeed, the release of all pituitary hormones can be promoted *in vitro* either by dibutyryl cyclic AMP alone or by dibutyryl cyclic AMP together with a phosphodiesterase inhibitors such as theophylline[150-152]. Theophylline alone can often enhance release. One would postulate that inhibiting factors would lower the cyclic AMP levels in the gland, but this has not been studied as yet in the absence of available purified or synthetic inhibiting factors. It would seem that nearly all of the criteria of Sutherland (see chapter by Robison and Strada) have been satisfied in order to draw the conclusion that cyclic AMP is indeed a second messenger to mediate releasing factor action. Cyclic AMP may not be the only cyclic nucleotide involved since purified GRF has been reported to increase cyclic GMP and not cyclic AMP in the pituitary and since cyclic GMP can also promote GH release[153].

If indeed cyclic AMP functions as a second messenger to mediate releasing factor effects, then the question would be raised as to how this is accomplished. Several possibilities suggest themselves. It is known that cyclic AMP acts in many tissues to activate a protein kinase and a cyclic AMP binding protein associated with this activity has been detected in the anterior pituitary[153a]. It is possible, as suggested by Labrie et al.[154] that the increased cyclic AMP levels act via protein kinase to alter the permeability of the cell membrane and allow uptake of calcium. Alternatively, the protein kinase may act in some manner to promote migration of secretory granules to the surface or to enhance synthesis of pituitary hormones.

Elevated medium potassium enhances release of pituitary hormones in the absence of any effect on cyclic AMP levels[155]. Consequently, the effect of elevated potassium must be after or independent of the cyclic AMP step and these findings are consistent with the hypothesis of Labrie et al.[154] that cyclic AMP acts to alter membrane permeability. Increased available calcium would then act either together with cyclic AMP or independently of it to promote release.

Microtubules are thought to be involved in bringing secretory granules to the cell surface in a number of endocrine tissues. Recently, Kraicer et al.[156] have reported that colchicine, which disrupts microtubules, can block the secretion of ACTH promoted by high potassium medium in vitro. On the other hand, Sundberg et al.[157] have not found any blocking ability of colchicine on the release of FSH, LH, prolactin, GH and TSH. In fact, colchicine can enhance release promoted by high potassium medium or by releasing factors. The role of microtubules in the secretory process remains to be elucidated.

In the present state of our knowledge the most likely hypothesis is that cyclic AMP plays a key role in mediating the action of the RFs and that this action is partially exerted on the cell membrane to alter permeability. In this respect it mimics the action of high potassium and this could reconcile the two hypotheses of secretion.

There may also be a role of prostaglandins in mediating release, perhaps as an intermediary between the releasing factor receptor complex and the activation of adenyl cyclase. For example, nearly all prostaglandins will increase the cyclic AMP in the pituitary[146], the most potent of these being prostaglandin E_1. This prostaglandin enhances the secretion of GH[158] but has little effect on the release of other pituitary hormones (Sundberg, unpublished observations). It is possible that a given prostaglandin may stimulate release of only a single pituitary hormone. If so, the possible role of prostaglandins could be cleared up by a systematic analysis of the effects of the different ones on the release of each pituitary hormone. There is some evidence that an inhibitor of prostaglandins, 7-oxyprostynoic acid, can inhibit the response of the pituitary to TRF[159] which would also fit with a role of prostaglandins.

2.8 INTERACTION OF RELEASING FACTORS AND TARGET GLAND HORMONES AT THE PITUITARY LEVEL

There is now no doubt that target gland hormones feed-back at the pituitary level to modify its response to releasing factors. This relationship has been apparent for many years but has been clearly elucidated with the availability of synthetic factors. For example, thyroid hormones can suppress the response to TRF and they are effective in physiological doses (for further review of the evidence, see section on TSH and thyroid control). A similar relationship has been shown for LRF. First, removal of the ovaries increases the sensitivity of the gland to LRF[160]. The effect is demonstrable within hours. In the ovariectomised animals, minute doses of intravenous oestrogen are capable of inhibiting the response to LRF administered either by an intravenous injection or by infusion in rats[161, 162] and man[163]. The interactions are complex since it has also been shown that large doses of oestrogen can sensitise the gland to LRF[164, 165]. Administration of 50 µg of oestradiol benzoate subcutaneously is followed 3 days later by an increase in sensitivity of the gland to LRF in ovariectomised animals[165]. The addition of a large dose of progesterone has little effect on the sensitivity in the presence or absence of oestrogen. More work is required to characterise fully these interactions; however, it is clear that they have physiological significance since sensitisation of the pituitary response to LRF has been shown to occur prior to ovulation in rats[166], hamsters[167], sheep[168] and humans[169]. Similarly, suppression of the response of the pituitary to CRF has been clearly demonstrated following dexamethasone treatment of rats[170]. The target gland feed-back at the pituitary level may require the synthesis of inhibitory peptides or proteins based on experiments, particularly with thyroid hormones, which indicated a lag for inhibition of the response to TRF and that the inhibition could be prevented by using drugs which inhibit protein synthesis[171, 172].

2.9 TARGET GLAND FEED-BACK AT THE HYPOTHALAMIC LEVEL

Although feed-back at the pituitary is now well established and has been shown to play a physiological role in the regulation of pituitary hormone release, there is no doubt that these feed-back actions also occur at the hypothalamic level. Earlier work with implants of hormones into the hypothalamus indicated a hypothalamic site for feed-back[173], but this work was criticised on the basis that the hormones might reach the portal vessels and be carried to the anterior lobe[174]. It has clearly been shown in studies with injections of CRF and TRF into the hypothalamus that the quantity of hormone injected into the hypothalamus which reaches the pituitary is quite small so it is likely that these early implants were actually acting at the hypothalamic level[175, 176]. Because of the high concentration of hormone at the feed-back site, it is impossible from this type of study to determine the physiological significance of such feed-backs .Further evidence to suggest that the hypothalamic site is of physiological significance was obtained by measuring the effects of systemic injection of hormone on the content of stored releasing factors in the median eminence[49]. Physiological levels of oestrogen can modify the content of FSH and LH-releasing activity and the content of prolactin-inhibiting activity in the hypothalamus[62]. It is also very likely that the ovulatory surge of gonadotrophins involves feed-back of oestrogen and/or progesterone at the hypothalamic level interacting with a cyclic clock mechanism in the rat. The evidence for this is the ability of drugs which act primarily at the CNS level to block the pro-oestrous discharge in the rat[177] and the increase in peripheral circulating LRF in humans prior to ovulation[178].

2.10 LOCALISATION OF RELEASING FACTORS

Early studies with implants of pituitaries to the hypothalamic region led to the conclusion that the releasing factors were restricted to a region known as the hypophysiotropic area[179]. This region which consists of the medial basal and anterior hypothalamus was identified on the basis of the fact that pituitary cell types remained differentiated when pituitary grafts were implanted into this area. A more direct approach was to extract particular regions of the hypothalamus and to assay them for releasing factor content. Extensive studies of this type have now been performed and it is clear that gonadotrophin-releasing activity can be extracted from a wide band of tissue extending from the medial preoptic area cuadally to the median eminence–arcuate region, where the bulk of the activity is stored[180, 181].

Since lesions in the suprachiasmatic region led to a reduction in stored LRF in the median eminence–arcuate region[182], we postulate that these lesions destroyed cell bodies of LRF neurones resulting in degeneration of the axons and loss of stored releasing factor. The remaining activity was presumably from neurones whose cell bodies lay more cuadally in anterior hypothalamus and median eminence–arcuate region. Thus, we postulate that there is a diverse population of neurosecretory cells synthesising LRF, the most rostral ones with cell bodies in the preoptic region and the more caudal ones with cell bodies located as far caudally as the arcuate nucleus.

Surprisingly, prolactin-inhibiting activity was found in the lateral preoptic area and lateral hypothalamus, whereas prolactin-releasing factor activity appeared in the medial suprachiasmatic region[181]. GH-releasing activity was concentrated in the lateral portion of the ventromedial nucleus which coincides with the areas which modify GH release when injured or stimulated. GH-inhibiting activity on the other hand was concentrated in the median eminence region[115]. The thyrotrophin-releasing activity of hypothalamic sections was most pronounced and extended from the bed nucleus of the stria terminalis caudally to the dorsomedial nucleus and ventrally to the median eminence region[181]. Thus, the releasing factors are not spread throughout the hypothalamus but are concentrated in specific regions which probably comprise the areas containing particular neurosecretory neurones specialised to synthesise and release particular neurohormones. So far, the data are largely consistent with lesions and stimulation studies; however, the effect of lesions as far forward as the bed nucleus of the stria terminalis on TSH release has not been evaluated, nor have the effects of lateral preoptic lesions on prolactin release been ascertained. The distribution of FSH and LH-releasing factor in a completely overlapping zone does not agree with stimulation[8] and lesion[183] experiments which seem to indicate that the LH-controlling region extends more rostrally than that controlling FSH, although the two regions overlapped caudally. It is interesting to note that the regions containing the releasing factors coincide with areas of the brain shown to take up oestrogen in the elegant autoradiographic studies of Pfaff[184] and of Stumpf[185]. This is perhaps not surprising since oestrogen can effect the release of nearly every pituitary hormone.

2.11 POSSIBLE SYNAPTIC TRANSMITTERS INVOLVED IN RELEASE OF THE FACTORS

Recently, a great deal of interest has been focused on putative synaptic transmitters which might mediate the relationship of the releasing factor neurones with the rest of the central nervous system. The histochemical fluorescence technique has revealed the presence of monoaminergic neurones in a variety of hypothalamic areas[186]. For example, there appears to be a dopaminergic pathway with neuronal cell bodies located in the arcuate nucleus and axons which project to the median eminence to terminate in close proximity to the hypophysial portal capillaries. In addition, there are many terminals which appear to contain norepinephrine located in the preoptic and anterior hypothalamic region. The suprachiasmatic region is rich in terminals of what appear to be serotonergic neurones.

The role of monoamines in releasing adenohypophysial hormones is being investigated extensively. Using an *in vitro* system in which pituitaries were incubated either alone or together with ventral hypothalamic fragments, it was possible to show that dopamine had no influence on the release of FSH and LH from pituitaries incubated alone, but that it could stimulate the release of FSH and LH-releasing factor from the ventral hypothalamus[187, 188]. On the other hand, small doses of either dopamine or norepinephrine were capable of inhibiting release of prolactin from the pituitary incubated alone *in vitro*[189-191]. Incubation of hypothalami with dopamine revealed that it could stimulate the release of PIF from these fragments[191].

To determine if the catecholamines were also active *in vivo*, they were injected into the third ventricle and shown to stimulate the release of FSH and LH and to inhibit that of prolactin[192-194]. This was accompanied by an increase in peripheral circulating LRF in hypophysectomised animals[195, 196] and by an increase in FSH and LH releasing activity and prolactin-inhibiting activity in portal blood[197]. Thus, it appeared that dopamine could function as a synaptic transmitter to enhance the release of gonadotrophin-releasing factors and PIF.

It was also shown that oestrogen could block the release of LRF induced by dopamine *in vitro*[198], suggesting that at least one site of the negative feed-back of oestrogen was on the releasing factor elements to block their response to dopamine. That this inhibitory effect might involve an inhibitory peptide or protein was suggested by experiments in which the oestrogen-induced blockade of the response to dopamine could be reversed by inhibitors of protein synthesis, such as puromycin or cycloheximide. The inhibitory effect of oestrogen on the response to dopamine was confirmed in *in vivo* experiments[196]. Injection of oestradiol into the third ventricle 2 h prior to injection of dopamine blocked the LRF release induced by the catecholamine.

Further studies were carried out to determine whether drugs which blocked catecholamine receptors or altered catecholamine synthesis could alter gonadotrophin and prolactin secretion. These studies clearly pointed once again to a role for dopamine as an inhibitory transmitter to inhibit prolactin release. For example, drugs such as *a*-methyl *p*-tyrosine, which inhibit catecholamine synthesis, resulted in a rapid elevation of prolactin which could be reversed by re-initiating catecholamine synthesis with L-DOPA[199]. On the other hand, drugs which blocked only norepinephrine synthesis, such as diethyldithiocarbamate, did not alter prolactin levels. There was some suggestion that an artificial elevation of norepinephrine levels could stimulate prolactin release since injection of dihydroxyphenylserine, which stimulates selectively norepinephrine synthesis, resulted in elevated levels of prolactin.

Thus, there is good evidence to support the hypothesis that dopamine may function as a synaptic transmitter to cause PIF discharge. That dopamine may also act at the pituitary level cannot be ruled out in view of its effect on the *in vitro* release of prolactin and the ability of L-DOPA to lower prolactin even in animals with hypothalamic lesions which appeared to block CNS control of the gland[200]. Against the possibility of a direct effect of dopamine at the pituitary level are the experiments of Kamberi *et al.*[194] in which infusions of dopamine into a cannulated hypophysial portal vessel failed to alter prolactin release.

Similar studies have pointed to a possible role of norepinephrine as a synaptic transmitter in the control of FSH and LH release by an *a*-adrenergic receptor. Phentolamine and phenoxybenzamine, drugs which block *a*-receptors, inhibited FSH and LH release as did haloperidol, a drug which apparently affects both *a*- and dopaminergic receptors[201, 202]. Pimozide, a drug which predominantly affects dopamine receptors, has blocked only FSH secretion in studies to date[202]. Using drugs to block catecholamine synthesis, blockade of FSH and LH release was obtained with drugs which interfered selectively with norepinephrine synthesis. Thus, it was possible to block the post-castration rise in gonadotrophins[202], the rise induced by progesterone[201] or oestrogen and the preovulatory surge of gonadotrophins using these drugs[203].

The noradrenergic synapse may lie in the preoptic or anterior hypothalamic area on the basis of the ability of drugs which block norepinephrine synthesis to interfere with the release of LH following electrochemical stimulation of the preoptic area, whereas similar drugs had no effect on the discharge which followed stimulation in the median eminence region[204]. This is consistent with the localisation of noradrenergic terminals in this region by the histochemical fluorescence technique.

We would visualise that the preovulatory surge of gonadotrophins in the rat is brought about by ovarian steroids acting to produce increased impulse traffic across this noradrenergic synapse at the time that the cyclic clock discharges on the afternoon of pro-oestrous. The post-castration rise in gonadotrophins may be brought about similarly by increased traffic across noradrenergic synapses but whether it involves a dopaminergic pathway as well has not yet been determined.

Similarly, there is evidence for an adrenergic link in the pathways controlling GH release. Unfortunately, the evidence is contradictory in that most work in humans suggests that an α-adrenergic receptor may be involved in stimulating GH release, whereas a β-adrenergic receptor may inhibit it[205]. This is consistent with work in the baboon in which norepinephrine can stimulate GH release when injected into the ventromedial nucleus[206]. It also fits with early work in which GH release was estimated by the pituitary depletion test and bioassay of GH in rats[207], but cannot be reconciled easily with recent studies utilising radioimmunoassay of GH which seem to indicate an inhibitory role for adrenergic mechanisms in GH control[208]. There also appears to be an inhibitory adrenergic pathway involved in the control of ACTH release from the extensive studies of Ganong, Scapagnini and their co-workers[209, 210].

Serotonin can clearly inhibit the release of gonadotrophins and stimulate the release of prolactin when injected into the third ventricle[192-197]; however its physiological significance in the control of these hormones remains to be established since injection of p-chlorophenylalanine, an inhibitor of serotonin biosynthesis, has not resulted in any alterations in gonadotrophin or prolactin release[199, 202]. In a recent abstract, it was claimed that p-chlorophenylalanine can interfere with the suckling-induced rise in prolactin[211].

Cholinergic mechanisms may also be involved in the release of gonadotrophins and prolactin since atropine given subcutaneously or intraventriculary can block the pro-oestrous surge of gonadotrophins and prolactin and interfere with the post-castration rise in gonadotrophins[212].

Although the precise details remain to be unravelled, it is clear that monoaminergic mechanisms are involved in the control of releasing and inhibiting factors. This is of potential clinical significance. L-DOPA has already been shown to lower prolactin in the human[213] just as in the rat and to be of possible value in the treatment of metastatic breast cancer[214].

2.12 CHEMISTRY AND BIOCHEMISTRY OF THE RELEASING FACTORS

The size of this section in the context of endocrine physiology is an indication of the scale of resources recently devoted to releasing-factor chemistry. The hypophysiotropic hormones of the hypothalamus (herein referred to as releasing factors) can now be divided into two main groups, those for which a chemical structure has been described and a synthetic version found to possess the biological activity of the natural preparations and those which remain a partially purified activity. In the former group now belong TRF, LRF, possibly FRF and possibly the MSH-controlling factors. The latest addition seems to be GIF. Those which remain in the latter group are CRF and the prolactin-controlling factors, with GRF lying uncomfortably somewhere in between. The following sections contain a summary of advances made in the last 3 years and the current status of the chemistry of each hormone.

2.12.1 CRF

The identification of a true CRF has been beset by more than an average amount of confusion, even for the hypophysiotropic-hormone field. We are therefore still faced with the possibility of the existence of CRF peptides with or without a disulphide structure as previously described[35-38, 215]. The recent discovery of the surprisingly high ACTH-releasing potency of pressinoic acid, even though in only a limited dose range[216], can be interpreted as a clue either to the nature of a true CRF or to that part of the vasopressin molecule responsible for its CRF-like activity*. However, it is surprising that deamino pressinoic acid and its amide had little or no activity while deaminolysine vasopressin has been found to have CRF activity almost equal to that of lysine vasopressin but a much higher CRF/pressor ratio[217]. The latter information was obtained in an assay system different from that in which the pressinoic acid peptides were tested.

The pioneering applications of the ultracentrifuge to this area of neuroendocrinology have also encountered the involvement of vasopressin[218, 219] as no secretory granule fraction with CRF activity was obtained free of pressor activity, although in one case[219] a distinct distribution of the two activities was obtained. Whether there is more than one CRF, whether it is an MSH-like peptide (a or β) as postulated earlier, or whether it is really related structurally to pressinoic and other disulphide peptides or disulphide-free peptides[220] are questions upon which little further light has been shed since this unfortunately confusing situation was last reviewed[221]. Reasonable assessment of all the evidence does tend to support the existence of at least two CRF peptides, of which one may have a disulphide component. One apparently has more acidic character at pH 6.5[215] and this is not easy (but not impossible) to reconcile with other reported cation exchange data[222, 223]. In view of the assay difficulties and the reported losses in activity and instability of CRF[215], only a confirmed optimist would predict that its (their) chemistry will be deciphered in the near future.

2.12.2 MIF and MRF

Interest in hypothalamic control of MSH has been rejuvenated recently by the discoveries of MIF and MRF activities of the fragments of the oxytocin molecule. New light was first shed on inhibition of MSH release by the observation that MIF activity was generated by the action of certain hypothalamic enzymes on oxytocin[224, 225]. The view that the active principle was Pro-Leu-GlyNH$_2$, the C-terminal tripeptide of oxytocin, appeared to have been confirmed by the activity of the synthetic tripeptide[226] and also by the identification of the MIF activity in ovine hypothalamic extracts with the same structure[227]. It was therefore quite extraordinary to read the report from another laboratory that this tripeptide had failed to cause any inhibition of MSH release, whereas tocinoic acid (the cyclic portion of oxytocin) was observed to cause quite clear inhibition[228]. This information followed closely the announcement of MRF activity at ng levels both *in vitro* and *in vivo*

* Further tests of more recent preparations of pressinoic acid have tended not to confirm its LRF activity (M. Saffran, personal communication).

of the reduced form of the pentapeptide corresponding to des-Cys-^{6} tocinoic acid [H-Cys-Tyr-Phe-Ileu-Gln-AspOH][229]. Explanation of these discrepancies, which are unusual in that they involve synthetic peptides, may involve in part the less than ideal characteristics of the various methods for measuring MSH release; however, they do require urgent resolution since tentative involvement of MIF in a new area is already being investigated. The observation of increased melanocyte-lightening activity in plasma of hypophysectomised rats has been somewhat tenuously related to the claimed but unsupported chromatographic detection of Pro-Leu-GlyNH$_2$ in plasma (together with melatonin). This observation was interpreted in terms of pineal–hypothalamo–pituitary interactions involving the action of MIF or MSH or both on the pineal gland[230]. Natriuresis in rats is another area in which a new role for MSH has been described[231], thus further warranting clarification of the MIF/MRF situation.

If physiologically important activities are eventually proved for these oxytocin fragments (and also the pressinoic acid peptide mentioned in the CRF section), then it is already tempting to speculate that the true substrate for the RF/IF forming enzymes may be the actual precursors of the neurohypophysial hormones[232] rather than the hormones themselves, i.e. there may be a common hypothalamic precursor of hypophysiotropic hormones and the disulphide peptides (and neurophysin) produced in several different types of secretory neurones which are cleaved according to the secretory speciality of the cell.

It should be noted that the oxytocin-cleaving enzymes involved here are not the same as the oxytocinase which occurs in pregnancy plasma[233] or the kidney enzyme which attacks oxytocin[234], but may well be the same as those previously investigated from the point of view of oxytocin inactivation in the hypothalamus during various stages of reproduction[235, 236].

This biochemical approach to the origins of these factors is more complex than at first appreciated since it has recently been reported that an enzyme in a 'mitochondrial' fraction from paraventricular tissue but not from the supraoptic locus is capable of producing an MRF from oxytocin and Lys-vasopressin and the activity was also found in median eminence tissue[237]. This may be the oestrous cycle-dependent mitochondrial enzyme formerly described as preventing the formation of MIF by competing for the same substrate[226]. The relations between reproductive states and enzyme levels have even led to the suggestion of the involvement of either these enzymes or oxytocin itself with releasing factor control of gonadotrophin release—an exciting speculation in terms of hypothalamic organisation[238].

2.12.3 GRF and GIF

Early purification of GRF[239] was eventually followed by its isolation. The sequence of the GRF peptide isolated by Schally *et al.* was determined to be H-Val-His-Leu-Ser-Ala-Glu-Glu-Lys-Glu-Ala-OH[240]. This was recognised as being very similar to the N-terminal sequence of the β-chain of porcine haemoglobin and eventually was found to be identical when the haemoglobin peptide was sequenced, synthesised and compared by chromatography and electrophoresis with natural GRF, even the possibility that position 9 was

-Gln- rather than -Glu- was apparently ruled out[241]. The synthetic and natural peptides each released GH *in vitro*[242], provided that GH was measured by the tibial plate method or by the sulphation factor assay, even though natural GRF had been isolated largely on the basis of the much-criticised pituitary-depletion test, with confirmation of its activity *in vitro*[243]. Unfortunately, neither the synthetic nor the natural peptide released GH when the hormone was measured by RIA[242]. As pointed out earlier, crude or partially purified hypothalamic fractions can increase GH release *in vitro* and *in vivo* as measured by RIA but there have been discrepancies between bio and immunoassay. The response of the aforementioned decapeptide *in vitro* with the sulphation factor and tibial-plate assays cannot be denied and although the sequence coincidence is suggestive of a GH-releasing artifact, one must begin to question just what these assays or the RIA are measuring, for instance, has a contribution from prolactin or another pituitary constituent been ruled out? Current opinion holds that another peptide will be isolated in the future which should be capable of releasing both bioassayable and immuno-assayable GH. This conclusion appears to have been reached even by the original perpetrators of the decapeptide work[244].

Evidence for the existence of a substance capable of inhibiting GH release *in vitro* was obtained by Krulich *et al.* with the aid of the tibia test[112]. Application of RIA for GH to detect changes in GH release *in vitro* induced by fractions from hypothalamic material purified by ultrafiltration and by gel-filtration again supplied convincing evidence for the existence of two GH-controlling factors which acted in opposing directions and it was pointed out that GIF might have a larger molecular weight than had been described for the hypophysiotropic hormones in general[115]. That this indeed might be the case has been shown by the report of the isolation and synthesis of an unusual tetradecapeptide claimed to have GIF activity[245]: H-Ala-Gly-Cys-Lys-Asn-Phe-Phe-Trp-Lys-Thr-Phe-Thr-Ser-Cys-OH. Confirmation of this report is awaited with interest, particularly with respect to its lack of effect on the release of the other pituitary hormones.

2.12.4 TRF

Establishment of the structure of TRF as pyroglutamyl-histidyl-prolineamide by synthesis and proof of chemical and biological identity was undoubtedly a landmark achievement in endocrinology[246, 247]. It is unfortunate that recognition of the simple structure was delayed by the mythical 'non-peptide' part of the molecule[248], and by the failure to recognise the formation of a pyroglutamyl ring after acetylation of the correct sequence[249]. Statements that 'p-Glu-His-ProNH$_2$ (and similar peptides) show spectral and chromatographic properties different from the natural hormone'[250] remain in the literature unexplained but overwhelmed by subsequent publications and perhaps are evidence of the race to achieve the first identification of a releasing factor (see also Ref. 221). Subsequently, many analogues of TRF were synthesised. The structure–activity studies using TRF analogues with amino acid substitutions have not yet yielded much useful information beyond the conclusion that 'like bradykinin and other peptide hormones its centre and two ends are also important for activity'[251]. As might have been expected intuitively, amino acid substitution for proline usually causes least reduction in activity; however, it should be realised that even a large reduction in specific activity of TRF, say 1000-fold, still results in a compound which is active in μg quantities. The tripeptides containing N-methyl imidazole are of some interest, both practical and theoretical. It has been shown that the N^{3-im} methyl histidine analogue is eight–tenfold more active than TRF itself whereas its N^{1-im} methyl isomer is almost without activity[252]. Whilst in general, investigation of the releasing activity of analogues has not yet given information worthy of the effort necessary to prepare and test them, investigations with the synthetic isotopically-labelled tripeptide promise to be much more fruitful. It has already been shown that some TRF does accumulate in the anterior pituitary, probably in the form of unchanged tripeptide p-Glu-His-Pro-NH$_2$ and P-Glu-His-Pro[253]. Investigation of the fate of injected labelled hormone indicates a very rapid disappearance of label ($t_{1/2} = 4$ min) but the labelled peptides found in plasma also indicate a rapid conversion to TRF fragments. Within one minute, half of the injected radioactivity was recovered in peptides resembling Glu-His-Pro and His-Pro-NH$_2$[254]. In contrast, incubation *in vitro* with plasma for 1 h at 37 °C caused a 72% decrease in activity, most of the TRF being deamidated to free acid[255].

It has also been possible to measure binding of labelled TRF to its presumed natural receptor on pituitary cells. Preparation of plasma membranes from bovine adenohypophyseal cells[132] and from mouse tumour thyrotrophs[133] bind [^{3}H-]TRF with dissociation constants of 4×10^{-7} and 4×10^{-8}, respectively. In each case the binding of labelled hormone was competitive with unlabelled TRF but not with other peptide hormones. Extension of studies of this type may reveal the nature of the membrane receptor and its relation to the postulated adenyl cyclase stage in the release process.

2.12.5 Gonadotrophin releasing factor(s)

Workers in this field are only too familiar with the erratic progress over the past 13 years towards identification of an LRF and FRF. This aim was realised finally in 1971 by the announcement of the structure of porcine 'LH and FSH-releasing hormone' by the group led by Schally[256], followed closely by the report of an identical structure for ovine LRF[257] as follows: p-Glu-His-Trp-Ser-Tyr-Gly-Leu-Arg-Pro-Gly-NH$_2$. The synthetic peptide releases LH and FSH *in vitro* at nanomolar concentrations, but definition of its true physiological action is not yet clear as an action on FSH is not readily observed *in vivo* where the pituitary is under the influence of various natural and artificial steroid profiles. Significant elevation of plasma FSH levels in untreated rats has been observed only when comparatively large doses are infused into immature males over several hours[258].

The occurrence of the p-Glu-His sequence in both TRF and LRF (also the C-terminal amide) has already led to speculation that thyrotroph and gonadotroph receptors have the common ability to recognise this terminus[259], a claim which might be the basis for the design of LRF inhibitors, although decapeptide analogues in which His is either missing or replaced by Gly have been found to have some antagonistic activity towards the decapeptide *in vitro*[260]. Of the many analogues already prepared and tested, these are the only ones which so far are of interest, although mention has been made of the 9-Pro-ethylamide, a nonapeptide which has been found to be five times more potent than the decapeptide in the ovulation test[261]. No dissociation between LH and FSH release by the analogues *in vitro* has yet been reported, and even the putative LRF tetrapeptide of Folkers *et al.*[262] which created temporary interest as a releaser of LH alone has been discounted as a meaningful stimulator of either[263, 164]. The report of sustained activity with the *N*-terminal tripeptide, p-Glu-His-Try-NH$_2$, following *oral* administration to ovariectomised oestrogen, progesterone-treated rats[265] requires further validation since this peptide was tested in our laboratory (actually before the decapeptide structure was known) and found inactive when given to these animals intravenously; this has been confirmed and the *N*-terminal tetrapeptide amide also found inactive[263].

The question of whether the decapeptide is the true and only gonadotrophin releaser is still very much a subject of debate in spite of the efforts of one group[266]. Identical dose-response curves for the synthetic and the highly purified porcine peptides have been obtained in one system *in vitro*[267] although from another system data indicating what may be slight differences in the responses given by synthetic and ovine LRF (with respect to LH/FSH stimulation ratio) have been reported without particular comment[268], which suggests that only experimental error may have been involved. Alternatively, this may be indicative of a slight species difference. Evidence for distinct guinea-pig and chicken LRFs has actually been reported[269, 270]. Suggestive evidence for the existence of more than one gonadotrophin-releasing factor in both ovine[271] and porcine extracts[272] has not yet been further substantiated. The imminent application of anti-sera to LRF should settle this question and possibly also the question of the existence of a separate FSH-RF. However, it is of some related concern that only recently it was found necessary to survey the evidence for the existence of LH and FSH as two separate entities on the grounds that there was sufficient uncertainty in the bioassay and radio-immunoassay procedures on which the hormone isolations (i.e. definitions) were based[273]. Refinement and extension of the ultracentrifugal separation of subcellular particles from hypothalamic tissue[274, 275] may well be a worth while approach to search for evidence of the existence of a separate FRF. At present we feel that there is insufficient data from experiments with the synthetic peptide to substantiate the claim that no other gonadotrophin-releasing factor exists.

Following the lead of the investigators of TRF biosynthesis[276] (for details, see chapter by Martin), incorporation *in vitro* of [^{14}C]-glutamic acid by hypothalamic tissue into a peptide having the chromatographic properties of synthetic LRF has been claimed[277]. Fractionation of this tissue also revealed that some of the label appeared to be associated with FSH- and LH-releasing activity, different from the synthetic peptide and with much greater capacity to stimulate FSH than LH release[278-280]. This was interpreted as evidence for the existence of a distinct FRF and is reminiscent of both the earlier separation of the two activities using bioassay[65] and also the more recent partial chromatographic separation of factors with different LH/FSH releasing ratio[281]. There is no doubt that resolution of this question deserves, and will probably obtain, high priority.

2.12.6 PRF and PIF

Availability of RIA for prolactin has not yet resulted in advances in the purification of PIF beyond the stage reached with the aid of bioassay[86]; however, it has been applied to the detection of prolactin-releasing activity in both crude and fractionated hypothalamic extracts[282]. It is of some interest that no good evidence for PIF activity was obtained in this particular study, whereas PIF activity is routinely detected in crude hypothalamic extracts and their ultrafiltrates in our own laboratory. This work may provide useful guidance for the anticipated attempts to isolate PRF.

References

1. Bailey, P. and Bremer, F. (1921). Experimental diabetes insipidus. *Arch. Intern. Med.*, **28**, 773
2. Smith, P. E. (1927). The disabilities caused by hypophysectomy and their repair. The tuberal syndrome in the rat. *J. Amer. Med. Ass.*, **88**, 158
3. Dey, F. L. (1943). Evidence of hypothalamic control of hypophysial gonadotropic functions in the female guinea pig. *Endocrinology*, **33**, 75
4. McCann, S. M. and Porter, J. C. (1969). Hypothalamic pituitary stimulating and inhibiting hormones. *Physiol. Rev.*, **49**, 240
5. Taleisnik, S. and McCann, S. M. (1961). Effects of hypothalamic lesions on the secretion and storage of hypophysial luteinizing hormone. *Endocrinology*, **68**, 263
6. Haterius, H. O. (1937). Studies on a neurohypophysial mechanism influencing gonadotrophic activity. *Cold Spring Harbor Symp. Quant. Biol.*, **5**, 280
7. Cramer, O. M. and Barraclough, C. A. (1971). Effect of electrical stimulation of the preoptic area on plasma LH concentrations in proestrous rats. *Endocrinology*, **88**, 1175
8. Kalra, S. P., Ajika, K., Krulich, L., Fawcett, C. P., Quijada, M. and McCann, S. M. (1971). Effect of hypothalamic and preoptic electrochemical stimulation on gonadotropin and prolactin release in proestrous rats. *Endocrinology*, **88**, 1150
9. Goldfien, A. and Ganong, W. F. (1962). Adrenal medullary and adrenal cortical response to stimulation of diencephalon. *Amer. J. Physiol.*, **202**, 205
10. Martin, J. B. and Reichlin, S. (1970). Thyrotropin secretion in the rat following hypothalamic stimulation or injection of synthetic TSH releasing factor. *Science*, **168**, 1366
11. Frohman, L. A., Bernardis, L. L. and Kant, K. J. (1968). Hypothalamic stimulation of growth hormone secretion. *Science*, **162**, 580
12. McCann, S. M. (1962). Effect of hypothalamic lesions on adrenal cortical response to stress. *Amer. J. Physiol.*, **171**, 746
13. Bogdanove, E. M. and Halmi, N. S. (1953). Effects of hypothalamic lesions and subsequent propylthiouracil treatment on pituitary function in the rat. *Endocrinology*, **53**, 274
14. Hinsey, J. C. and Markee, J. E. (1933). Pregnancy following bilateral section of the cervical sympathetic trunks in the rabbit. *Proc. Soc. Exp. Biol. Med.*, **31**, 270
15. Popa, G. and Fielding, U. (1930). A portal circulation from the pituitary to the hypothalamic region. *J. Anat.*, **65**, 88
16. Wislocki, G. B. and King, L. S. (1936). The permeability of the hypophysis and hypothalamus to vital dyes with the study of the hypophysial vascular supply. *Amer. J. Anat.*, **58**, 421

17. Houssay, B. A., Biasotti, A. and Sammartino. (1935). Modifications fonctionnelles de l'hypophyse après les lésions infundibulotubériennes chez le carpaud. *Compt. Rend. Soc. Biol.*, **120**, 725

18. Green, J. D. and Harris, G. W. (1949). Observation of the hypophysioportal vessels of the living rat. *J. Physiol. (London)*, **108**, 359

19. Friedgood, H. B. (1970). The nervous control of the anterior hypophysis. *J. Reprod. Fert.*, **10**, 3

20. Hinsey, J. C. (1937). The relation of the nervous system to ovulation and other phenomena of the female reproductive tract. *Cold Spring Harbor Symp. Quant. Biol.*, **5**, 269

21. Harris, G. W. (1937). The induction of ovulation in the rabbit by electrical stimulation of the hypothalamo-hypophysial mechanism. *Proc. Roy. Soc. (London)*, **B122**, 374

22. Markee, J. E., Sawyer, C. H. and Hollinshead, W. H. (1946). Activation of the anterior hypophysis by electrical stimulation in the rabbit. *Endocrinology*, **38**, 345

23. Harris, G. W. (1950). Oestrous rhythm. Pseudopregnancy and the pituitary stalk in the rat. *J. Physiol. (London)*, **111**, 347

24. Harris, G. W. and Jacobsohn, D. (1952). Functional grafts of the anterior pituitary gland. *Proc. Roy. Soc. (London)*, **B139**, 263

25. Sayers, M. A., Sayers, G. and Woodbury, L. A. (1948). The assay of adrenocorticotrophic hormone by the adrenal ascorbic acid-depletion method. *Endocrinology*, **42**, 379

26. Briggs, F. N. and Munson, P. L. (1955). Studies on the mechanism of stimulation of the ACTH secretion with the aid of morphine as a blocking agent. *Endocrinology*, **57**, 205

27. Porter, J. C. and Runsfeld, H. W. (1956). Effect of lyophilized plasma and plasma fractions from hypophyseal-portal vessel blood on adrenal ascorbic acid. *Endocrinology,*, **58**, 359

28. McCann, S. M. (1957). The ACTH-releasing activity of extracts of the posterior lobe of the pituitary *in vivo*. *Endocrinology*, **60**, 664

29. Saffran, M., Schally, A. V. and Benfey, B. G. (1955). Stimulation of release of corticotropin from the adenohypophysis by a neurohypophysial factor. *Endocrinology*, **57**, 439

30. Guillemin, R., Hearn, W. R., Cheek, W. R. and Householder, D. D. (1957). Control of corticotrophin release: further studies with *in vitro* methods. *Endocrinology*, **60**, 488

31. McCann, S. M. and Haberland, P. (1959). Relative abundance of vasopressin and corticotrophin-releasing factor in neurohypophyseal extracts. *Proc. Soc. Exp. Biol. Med.*, **102**, 319

32. Guillemin, R. (1964). Hypothalamic factors releasing pituitary hormones. *Recent. Progr. Horm. Res.*, **20**, 89

33. Rumsfeld, H. W. and Porter, J. C. (1962). ACTH-releasing activity of bovine posterior pituitaries. *Endocrinology*, **70**, 62

34. Royce, P. C. and Sayers, G. (1958). Corticotropin-releasing activity of a pepsin labile factor in the hypothalamus. *Proc. Soc. Exp. Biol. Med.*, **98**, 677

35. Royce, P. C. and Sayers, G. (1960). Purification of hypothalamic corticotrophin-releasing factor. *Proc. Soc. Exp. Biol. Med.*, **103**, 447

36. Rumsfeld, H. W. and Porter, J. C. (1959). ACTH-releasing activity in an acetone extract of beef hypothalamus. *Arch. Biochem. Biophys.*, **82**, 473

37. Dhariwal, A. P. S., Antunes-Rodrigues, J., Reeser, F., Chowers, I. and McCann, S. M. (1966). Purification of hypothalamic corticotrophin-releasing factor (CRF) of ovine origin. *Proc. Soc. Exp. Biol. Med.*, **121**, 8

38. Schally, A. V., Arimura, A., Bowers, C. Y., Kastin, A. J., Sawano, S. and Redding, T. W. (1968). Hypothalamic neurohormones regulating anterior pituitary function. *Recent Progr. Horm. Res.*, **24**, 497

39. Porter, J. C. and Rumsfeld, H. W. (1959). Further study of an ACTH-releasing protein from hypophyseal portal vessel plasma. *Endocrinology*, **64**, 948

40. Daniel, P. M. (1966). The anatomy of the hypothalamus and pituitary gland. *Neuroendocrinology*, Vol. 1, 15 (L. Martini and W. F. Ganong, editors) (New York: Academic Press)

41. Török, B. (1954). Lebendbeobachtung des hypophysenkreislaufes an hunden. *Acta Morphol. Acad. Sci. Hung.*, **4**, 83

42. Adams, J. H., Daniel, P. M. and Prichard, M. M. L. (1964). Distribution of hypophysial portal blood in the anterior lobe of the pituitary gland. *Endocrinology*, **75**, 120
43. Porter, J. C., Mical, R. S., Ondo, J. G. and Kamberi, I. A. (1971). Perfusion of the rat anterior pituitary via a cannulated portal vessel. *Karolinska Symposia on Research Methods in Reproductive Endocrinology. 4th Symposium: Perfusion Techniques*, 249 (Karolinska Institutet 1971: Stockholm)
44. Porter, J. C., Hines, M. F. M., Smith, K. R., Repass, R. L. and Smith, A. J. K. (1967). Quantitative evaluation of local blood flow of the adenohypophysis in rats. *Endocrinology*, **80**, 583
45. Goldman, H. (1965–1966). Vasopressin modulation of the distribution of blood flow in the unanesthetized rat. *Neuroendocrinology*, **1**, 23
46. Farquhar, M. G. (1961). Fine structure and function in capillaries of the anterior pituitary gland. *Angiology*, **12**, 270
47. Porter, J. C., Dhariwal, A. P. S. and McCann, S. M. (1967). Response of the anterior pituitary–adrenocortical axis to purified CRF *Endocrinology*, **80**, 679
48. McCann, S. M. and Dhariwal, A. P. S. (1966). Hypothalamic releasing factors and the neurovascular link between brain and anterior pituitary. *Neuroendocrinology*, Vol. 1, 261 (L. Martini and W. F. Ganong, editors) (New York: Academic Press)
49. Meites, J. (1970). Direct studies of the secretion of the hypothalamic hypophysiotropic hormones (HHH). *Hypophysiotropic Hormones of the Hypothalamus: Assay and Chemistry*, 261 (J. Meites, editor) (Baltimore: Williams and Wilkins)
50. Guillemin, R. and Vale, W. (1970). Bioassay of the hypophysiotropic hormones: *In Vitro* Systems. *Hypophysiotropic hormones of the hypothalamus: Assay and Chemistry* 21 (J. Meites, editor) (Baltimore: Williams and Wilkins)
51. Serra, G. B. and Midgley, A. R. Jr. (1970). The *in vitro* release of LH during continuous superfusion of single rat anterior pituitary glands. *Proc. Soc. Exp. Biol. Med.* **133**, 1370
52. Sayers, G., Portanova, R., Beall, R. J. and Malamed, S. (1971). Techniques for the isolation of cells of the adrenal cortex, the anterior pituitary and the corpus luteum: Morphological and functional evaluation of the isolated cells. *Karolinska Symposia on Research Methods in Reproductive Endocrinology, 3rd Symposium In vitro methods in reproductive cell biology*, 11 (Karolinksa Institutet 1971: Stockholm)
53. Vale, W., Grant, G., Amoss, M., Blackwell, R. and Guillemin, R. (1972). Culture of enzymatically dispersed pituitary cells. *J. Clin. Exp. Med.*, **91**, 562
54. Dhariwal, A. P. S., Russell, S., McCann, S. M. and Yates, F. E. Assay of corticotrophin releasing factors by injection into the anterior pituitary of intact rats. *Endocrinology*, **84**, 544
55. Brodish, A. and Long, C. N. H. (1962). ACTH-releasing hypothalamic neurohumor in peripheral blood. *Endocrinology*, **71**, 298
56. Vernikos-Danellis, J. (1965). Effect of stress, adrenalectomy, hypophysectomy and hydrocortisone on the corticotropin-releasing activity of rat median eminence. *Endocrinology*, **76**, 122
57. McCann, S. M. and Taleisnik, S. and Friedman, H. M. (1960). LH-releasing activity in hypothalamic extracts. *Proc. Soc. Exp. Biol. Med.*, **104**, 432
58. Schally, A. V. and Bowers, C. Y. (1964). *In vitro* and *in vivo* stimulation of the release of luteinising hormone. *Endocrinology*, **75**, 312
59. McCann, S. M. (1962). A hypothalamic luteinising-hormone-releasing factor. *Amer. J. Physiol.*, **202**, 395
60. Schneider, H. P. G. and McCann, S. M. (1970). Release of LRF into the peripheral circulation of hypox rats by dopamine and its blockade by oestradiol. *Endocrinology*, **87**, 249
61. Kamberi, I. A., Mical, R. S. and Porter, J. C. (1969). Luteinising hormone-releasing activity in hypophysial stalk blood and elevation by dopamine. *Science*, **166**, 388
62. Ajika, K., Krulich, L., Fawcett, C. P. and McCann, S. M. (1972). Effects of oestrogen on plasma and pituitary gonadotropins and prolactin, and on hypothalamic releasing and inhibiting factors. *Neuroendocrinology*, **9**, 304
63. Igarashi, M., Nallar, R. and McCann, S. M. (1964). Further studies on the follicle stimulating hormone-releasing action of hypothalamic extracts. *Endocrinology*, **75**, 901
64. Mittler, J. C. and Meites, J. (1964). *In vitro* stimulation of pituitary follicle-stimulating-hormone release by hypothalamic extract. *Proc. Soc. Exp. Biol. Med.*, **117**, 309

65. Dhariwal, A. P. S., Nallar, R., Batt, M. and McCann, S. M. (1965). Separation of FSH-releasing factor from LH-releasing factor. *Endocrinology*, **76**, 290
66. Dhariwal, A. P. S., Watanabe, S., Antunes-Rodrigues, J. and McCann, S. M. (1967). Chromatographic behaviour of follicle stimulating hormone-releasing factor on Sephadex and carboxy methyl cellulose. *Neuroendocrinology*, **2**, 294
67. Schally, A. V., Saito, T., Arimura, A., Sawano, S. and Bowers, C. Y. (1967). Purification and *in vitro* and *in vivo* studies with porcine hypothalamic follicle-stimulating hormone-releasing factor. *Endocrinology*, **81**, 882
68. Jutisz, M. (1970). Purification and chemistry of gonadotropin releasing factors. *The Human Testis*, 207 (E. Rosemberg and C. A. Paulsen, editors) (New York: Plenum Press)
69. Negro-Vilar, A., Dickerman, E. and Meites, J. (1968). Effects of continuous light on hypothalamic FSH-releasing factor and pituitary FSH levels in rats. *Proc. Soc. Exp. Biol. Med.*, **126**, 751
70. Watanabe, S. and McCann, S. M. (1969). The effects of castration or treatment with testosterone on the content of pituitary FSH and hypothalamic FSH-releasing factor in the male rat. *Proc. Soc. Exp. Biol. Med.*, **130**, 1075
71. Kamberi, I. A., Mical, R. S. and Porter, J. C. (1970). FSH-releasing activity in hypophyseal portal blood and elevation by dopamine. *Nature (London)*, **227**, 714
72. Negro-Vilar, A., Dickerman, A. E. and Meites, J. (1968). FSH-releasing factor activity in plasma of rats after hypophysectomy and continuous light. *Endocrinology*, **82**, 939
73. Shibusawa, K., Saito, S. Nishi, K., Yamamoto, T., Tomisawa, K. and Abe, C. (1956). Hypothalamic control of thyrotroph-thyroidal function. *Endocrinol., Jap.*, **3**, 116
74. Schreiber, V. (1963). *The Hypothalamo-Hypophysial System*, (Prague: Czechoslovak Academy of Sciences)
75. Guillemin, R., Yamazaki, E., Jutisz, M. and Sakiz, E. (1962). Présence dans un extrait de tissus hypothalamiques d'une substance stimulant la sécrétion de l'hormone hypophysaire thyréotrope (TSH). Première purification par filtration sur gel Sephadex. *C. R.*, **255**, 1018
76. Schally, A. V., Bowers, C. Y. and Redding, T. W. (1966). Purification of thyrotropic hormone releasing factor from bovine hypothalamus. *Endocrinology*, **78**, 726
77. Bassiri, R. and Utiger, R. D. (1972). Serum inactivation of immunological and biological activity of TRF. *Endocrinology*, **91**, 657
78. Sinha, D. and Meites, J. (1965–1966). Effects of thyroidectomy and thyroxine on hypothalamic concentration of 'thyrotropin releasing factor' and pituitary content of thyrotropin in rats. *Neuroendocrinology*, **1**, 4
79. Porter, J. C., Vale, W., Burgus, R., Mical, R. S. and Guillemin, R. (1971), Release of TSH by TRF infused directly into a pituitary stalk portal vessel. *Endocrinology*, **89**, 1054
80. Bishop, W., Fawcett, C. P., Krulich, L. and McCann, S. M. (1972). Acute and chronic effects of hypothalamic lesions on the release of FSH, LH and prolactin in intact and castrated rats. *Endocrinology*, **91**, 643
81. Talwalker, P. K., Ratner, A. and Meites, J. (1963). *In vitro* inhibition of pituitary prolactin synthesis and release by hypothalamic extract. *Amer. J. Physiol.*, **205**, 213
82. Pasteels, J. L. (1961). Premiers resultats de culture combinee *in vitro* d'hypophyse et d'hypothalamus dans le but d'en apprecier la sécrétion de prolactine. *C.R. Acad. Sci. Paris*, **253**, 3074
83. Watson, J. T., Krulich, L. and McCann, S. M. (1971). Effect of crude rat hypothalamic extract on serum gonadotropin and prolactin levels in normal and orchidectomized male rats. *Endocrinology*, **89**, 1412
84. Kamberi, I. A., Mical, R. S. and Porter, J. C. (1971). Hypophyseal portal vessel infusion: *In vivo* demonstration of LRF, FRF and PIF in stalk plasma. *Endocrinology*, **89**, 1042
85. Malacara, J. M., Valverde-R., Reichlin, S. and Bollinger, J. (1972). Elevation of plasma radioimmunoassayable growth hormone in the rat induced by porcine hypothalamic extract. *Endocrinology*, **91**, 1189
86. Dhariwal, A. P. S., Antunes-Rodrigues, J., Grosvenor, C. and McCann, S. M. (1968). Purification of ovine prolactin-inhibiting factor (PIF). *Endocrinology*, **82**, 1236
87. Nicoll, C. S., Fiorindo, R. P., McKennee, C. T. and Parsons, J. A. (1970). Assay

of hypothalamic factors which regulate prolactin secretion. *Hypophysiotropic Hormone of the Hypothalamus: Assay and Chemistry*, 115 (J. Meites, editor) (Baltimore: William and Wilkins)

88. Kragt, C. L. and Meites, J. (1965). Stimulation of pigeon pituitary prolactin release by pigeon hypothalamic extract *in vitro*. *Endocrinology*, **76**, 1169

89. Etkin, W. (1962). Hypothalamic inhibition of pars intermedia activity in the frog. *Gen. Comp. Endocrinol., Suppl.*, **1**, 148

90. Kastin, A. J. and Ross, G. T. (1965). Melanocyte-stimulating hormone activity in pituitaries of frogs with hypothalamic lesions. *Endocrinology*, **77**, 45

91. Kastin, A. J., Viosca, S. and Schally, A. V. (1970). Assay of mammalian MSH release-regulating factor(s). *Hypophysiotropic Hormones of the Hypothalamus: Assay and Chemistry*, **171**, (J. Meites, editor) (Baltimore: Williams and Wilkins)

92. Taleisnik, S. and Orias, R. A. (1965). A melanocyte stimulating hormone-releasing factor in hypothalamic extracts. *Amer. J. Physiol.*, **208**, 293

93. Reichlin, S. (1961). Growth hormone content of pituitaries from rats with hypothalamic lesions. *Endocrinology*, **69**, 225

94. Krulich, L., Dhariwal, A. P. S. and McCann, S. M. (1965). Hypothalamic control of growth hormone (GH) secretion. *Program of the 47th Endocrine Society Meeting*, 21

95. Glick, S. M. (1969). Regulation of GH secretion. *Frontiers in Neuroendocrinology*, 141 (W. F. Ganong and L. Martini, editors) (London: Oxford Univerity Press)

96. Franz, J., Haselbach, C. H. and Libert, O. (1962). Studies of the effect of hypothalamic extracts on somatotrophic pituitary function. *Acta Endocrinol.*, **41**, 336

97. Deuben, R. R. and Meites, J. (1964). Stimulation of pituitary growth hormone release by a hypothalamic extract *in vitro*. *Endocrinology*, **74**, 408

98. Müller, E. E. and Pecile, A. (1965). Growth hormone releasing factor of a guinea-pig hypothalamic extract: its activity in guinea-pig and rat. *Proc. Soc. Exp. Biol. Med.*, **119**, 1191

99. Krulich, L., Dhariwal, A. P. S. and McCann, S. M. (1965). Growth hormone-releasing activity of crude ovine hypothalamic extracts. *Proc. Soc. Exp. Biol. Med.*, **120**, 180

100. Katz, S., Dhariwal, A. P. S. and McCann, S. M. (1967). Effect of hypoglycemia on the content of pituitary growth hormone and hypothalamic growth hormone-releasing factor in the rat. *Endocrinology*, **81**, 333

101. Pecile, A., Müller, E. E., Falconi, G. and Martini, L. (1965). Growth hormone-releasing activity of hypothalamic extracts at different ages. *Endocrinology*, **77**, 241

102. Krulich, L. and McCann, S. M. (1966). Evidence for the presence of growth hormone-releasing factor in blood of hypoglycemic, hypophysectomised rats. *Proc. Soc. Exp. Biol. Med.*, **122**, 668

103. Müller, E. E., Arimura, A., Sawano, S., Saito, T. and Schally, A. V. (1967). Growth hormone-releasing activity in hypothalamus and plasma of rats subjected to stress. *Proc. Soc. Exp. Biol. Med.*, **125**, 874

104. Müller, E. E., Arimura, A., Saito, T. and Schally, A. V. (1967). Growth hormone-releasing activity in plasma of normal and hypophysectomised rats. *Endocrinology*, **80**, 77

105. Hagen, T. C., Lawrence, A. M. and Kirsteris, L. (1971). *In vitro* release of monkey pituitary growth hormone by acromegalic plasma. *J. Clin. Endocrinol.*, **33**, 448

106. Wilber, J. F. and Porter, J. C. (1970). Thyrotropin and growth hormone releasing activity in hypophysial portal blood. *Endocrinology*, **87**, 807

107. Worthington, W. C., Folsom, S. E. Jr. and Buse, M. G. (1972). Pituitary growth hormone 'synthesising factor' in hypophysial portal blood. *Endocrinology*, **90**, 1664

108. Reichlin, S. and Schalch, D. S. (1969). Growth hormone releasing factor. *Progress in Endocrinology*, 584 (C. Gual, editor) (Amsterdam: Excerpta Medica)

109. Frohman, L. A., Maran, J. W. and Dhariwal, A. P. S. (1971]. Plasma growth hormone responses to intra-pituitary injections of growth hormone releasing factor (GRF) in the rat. *Endocrinology*, **88**, 1483

110. Machlin, L. J., Horino, M., Kipnis, D. M., Philips, S. L. and Gordon, R. S. (1967). Stimulation of growth hormone secretion by median eminence extracts in the sheep. *Endocrinology*, **80**, 205

111. Smith, G. P., Katz, S., Root, A. W., Dhariwal, A. P. S., Bongiovanni, A., Eberlein, W. and McCann, S. M. (1968). Growth hormone releasing activity of crude ovine SME extracts in Rhesus monkeys. *Endocrinology*, **83**, 25

112. Krulich, L., Dhariwal, A. P. S. and McCann, S. M. (1968). Stimulatory and inhibitory effects of purified hypothalamic extracts on growth hormone release from rat pituitary *in vitro*. *Endocrinology*, **83**, 783
113. Dhariwal, A. P. S., Krulich, L. and McCann, S. M. (1969). Purification of a growth hormone inhibiting factor (GIF) from sheep hypothalamus. *Neuroendocrinology*, **4**, 282
114. Krulich, L. and McCann, S. M. (1969). Effect of GRF and GIF on the release and concentration of GH in pituitaries incubated *in vitro*. *Endocrinology*, **85**, 319
115. Krulich, L., Illner, P., Fawcett, C. P., Quijada, N. and McCann, S. M. (1972). Dual hypothalamic regulation of growth hormone secretion. *Growth and Growth Hormone*, 306 (A. Pecile and E. E. Müller, editors) (Amsterdam: Excerpta Medica)
116. Stachura, M. E., Dhariwal, A. P. S. and Frohman, L. A. (1972). Inhibitory effects of purified hypothalamic extract (HTE) on rat growth hormone synthesis and release *in vitro*. *IVth Int. Cong. Endocrinol.*, ICS **256**, 83 (Amsterdam: Excerpta Medica)
117. Brazeau, P., Vale, W., Burgus, R., Ling, M., Butcher, M., Rivier, J. and Guillemin, R. (1973). Hypothalamic polypeptide that inhibits the secretion of immunoreactive pituitary growth hormone. *Science*, **179**, 77
118. McCann, S. M. (1971). Mechanism of action of hypothalamic hypophyseal stimulating and inhibiting hormones. *Frontiers in Neuroendocrinology*, *1971*, 209 (L. Martini and W. F. Ganong, editors) (New York: Oxford)
119. Gay, V. L., Niswender, G. D. and Midgley, A. R. Jr. (1970). Response of individual rats and sheep to one or more injections of hypothalamic extract as determined by radioimmunoassay of plasma LH. *Endocrinology*, **86**, 1305
120. Orias, R. and Libertun, C. (1973). Effects of synthetic LRF infusion on gonadotropin release and inhibition of these effects by oestrogen (E_2) and progesterone (P). *Program of the 55th Meeting of Endocrine Society*, **57**
121. Stachura, M. E., Dhariwal, A. P. S. and Frohman, L. A. (1972). Growth hormone synthesis and release *in vitro*: Effects of partially purified ovine hypothalamic extract. *Endocrinology*, **91**, 1071
122. Motta, M., Piva, F., Fraschini, F. and Martini, L. (1970). 'Pituitary depletion methods for the bioassay of hypothalamic releasing factors. *Hypophysiotropic Hormones of the Hypothalamus: Assay and Chemistry*, 44 (J. Meites, editor) (Baltimore: Williams and Wilkins)
123. Wakabayashi, K. and McCann, S. M. (1970). *In vitro* responses of anterior pituitary glands from normal, castrated and androgen treated male rats to LH-releasing factor (LRF) and high potassium medium. *Endocrinology*, **87**, 771
124. Krulich, L. and McCann, S. M. (1969). Effect of GRF and GIF on the release and concentration of GH in pituitaries incubated *in vitro*. *Endocrinology*, **85**, 319
125. Mittler, J. C., Arimura, A. and Schally, A. V. (1970). Release and synthesis of luteinising hormone and follicle-stimulating hormone in pituitary cultures in response to hypothalamic preparations. *Proc. Soc. Exp. Biol. Med.*, **133**, 1321
126. Crighton, D. B., Schneider, H. P. G. and McCann, S. M. (1969). A study of the possible interaction of LRF with other hypothalamic releasing factors at the level of the pituitary gland. *J. Endocrinol.*, **44**, 405
127. Bowers, C. Y. and Schally, A. V. (1970). Assay of thyrotropin release hormone. *Hypophysiotropic Hormones of the Hypothalamus: Assay and Chemistry*, 74 (J. Medies, editor) (Baltimore: Williams and Wilkins)
128. Bowers, C. H., Friesen, H. G., Hwang, P., Gyuda, H. J. and Folkers, K. (1971). Prolactin and thyrotropin release in man by synthetic pyroglutamyl-histidyl-prolinamide. *Biochem. Biophys. Res. Commun.*, **45**, 1033
129. Jacobs, L. S., Snyder, P.J., Wilbur, J. F., Utiger, R. D. and Daughaday, W. H. (1971). Increased serum prolactin after administration of synthetic TRF in man. *J. Clin. Endocrinol. Metab.*. **33**, 996
130. Lu, K. H., Shaar, C. J., Kortnight, K. H. and Meites, J. (1972). Effects of synthetic TRH on *in vitro* and *in vivo* prolactin release in the rat. *Endocrinology*, **91**, 1540
131. Tashjian, A. H., Barofsky and Jensen, D. K. (1971). Thyrotropin-releasing hormone: direct evidence for stimulation of prolactin production by pituitary cells in culture. *Biochem. Biophys. Res. Commun.*, **43**, 516
132. Labrie, F., Barden, N., Poirier, G. and DeLean, A. (1972). Binding of thyrotropin-releasing hormone to plasma membranes of bovine anterior pituitary gland. *Proc. Nat. Acad. Sci. USA*, **69**, 283

133. Grant, G., Vale, W. and Guillemin, R. (1972). Interaction of thryotropin releasing factor with membrane receptors of pituitary cells. *Biochem. Biophys. Res. Commun.*, **46**, 28
134. Wilbur, J. F. and Seibel, J. (1973). TRH binding to a thyrotroph receptor: the primary events in releasing hormone action. *Serono Conference on Releasing Factors*, (E. Rosemberg and C. Gual, editors) (in the press)
135. Douglas, W. W. and Poisner, A. M. (1964). The role of calcium in the release of vasopressin from the neurohypophysis. *J. Physiol.*, **172**, 1
136. Coates, P. W., Ashby, E., Krulich, L., Dhariwal, A. P. S. and McCann, S. M. (1970). Morphological alterations in somatotrophs of the rat adenohypophysis following administration of hypothalamic extracts. *Amer. J. Anat.*, **128**, 389
137. de Virgiliis, G., Meldolesi, J. and Clementi, F. (1968). Ultrastructure of growth hormone-producing cells of rat pituitary after injection of hypothalamic extract. *Endocrinology*, **83**, 1278
138. Samli, M. H. and Geschwind, I. I. (1968). Some effects of energy transfer inhibitors and of Ca^{2+}-free or K^+ enhanced media on the release of luteinising hormone (LH) from the rat pituitary gland *in vitro. Endocrinology*, **82**, 225
139. Wakabayashi, K., Kamberi, I. A. and McCann, S. M. (1969). *In vitro* response of the rat pituitary to gonadotropin-releasing factors and to ions. *Endocrinology*, **85**, 1046
140. MacLeod, R. M. and Fontham, E. H. (1970). Influence of ionic environment on the *in vitro* synthesis and release of pituitary hormones. *Endocrinology*, **86**, 863
141. Ashworth, R., Wakabayashi, K., McGavren, W., Dhariwal, A. P. S. and McCann, S. M. (1968). The possible relationship between membrane depolarisation and the action of hypothalamic-releasing factors on the pituitary cell. *Proc. 24th Int. Cong. Physiol. Sci.*, **2**, 19
142. Milligan, J. V. and Kraicer, J. (1970). Adenohypophysial transmembrane potentials: Polarity reversed by elevated external potassium ion concentration. *Science*, **167**, 182
143. Peake, G. T. (1973). The role of cyclic nucleotides in secretion of pituitary GH. *Frontiers in Neuroendocrinology*, (W. F. Ganong and L. Martini, editors) (New York: Oxford University Press) (in the press)
144. Parsons, J. A. (1969). Calcium ion requirement for prolactin secretion by rat adenohypophyses *in vitro. Amer. J. Physiol.*, **217**, 1599
145. Milligan, J. V., Kraicer, J., Illner, P. and Fawcett, P. (1972). Purified growth hormone releasing factor increased ^{45}Ca uptake into pituitary cells. *Canad. J. Physiol. Pharm.*, **50**, 613
146. Zor, U., Kaneko, T., Schneider, H. P. G., McCann, S. M., Lowe, I., Bloom, G., Borland, B. and Field, J. B. (1969). Stimulation of anterior pituitary adenyl cyclase activity and adenosine 3',5'-cyclic phosphate by hypothalamic extract and prostaglandin E_1. *Proc. Nat. Acad. Sci. USA*, **63**, 918
147. Steiner, A. L., Peake, G. T., Utiger, R. D., Karl, I. E. and Kipnis, D. M. (1970). Hypothalamic stimulation of GH and TSH release *in vitro* and pituitary 3',5'-adenosine cyclic monophosphate. *Endocrinology*, **86**, 1354
148. Labrie, F., Beraud, G., Gauthier, M. and Lemay, A. (1971). Actinomycin-insensitive stimulation of protein synthesis in rat anterior pituitary *in vitro* by dibutyryl adenosine 3'5'-monophosphate. *J. Biol. Chem.*, **246**, 1902
149. Borgeat, P., Chavaucy, G. and Labrie, F. (1973). Stimulation of adenohypophyseal adenyl cyclase activity by synthetic LRF and purified GRF *in vitro. Serono Conference on releasing factors*. (E. Rosemberg and C. Gual, editors)
150. Scofield, G. H. (1970). Role of cyclic 3',5'-AMP in the release of GH *in vitro. Nature (London)*, **215**, 1382
151. Wilber, J. F., Peake, G. T., and Utiger, R. D. (1969). Thyrotropin release *in vitro*: Stimulation of 3'-5'-adenosine monophosphate. *Endocrinology*, **84**, 758
152. Wakabayashi, K., Antunes-Rodrigues, J., Tamaoki, B.-I. and McCann, S. M. (1972). *In vitro* effect of hypothalamic extract and other stimulating agents on glucose oxidation and luteinising hormone (LH) release from rat anterior pituitary glands. *Endocrinology*, **90**, 690
153. Peake, G. T., Steiner, A. L. and Daughaday, W. H. (1972). Guanosine 3',5'-cyclic monophosphate is a potent pituitary growth hormone secretogogue. *Endocrinology*, **90**, 212

153a. Howell, S. L. and Montague, W. (1971). The mode of action of cyclic AMP in the rat anterior pituitary. *FEBS Lett.*, **18**, 293

154. Labrie, F., Lemay, A., Lemaire, S., Poirier, G., Boucher, R., Barden, M., De Léan, A. and Gauthier, M. (1971). Cyclic AMP and control of pituitary protein synthesis and release. *Proc. of the 25th Int. Cong. Physiol. Sci.*, **9**, 331 (German Physiological Society) 1971: Munich

155. Zor, U., Kaneko, T., Schneider, H. P. G., McCann, S. M. and Field, J. B. (1970). Further studies of stimulation of anterior pituitary cyclic adenosine 3′,5′-monophosphate by hypothalamic extract and prostaglandins. *J. Biol. Chem.* **245**, 2883

156. Kraicer, J. and Milligan, J. V. (1971). Effect of colchicine on *in vitro* ACTH release induced by high K^+ and by hypothalamus-stalk-median eminence extract. *Endocrinology*, **89**, 408

157. Sundberg, D. K., Krulich, L., Fawcett, C. P., Illner, P. and McCann, S. M. (1973). The effect of colchicine on the release of rat anterior pituitary hormones *in vitro*. *Proc. Soc. Exp. Biol. Med.*, **142**, 1097

158. MacLeod, R. M. and Lehmeyer, J. E. (1970). Release of pituitary growth hormone by prostaglandins and dibutryryl adenosine cyclic 3′,5′-monophosphate in the absence of protein synthesis. *Proc. Nat. Acad. Sci. USA*, **67**, 1172

159. Vale, W., Rivier, C. and Guillemin, R. (1971). A 'prostaglandin receptor' in the mechanisms involved in the secretion of anterior pituitary hormones. *Fed. Proc. (Fed. Amer. Soc. Exp. Biol.)*, **30**, 363

160. Cooper, K., Fawcett, C. P. and McCann, S. M. (in preparation). Increased sensitivity to LRF in acutely ovariectomised rats

161. Negro-Vilar, A., Orias, R. and McCann, S. M. (1973). Evidence for a pituitary site of action for the acute inhibition of LH release by oestrogen in the rat. *Endocrinology*, **92**, 1680

162. Libertun, C., Orias, R. and McCann, S. M. (in preparation). Infusion of synthetic LRF: inhibition of effects by steroids

163. Yen, S. S. C. (1973). *Proc. of the IPPF Symp. on Hypothalamic Control of Fertility*, (in the press)

164. Arimura, A. and Schally, A. V. (1971). Augmentation of pituitary responsiveness to LH-releasing hormone (LH-RH) by oestrogen. *Proc. Soc. Exp. Biol. Med.*, **136**, 290

165. Libertun, C., Cooper, K. J., Fawcett, C. P. and McCann, S. M. (1973). Effects of ovariectomy and steroid treatment on hypophyseal sensitivity to purified LRF. *Endocrinology*, (in the press)

166. Cooper, K. J., Fawcett, C. P. and McCann, S. M. (1973). Variations in pituitary responsiveness to luteinising hormone releasing factor during the rat oestrous cycle. *J. Endocrinol.*, **57**, 107

167. Arimura, A., Debeljuk, L. and Schally, A. V. (1972). LH release by LH-releasing hormone in golden hamsters at various stages of oestrous cycle. *Proc. Soc. Exp. Biol. Med.* **140**, 609

168. Reeves, J. J., Arimura, A. and Schally, A. V. (1971). Pituitary responsiveness to purified luteinising hormone-releasing hormone (LH-RH) at various stages of the oestrous cycle in sheep. *J. Anim. Sci.*, **32**, 123

169. Yen, S. S. C., Van den Berg, G., Rebar, R. and Ehara, Y. (1972). Variation of pituitary responsiveness to synthetic LRF during different phases of the menstrual cycle. *J. Clin. Endocrinol. Med.*, **35**, 931

170. Russell, S. M., Dhariwal, A. P. S., McCann, S. M. and Yates, F. E. (1969). Inhibition by dexamethoasone of the *in vivo* pituitary response to corticotropin-releasing factor (CRF). *Endocrinology*, **85**, 512

171. Vale, W., Burgus, R. and Guillemin, R. (1968). On the mechanism of action of TRF. *Neuroendocrinology*, **3**, 34

172. Bowers, C. Y., Lee, K. L. and Schally, A. V. (1968). A study of the interaction of the TRF and T_3: effects of puromycin and cycloheximide. *Endocrinology*, **82**, 75

173. Davidson, J. M. (1969). Feedback control of gonadotropin secretion. *Frontiers in Neuroendocrinology, 1969*, 343 (W. F. Ganong and L. Martini, editors) (New York: Oxford University Press)

174. Bogdanove, E. M. (1963). Direct gonad–pituitary feedback: an analysis of effects of intracranial oestrogenic depots on gonadotrophin secretion. *Endocrinology*, **73**, 696

175. Dhariwal, A. P. S., Russell, S. M., McCann, S. M. and Yates, F. E. (1969). Assay

of corticotropin-releasing factors by injection into the anterior pituitary of intact rats. *Endocrinology*, **84**, 544

176. Brown, M. R. and Hedge, G. A. (1972). TSH and ACTH secretion after intrapituitary injection of synthetic TRF. *Endocrinology*, **91**, 206

177. Blake, C. A. and Sawyer, C. H. (1972). Ovulation blocking actions of urethane in the rat. *Endocrinology*, **91**, 87

178. Malacara, J. M., Seyler, L. E. and Reichlin, S. (1972). Luteinising hormone releasing factor activity in peripheral blood from women during the midcycle luteinising hormone ovulatory surge. *J. Clin. Endocrinol. Metabol.*, **34**, 271

179. Halasz, B., Pupp, L., Uhlarik, S. and Tima, L. (1965). Further studies on the hormone secretion of the anterior pituitary transplanted into the hypophysiotropic area of the rat hypothalamus, *Endocrinology*, **77**, 343

180. Crighton, D. B., Schneider, H. P. G. and McCann, S. M. (1970). Localisation of LH-releasing factor in the hypothalamus and neurohypophysis as determined by *in vitro* assay. *Endocrinology*, **87**, 323

181. Krulich, L., Quijada, M., Illner, P. and McCann, S. M. (1971). The distribution of hypothalamic hypophysiotropic factors in the hypothalamus of the rat. *Proc. of the 25th Int. Cong. Physiol. Sci.*, **9**, 326 (German Physiological Society 1971: Munich)

182. Schneider, H. P. G., Crighton, D. B. and McCann, S. M. (1969). Suprachiasmatic LH-releasing factor. *Neuroendocrinology*, **5**, 271

183. Bishop, W., Kalra, P. S., Fawcett, C. P., Krulich, L. and McCann, S. M. (1972). The effects of hypothalamic lesions on the release of gonadotropins and prolactin in response to oestrogen and progesterone treatment in female rats. *Endocrinology*, **91**, 1404

184. Pfaff, D., Lewis, C., Diakow, C. and Keiner, M. (1973). Neurophysiological analysis of mating behaviour responses as hormone-sensitive reflexes. *Progress in Physiological Psychology*, **5**, (in press) (E. Stellar and J. Sprague, editors) (New York: Academic Press)

185. Stumpf, W. (1968). Estradiol-concentrating neurones: topography in the hypothalamus by dry-mount autoradiography. *Science*, **162**, 1001

186. Fuxe, K. and Hökfelt, T. (1969). Catecholamines in the hypothalamus and the pituitary gland. *Frontiers in Neuroendocrinology, 1969*, 47 (W. F. Ganong and L. Martini, editors) (New York: Oxford)

187. Schneider, H. P. G. and McCann, S. M. (1969). Possible role of dopamine as transmitter to promote discharge of LH-releasing factor. *Endocrinology*, **85**, 121

188. Kamberi, I. A., Schneider, H. P. G. and McCann, S. M. (1970). Action of dopamine to induce release of FSH-releasing factor (FRF) from hypothalamic tissue *in vitro*. *Endocrinology*, **86**, 278

189. MacLeod, R. M. (1969). Influence of norepinephrine and catecholamine-depleting agents on the synthesis and release of prolactin and growth hormone. *Endocrinology*, **85**, 916

190. Birge, C. A., Jacobs, L. S., Hameo, C. T. and Daughaday, W. H. (1970). Catecholamine inhibition of prolactin secretion by isolated rat adenohypophyses. *Endocrinology*, **86**, 120

191. Quijada, M., Illner, P., Krulich, L. and McCann, S. M. (1973). The effect of catecholamines on hormone release from anterior pituitaries and ventral hypothalamic incubated *in vitro*. *Neuroendocrinology*, (in the press)

192. Schneider, H. P. G. and McCann, S. M. (1970). Mono- and indol-amines and control of LH-secretion. *Endocrinology*, **86**, 1127

193. Kamberi, I. A., Mical, R. S. and Porter, J. C. (1971). Effect of anterior pituitary perfusion and intraventricular injection of catecholamines on FSH release. *Endocrinology*, **88**, 1003

194. Kamberi, I. A., Mical, R. and Porter, J. C. (1971). Effect of anterior pituitary perfusion and intraventricular injection of catecholamines on prolactin release. *Endocrinology*, **88**, 1012

195. Schneider, H. P. G. and McCann, S. M. (1970). LH-releasing factor discharged by dopamine in rats. *J. Endocrinol.*, **46**, 555

196. Schneider, H. P. G. and McCann, S. M. (1970). Release of LRF into the peripheral circulation of hypox rats by dopamine and its blockade by oestradiol. *Endocrinology*, **87**, 249

197. Porter, J. C., Kamberi, I. A. and Ondo, J. G. (1972). Role of biogenic amines and cerebrospinal fluid in the neurovascular transmittal of hypophysiotrophic substances.

Brain–Endocrine Interaction. Median Eminence: Structure and Function, 245 (K. M. Knigge, D. E. Scott and A. Weindl, editors) (Basel: S. Karger)

198. Schneider, H. P. G. and McCann, S. M. (1970). Estradiol and the neuroendocrine control of LH-release *in vitro. Endocrinology*, **87**, 330

199. Donoso, A. O., Bishop, W., Fawcett, C. P. Krulich, L. and McCann, S. M. (1971). Effects of drugs that modify brain monoamine concentrations on plasma gonadotropin and prolactin levels in the rat. *Endocrinology*, **89**, 774

200. Donoso, A. O., Bishop, W. and McCann, S. M. (1973). The effects of drugs which modify catecholamine synthesis on serum prolactin in rats with median eminence lesions. *Proc. Soc. Exp. Biol. Med.*, **143**, 360

201. Kalra, P. S., Kalra, S. P., Krulich, L., Fawcett, C. P. and McCann, S. M. (1972). Involvement of norepinephrine in transmission of the stimulatory influence of progesterone on gonadotropin release. *Endocrinology*, **90**, 1168

202. Ojeda, S. R. and McCann, S. M. (1973). Evidence for participation of a catecholaminergic mechanism in the post-castration rise in plasma gonadotropins. *Neuroendocrinology*, **12**, 295

203. Kalra, P. S. and McCann, S. M. (1973). Involvement of catecholamines in feedback mechanisms. *Proc. of the Symp. on Drug Effects on Neuroendocrine Regulation*, (in the press) (Amsterdam: Elsevier)

204. Kalra, S. P. and McCann, S. M. (1972). Modification of brain catecholamine levels and LH release by preoptic stimulation. *Proc. the 4th Int. Cong. of Endocrinology* 508

205, Blackard, W. G. and Heidingsfelder, S. A. (1968). Adrenergic receptor control mechanism for growth hormone secretion. *J. Clin. Invest.*, **47**, 1407

206. Toivola, P., Gale, C. C., Werrbach, J. and Goodner, C. J. (1969). Intrahypothalamic infusion of biogenic amines: effect on temperature regulation and neuroendocrine function in baboons. *The Physiologist*, **12**, 377

207. Müller, E. E., Dal Pra, P. and Pecile, A. (1968). Influence of brain neurohumor injected into the lateral ventricle of the brain on growth hormone release. *Endocrinology*, **83**, 893

208. Collu, R., Fraschini, F., Visconti, P. and Martini, L. (1972). Adrenergic and serotoninergic control of growth hormone secretion in adult male rats. *Endocrinology*, **90**, 1231

209. Scapagnini, U., Van Loon, G. R., Moberg, G. P. and Ganong, W. F. (1970). Effect of α-methyl-*p*-tyrosine on the circadian variation of plasma corticosterone in rats. *Europ. J. Pharmacol.*, **11**, 266

210. Van Loon, G. R., Scapagnini, U., Moberg, G. P. and Ganong, W. F. (1971). Evidence for central adrenergic neural inhibition of ACTH secretion in the rat. *Endocrinology*, **89**, 1464

211. Kordon, C. A., Blake, C. A. and Sawyer, C. H. (1972). Participation of serotonin-containing neurones in suckling-induced rise in plasma prolactin. *Proc. 4th Int. Cong. of Endocrinology*, 51a

212. Libertun, C. and McCann, S. M. (1973). Blockade of the release of gonadotropins and prolactin by subcutaneous or intraventricular injection of atropine in male and female rats. *Endocrinology*, **92**, 1714

213. Frantz, A. (1973). *Proc. of the Symp. on Drug Effects on Neuroendocrine Regulation*, (in the press) (Amsterdam: Elsevier)

214. Frantz, A. personal communication

215. Chan, L. T., Schaal, S. M. and Saffran, M. (1969). Properties of the corticotrophin-releasing factor of the rat median eminence. *Endocrinology*, **85**, 644

216. Saffran, M. Pearlmutter, A. F., Rapino, E. and Upton, G. V. (1972). Pressinoic acid: a peptide with potent corticotrophin-releasing activity. *Biochem. Biophys. Res. Commun.* **49**, 748

217. Arimura, A., Schally, A. V. and Bowers, C. Y. (1969). Corticotrophin releasing activity of lysine vasopressin analogues. *Endocrinology*, **84**, 579

218. Ishii, S., Zwata, T. and Kobayashi, H. (1969). Granular localisation of corticotrophin releasing activity in horse hypophysial stalk homogenate. *Endocrinol. Jap.*, **16**, 171

219. Maiden, A. H., Geuze, J. J. and DeWied, D. (1970). Studies on the subcellular localisation of corticotrophin releasing factor (CRF) and vasopressin in the median eminence of the rat. *Endocrinology*, **87**, 61

220. Ramirez, V. D. and McCann, S. M. (1964). Thioglycollate-stable luteinising hormone

and corticotrophin-releasing factors in beef hypothalamic extract. *Amer. J. Physiol.*, **207**, 441

221. Burgus, R. and Guillemin, R. (1970). Hypothalamic releasing factors. *Ann. Rev. Biochem.*, **39**, 499
222. Dhariwal, A. P. S., Antines-Rodrigues, J., Krulich, L. and McCann, S. M. (1966). Separation of growth hormone-releasing factor (GHRF) from corticotrophin-releasing factor (CRF). *Neuroendocrinology*, **1**, 341
223. Schally, A. V., Lipscomb, H. S., Long, J. M., Dear, W. E. and Guillemin, R. (1962). Chromatography and hormonal activities of dog hypothalamus. *Endocrinology*, **70**, 478
224. Celis, M. E. and Taleisnik, S. (1971). *Int. J. Neuroscience*, **1**, 223
225. Celis, M. E., Taleisnik, S., Schwartz, L. L. and Walter, R. (1971). Proposed structure of melanocyte-stimulating hormone-release-inhibiting factor. *Biophys. J.* (*Abstracts*), **11**, 98a
226. Celis, M. E., Taleisnik, S. and Walter, R. (1971). Regulation of formation and proposed structure of the factor inhibiting the release of melanocyte-stimulating hormone. *Proc. Nat. Acad. Sci. USA*, **68**, 1428
227. Nair, R. M. G., Kastin, A. J. and Schally, A. V. (1971). Isolation and structure of hypothalamic MSH release-inhibiting hormone. *Biochem. Biophys. Res. Commun.*, **43**, 1376
228. Bower, A., Hadley, M. E. and Hruby, V. J. (1971). Comparative MSH release-inhibiting activities of tocinoic acid (the ring of ocytocin) and L-PRO-L-LEU-GLY-NH$_2$ (the side chain of oxytocin). *Biochem. Biophys. Res. Commun,*, **45**, 1185
229. Celis, M. E., Taleisnik, S. and Walter, R. (1971). Release of pituitary melanocyte-stimulating hormone by the oxytocin fragment H-Cys-TYR-ILE-GLN-ASN-OH. *Biochem. Biophys. Res. Commun.*, **45**, 564
230. Kastin, A. J., Viosca, S., Nair, R. M. G., Schally, A. V. and Miller, M. E. (1972). Interactions between pineal, hypothalamus and pituitary involving melatonin MSH release-inhibiting factor and MSH. *Endocrinology*, **91**, 1323
231. Orias, R. and McCann, S. M. (1972). Natriuresis induced by.alpha and beta melanocyte stimulating hormone (MSH) in rats. *Endocrinology*, **90**, 700
232. Sachs, H., Fawcett, C. P., Takabatake, Y. and Portanova, R. (1969). Biosynthesis and release of vasopressin and neurophysin. *Recent Progr. Horm. Res.*, Vol. 25, 447 (E. B. Astwood, editor) (New York: Academic)
233. Tuppy, H. (1968). The influence of enzymes on neurohypophysial hormones and similar peptides. *Handb. Exp. Pharmacol.*, Vol. 23, 67 (B. Berde, editor) (Berlin: Springer-Verlag)
234. Koida, M., Glass, J. D., Schwartz, I. L. and Walter, R. (1970). Mechanism of inactivation of oxytocin by rat kidney enzymes. *Endocrinology*, **88**, 633
235. Hooper, K. E. (1966). Some observations on the behaviour of hypothalamic enzymes during the time of blastocyst implantation in the rabbit. *Biochem. J.*, **99**, 128
236. Hooper, K. E. (1967). The metabolism of oxytocin during lactation in the rabbit. *Biochem. J.*, **100**, 823
237. Celis, M. and Taleisnik, S. (1971). *In vitro* formation of a MSH-releasing agent by hypothalamic extracts. *Experientia*, **27**, 1481
238. Frith, D. A. and Hooper, K. C. (1972). The action of progestational agents on oxytocinase activity in the female rabbit hypothalamus. *Acta Endocrinol.*, **10**, 429
239. Dhariwal, A. P. S., Krulich, L., Katz, S. and McCann, S. M. (1965). Purification of growth hormone-releasing factor (GH-RF). *Endocrinology*, **77**, 932
240. Schally, A. V., Baba, Y., Nair, R. M. G. and Bennet, C. D. (1971). The amino acid sequence of a peptide with growth hormone-releasing activity isolated from porcine hypothalamus. *J. Biol. Chem.*, **246**, 6647
241. Veber, D. F., Bennett, C. D., Milkowski, J. D., Gal, G., Denkewalter, R. G. and Hirschmann, R. (1971). Synthesis of a proposed growth hormone releasing factor. *Biochem. Biophys. Res. Commun.*, **45**, 235
242. Schally, A. V., Arimura, A., Wakabayashi, I., Redding, T. W., Dickerman, E. and Meites, J. (1972). Biological activity of a synthetic decapeptide corresponding to the proposed growth hormone-releasing hormone. *Experientia*, **28**, 205
243. Muller, E. E., Schally, A. V. and Cocehi, D. (1971). Increase in plasma growth hormone (GH)-like activity after administration of porcine GH-releasing hormone. *Proc. Soc. Exp. Biol. Med.*, **137**, 489

244. Sandow, J., Arimura, A. and Schally, A. V. (1972). Stimulation of growth hormone release by anterior pituitary perfusion in the rat. *Endocrinology*, **90**, 1315

245. Brazeau, P., Vale, W., Burgus, R., Ling, N., Butcher, M., Rivier, J. and Guillemin, R. (1973). Hypothalamic polypeptide that inhibits the secretion of immunoreactive pituitary growth hormone. *Science*, **179**, 77

246. Bøler, J., Enzmann, F., Folkers, K., Bowers, C. Y. and Schally, A. V. (1969). The identity of chemical and hormonal properties of the thyrotopin releasing hormone and pytoglutamyl-histidyl-proline amide. *Biochem. Biophys. Res. Commun.*, **37**, 705

247. Burgus, R., Dunn, T. F., Desiderio, D. and Guillemin, R. (1969). Structure moléculaire du facteur hypothalamique hypophysiotrope TRF d'origine ovine: mise en évidence por spectrométrie de masse de la séquence PCA-His-Pro-NH₂. *C.R. Acad. Sci. Paris*, **269**, 1870

248. Schally, A. V., Arimura, A., Bowers, C. Y., Kastin, A. J., Sawano, S. and Redding, T. W. (1968). Hypothalamic neurohormones regulating anterior pituitary function. *Recent Prog. Horm. Res.*, Vol. 24, 497 (E. B. Astwood, editor) (New York: Academic)

249. Burgus, R., Dunn, R. F., Ward, D. N., Vale, W., Amoss, M. and Guillemin, R. (1969). Dérivés polypeptideques de synthese doués d'activité hypophysiotrope. *C.R. Acad. Sci. Paris*, **268**, 2116

250. Burgus, R., Dunn, T. F., Desiderio, D., Vale, W. and Guillemin, R. (1969). Derives polypeptidiques de synthese doués d'activité hypophysiotrope TRF. Nouvelles observations. *C.R. Acad. Sci. Paris*, **269**, 226

251. Bowers, C. Y., Weil, A., Chang, J. K., Sievertsson, H. Enzmann and Folkers, K. (1970). Activity-structure relationships of the thyrotropin releasing hormone. *Biochem. Biophys. Res. Commun.*, **40**, 683

252. Vale, W., Rivier, J. and Burgus, R. (1971). Synthetic TRF (thyrotropin releasing factor) analogues: II. pGlu-N-^{3im}Me-His-Pro-NH₂: A synthetic analogue with specific activity greater than that of TRF. *Endocrinology*, **89**, 1485

253. Redding, T. W. and Schally, A. V. (1971). The distribution of radioactivity following the administration of labelled thyrotropin-releasing hormone (TRH) in rats and mice. *Endocrinology*, **89**, 875

254. Redding, T. W. and Schally, A. V. (1972). On the half life of thyrotropin releasing hormone in rats. *Neuroendocrinology*, **9**, 250

255. Nair, R. M. G., Redding, T. W. and Schally, A. V. (1971). Site of inactivation of thyrotropin-releasing hormone by human plasma. *Biochemistry*, **10**, 3621

256. Matsuo, H., Baba, Y., Nair, R. M. G., Arimura, A. and Schally, A. V. (1971). Structure of the porcine LH- and FSH-releasing hormone. I. The proposed amino acid sequence. *Biochem. Biophys. Res. Commun.*, **43**, 1334

257. Burgus, R., Butcher, M., Amoss, M., Ling, N., Monahan, M., Rivier, J., Fellows, R., Blackwell, R., Vale, W. and Guillemin, R. (1972). Primary structure of the ovine hypothalamic luteinising hormone-releasing factor (LRF) *Proc. Nat. Acad. Sci.*, **69**, 278

258. Arimura, A., Debeljuk, L. and Schally, A. V. (1972). Stimulation of FSH release *in vivo* by prolonged infusion of synthetic LH-RH. *Endocrinology*, **91**, 529

259. Grant, G. and Vale, W. (1972). Speculations on structural relationships between the hypothalamic releasing factors of pituitary hormones. *Nature New Biol.*, **237**, 182

260. Monahan, M., Rivier, J., Vale, W., Guillemin, R. and Burgus, R. (1972). [Gly²] LRF and des-His²-LRF. The synthesis, purification and characterisation of two LRF analogues antagonistic to LRF. *Biochem. Biophys. Res. Commun.*, **47**, 551

261. Fugino, M., Kobayashi, S., Obayashi, M., Shiuagawa, S., Fukada, T., Kitada, C., Nakayama, R. and Yamazaki, I. (1972). Structure–activity relationships in the C-terminal part of luteinising hormone releasing hormone (LH-RH) *Biochem. Biophys. Res. Commun.*, **49**, 863

262. Chang, J. K., Sieventsson, H., Bogentoft, C., Currie, B. L., Folkers, K. and Bowers, E. Y. (1971). Discovery of a new synthetic tetrapeptide having luteinising releasing hormone (LRH) activity. *Biochem. Biophysl Res. Commun.*, **44**, 409

263. Schally, A. V., Arimura, A., Carter, W. H., Redding, T. W., Geiger, R., Konig, W., Wissman, H., Gaeger, G., Sandow, J., Yanihara, W., Yanihara, E., Hashimoto, T. and Sakagani, M. (1972). Luteinising hormone-releasing hormone (LH-RH) activity of some synthetic polypeptides. I. Fragments shorter than decapeptide. *Biochem. Biophys. Res. Commun.*, **48**, 366

264. Guillemin, R., Amoss, M., Blackwell, R., Rivier, J., Ling, N. and Vale, W. (1972). On the biological activities of the synthetic tetrapeptide pyroglutamyl-tyrosylarginyl-tryptophenyl-amide. *Biochem. Biophys. Res. Commun.*, **48**, 1093

265. Amoss, M., Rivier, J. and Guillemin, R. (1972). Release of gonadotropins by oral administration of synthetic LRF or a tripeptide fragment of LRF. *J. Clin. Endocrin. Metab.*, **35**, 16

266. Schally, A. V., Arimura, A., Kastin, A. J., Matsuo, H., Baba, R., Redding, T. W., Nair, R. M. G. and Debeljuk, L. (1971). Gonadotropin-releasing hormone: one polypeptide regulates secretion of luteinising and follicle stimulating hormones. *Science*, **173**, 1036

267. Schally, A. V., Redding, T. W., Matsuo, H. and Arimura, A. (1972). Stimulation of FSH and LH release *in vitro* by natural and synthetic LH and FSH-releasing hormone. *Endocrinology*, **90**, 156

268. Vale, W., Grant, G., Amoss, M., Blackwell, R. and Guillemin, R. (1972). Culture of enzymatically dispersed anterior pituitary cells: functional validation of a method. *Endocrinology*, **91**, 562

269. Moschetto, Y., Leonardelli, J. and Barry, J. (1971). Composition en acides aminés de l'hormone hypothalamique contrôlant la sécrétion de LH-ICSH chez le Cobaye. Noveau protocole de fractionnement rapide et non contaminant, par MM. *C.R. Acad. Sci. Paris*, **272**, 1902

270. Jackson, G. L. (1971). Partial purification and characterisation of chicken and rat follicle stimulating hormone-releasing factors. *Endocrinologh*, **91**, 1090

271. Geiger, R., Konig, W., Wissman, H., Geissen, K., Enzman, F. (1972). Synthesis and characterisation of a decapeptide having LH-RH/FSH-RH activity. *Biochem. Biophys. Res. Commun.*, **45**, 767

272. Shin, S. and Fawcett, C. P. (1971). Biochemical properties of LRF and FRF. *Program of the 53rd Endocrine Society Meeting*, ♯56

273. Schwartz, N. B. and McCormack, C. E. (1972). Reproduction: gonadal function and its regulation. *Ann. Rev. Physiol.*, Vol. 34, 425 (J. H. Comroe, Jr., editor) (Palo Alto: Annual Review Inc.)

274. Ishii, S. (1970). Association of luteinising hormone-releasing factor with granules separated from equine hypophysial stalk. *Endocrinology*, **86**, 207

275. Fink, G., Smith, G. C. and Tibballs, J. (1972). LRF and CRF release in subcellular fractions of bovine median eminence. *Nature New Biol.*, **239**, 57

276. Mitnick, M. and Reichlin, S. (1972). Enzymatic synthesis of thyrotropin-releasing hormone (TRH) by hypothalamic TRH synthetase. *Endocrinology*, **91**, 1145

277. Johansson, K. N. G., Hooper, F., Sieventson, H., Currie, B. L. and Folkers, K. (1972). Biosynthesis *in vitro* of the luteinising releasing hormone by hypothalamic tissue. *Biochem. Biophys. Res. Commun.*, **49**, 656

278. Johansson, K. N. G., Currie, B. L., Folkers, K. and Bowers, C. Y. (1973). Biosynthesis and evidence of the existence of the follicle stimulating hormone releasing hormone. *Biochem. Res. Commun.*, **50**, 8

279. Johansson, K. N. G., Currie, B. L., Folkers, K. and Bowers, C. Y. (1973). On the chemical existence and partial purification of the hypothalamic follicle stimulating hormone-releasing hormone. *Biochem. Biophys. Res. Commun.*, **50**, 14

280. Johansson, K. N. G., Currie, B. L., Folkers, K. and Bowers, C. Y. (1973). Biological evidence that separate hypothalamic hormones release the follicle stimulating and luteinising hormones. *Biochem. Biophys. Res., Commun.*, **50**, 20

281. Fawcett, C. P. (1972). Discussion of paper ♯24. *Serono Foundation Conference, Acapulco, Mexico.* (in the press). (E. Rosemberg, editor) (Amsterdam: Excerpta Medica)

282. Valverde-R., C., Chieffo, V. and Reichlin, S. (1972). Prolactin-releasing factor in porcine and rat hypothalamic tissue. *Endocrinology*, **91**, 982

3
Regulation of the Pituitary–Thyroid Axis

J. B. MARTIN
Montreal General Hospital and McGill University, Montreal

3.1   INTRODUCTION

Of hormone regulatory systems, that of the pituitary-thyroid axis has received the most penetrating analysis. First elaborated as a negative feedback self-regulatory system by Hoskins in 1949[1], it has become possible in recent years to formulate a rather precise description of the various interactions which occur to achieve this regulation because each component of the system has now been characterised. Of particular importance in this regard has been (a) the development of methodology permitting more detailed quantitation of interactions at each level of the system and (b) the discovery of the structure and the subsequent synthesis of the hypothalamic hypophysiotropic substance, thyrotropin releasing hormone (TRH)*.

In the present review, certain selected areas of pituitary–thyroid regulation, which have been the subject of substantial advances in the last few years have been chosen for preferential consideration. A strong bias has been taken toward a conceptualisation of the neural and feed-back interactions which are important in the control of this system. In particular, priority has been given to (a) the neural regulatory mechanisms for TSH secretion; (b) a consideration of TRH—its structure, biosynthesis and mechanisms of action; (c) an analysis of feed-back control mechanisms including TRH-thyroid hormone interactions at both the pituitary and hypothalamic level; (d) mechanisms of TSH action on the thyroid and the interactions of this control with that of the sympathetic nervous system and monoamines; and (e) a consideration of the role of T_3 in the metabolic actions of the thyroid hormones.

A number of excellent reviews on various aspects of pituitary–thyroid regulation have appeared in the past decade. These include detailed accounts of the control of TSH secretion[2-7], the mechanisms of TSH action[8-11], and the role of T_3 in the metabolic action of the thyroid hormones (TH)[12].

3.2   THE HYPOTHALAMIC–PITUITARY–THYROID AXIS

The regulation of thyroid hormone (TH) secretion by the thyroid gland is achieved by the interaction of three groups of hormones (see Figure 3.1).

* The terms thyrotropin releasing hormone (TRH) and thyrotropin-releasing factor (TRF) are used interchangeably in the present review.

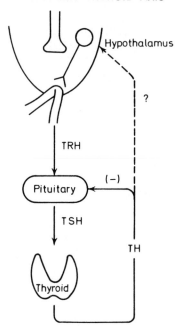

Figure 3.1 The hypothalamic–
pituitary–thyroid axis

Thyrotropin-releasing hormone (TRH) stimulates the release (and probably synthesis) of thyrotropin-stimulating hormone (TSH) by the pituitary thyrotrope. TSH, in turn, activates iodide uptake, hormonogenesis and release of the thyroid hormones thyroxine (T_4) and tri-iodothyronine (T_3). Circulating TH has important feed-back effects upon the pituitary (and possibly also the hypothalamus) to regulate further secretion of TSH and TRH. The interaction of the negative feed-back effects of TH on the pituitary with the stimulatory effects of TRH appears to be the primary determining factor in regulation of TSH secretion. Thus, pituitary TSH secretion is regulated by the interactions of two components, a neural component mediated by a neurohormone and a feed-back component mediated by circulating levels of plasma TH.

3.3 NEURAL REGULATION OF TSH SECRETION

3.3.1 Hypothalamic control of TSH secretion

The importance of intact hypothalamic–pituitary relationships for the maintenance of basal pituitary–thyroid function has been documented by a number of experimental manipulations. Anatomical disconnection of the pituitary from the hypothalamus (by either stalk section or transplantation) decreases basal pituitary TSH secretion resulting in a hypothyroid state (see Ref. 2 for a review). These studies imply a tonic drive by the hypothalamus which is necessary for the maintenance of basal TSH secretion.

The hypothalamic deafferentation experiments of Halasz et al.[13] indicate that near normal basal TSH secretion occurs in rats with hypothalamic islands in which the entire medial basal (hypophysiotropic area) of the hypothalamus remains in contact with the pituitary. Such lesions caused only a small decrease in plasma PBI levels and ^{131}I uptake. Knigge and his co-workers[14, 15] reported that even smaller conical hypothalamic islands containing only the ventromedial and arcuate nuclei attached to the pituitary stalk were also capable of maintaining normal thyroid size and radioiodide uptake in the rat[14] and the cat[15]. These studies suggest that hypothalamic-pituitary islands can maintain basal pituitary-thyroid functional capacity.

3.3.1.1 Effects of hypothalamic lesions

There is extensive evidence (see Ref. 2 for a review) to indicate that lesions placed in the vicinity of the paraventricular nuclei result in a decrease in pituitary–thyroid function without any definite direct effects on other pituitary tropic hormones. Anterior hypothalamic lesions in the paraventricular region cause a reduction in plasma PBI levels and a fall in both plasma and pituitary TSH levels[16, 17]. In one study of the effects of such lesions on feedback regulation of TSH secretion, it was shown that lesions resulted in a fall in plasma PBI from 3.0 ± 1.0 to 1.7 ± 0.2 μg $(100 \text{ ml})^{-1}$ and plasma TSH levels, as measured by radioimmunoassay, became undetectable[17]. Pituitary TSH levels were reduced to one-third of control levels. Although TSH levels were undetectable in the plasma of hypothalamic-lesioned rats, such animals were capable of increased TSH secretion following a further reduction in plasma TH after thyroidectomy. Hypothalamic-lesioned rats were also shown to be more sensitive than intact controls to the feedback effects of small doses of T_4. These studies were interpreted to indicate that anterior hypothalamic lesions lower basal TSH secretion and modify, but do not prevent, qualitatively normal secretory responses to alterations in plasma TH levels. The hypothalamus thus acts to determine the sensitivity of the pituitary to feed-back inhibition, presumably by reducing the quantity of TRH which reaches the pituitary. Additional evidence for the importance of an anterior hypothalamic region in TSH control has been provided by the segmental deafferentation experiments of Halasz et al.[13]. These investigators observed that a coronal section through the mid-hypothalamus anterior to the arcuate nucleus and posterior to the paraventricular nuclei caused a marked decrease in plasma PBI levels from 4.0 ± 0.2 to 1.6 ± 0.2 μg $(100 \text{ ml})^{-1}$.

Although the exact locality of the TRH-producing neurones has not been demonstrated, it seems likely that TRH-synthesising cells are distributed widely within the medial basal hypothalamus in the rat. TRH, as measured by bioassay, is reported to be detectable in hypothalamic fragments obtained from the entire hypophysiotropic area[18] which, as originally defined by Halasz[13], extends from the anterior hypothalamus and paraventricular region anteriorly to the mammillary bodies posteriorly. Moreover, hypothalamic tissue from a similar distribution is capable of in vitro synthesis of TRH[7] (see p. 84). Anatomical[19] and electrophysiological[20] studies support the concept that tuberohypophysial neurones are indeed located over this entire region, although restricted to the medial zone which extends 1.0–1.5 mm on either side of the third ventricle.

The repeated observations of the importance of the paraventricular area in thyroid regulation suggest that either there is an accumulation of TRH containing neurones in this region or that a functional 'centre' exists which secondarily connects with large numbers of releasing factor neurones. Martini et al.[21] attempted to answer this question by determining the residual content of hypothalamic TRH after the placement of small hypothalamic lesions. They found that lesions localised to either the suprachiasmatic, paraventricular or arcuate–ventromedial regions resulted in comparable decreases in TRH content as determined by a pituitary-depletion bioassay. These results did not indicate any regional disparities in TRH content. Flament-Durand[22], using electron microscopic and autoradiographic techniques, observed that the small neurones of the paraventricular nuclei (which comprise ca. 25% of the total population of this nuclear group) contain granules of a different size and morphology than those implicated as storage sites for oxytocin and suggested that these cells may produce TRF.

3.3.1.2 Effects of electrical stimulation

Over the years, several attempts have been made to define the hypophysio-tropic region of the hypothalamus by utilising electrical stimulation techniques. Prior to development of radioimmunoassay methods most of such studies used evidence of thyroid activation as a parameter of TSH release, although a few reports appeared in which TSH was measured by bioassay. Elevated levels of TSH have now been reported following electrical stimulation in the rat[23-25], dog[26] and rabbit[27]. In stimulation studies in the rat[24, 25], radioimmunoassayable plasma TSH levels rose rapidly (in pentobarbital-anaesthetised rats) after hypothalamic stimulation, whereas in sham-stimulated animals, plasma TSH levels fell during the period of observation. The area from which positive responses were obtained was extensive, including the anterior hypothalamus and preoptic area, the paraventricular nuclei and the dorsomedial, ventromedial and arcuate nuclei (Figure 3.2). A similar distribution of effective stimulation sites for TSH release was found by Averill and Salaman[27] in the rabbit using a TSH bioassay. Interestingly, the largest responses in the rat occurred with stimulation of the anterior hypothalamus in the vicinity of the paraventricular nuclei[25]. Negative responses occurred with stimulation of the lateral hypothalamus, thalamus and mammillary bodies.

As the currents used in these experiments were large, the possibility was considered that the localities were non-specific. Arguing against this fact was the observation that parallel studies of plasma GH levels in the same rats indicated that GH responses were strictly limited to the ventromedial and arcuate regions[28]. These results would seem to be of valid localising value since bioassay determinations of releasing factor concentrations have shown that TRH is present in a distribution similar to that defined by electrical stimulation, whereas GRF is restricted to the ventromedial nucleus[29].

The time course of electrically-induced TSH release in the rat was compared with that which followed intravenous administration of synthetic TRH[24, 25]. In each case, plasma TSH levels were significantly elevated within 5 min; the electrically-induced response was slightly more sustained probably because stimulation was continued for 5–10 min, whereas TRF was administered in

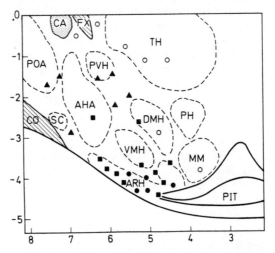

Figure 3.2 Anatomical localisation of electrical stimulation points in 30 animals. Positive responses (solid symbols) extend over an area which corresponds closely to the 'hypophysiotropic' area. Largest responses occurred in two animals stimulated in the paraventricular nucleus (PVH). Negative responses are indicated by open circles

Abbreviations: CA = anterior commissure; FX = fornix; POA = preoptic area; PVH = paraventricular nucleus; TH = thalamus; AHA = anterior hypothalamic area; SC = suprachiasmatic nucleus; CO = optic chiasm; DMH = dorsomedial hypothalamic nucleus; PH = posterior hypothalamus; VMH = ventromedial hypothalamic nucleus; ARH = arcuate nucleus; MM = mammillary body; PIT = pituitary. The numbers indicate deGroot coordinates. (From Martin and Reichlin[25], by courtesy of *Endocrinology*)

a single injection. Although the effects of incremental doses of TH on electrically-induced TSH release were not examined, it was found that T_4 in a dose of 50 µg (100 g)$^{-1}$ body weight administered 2 h before the experiment was effective in blocking TSH release to both electrical stimulation and synthetic TRH[25]. As will be considered below, it is likely that this effect was due to a blockade of the TRH effect at the pituitary level.

The similarity of the time course of TSH release following electrical stimulation and TRH administration and its prevention by T_4 pretreatment suggests that hypothalamic electrical stimulation is effective by causing release of stored TRH. Wilber and Porter[30] have reported that bioassayable

TRH activity appears in the portal blood after electrical stimulation of the anterior hypothalamus. Prior T_4 administration had no effect on this response.

3.3.1.3 Hypothalamic inhibition of TSH secretion

The observation that certain stimuli, such as stress, cause a rapid reduction in plasma TSH levels raises the question of whether such an effect is mediated by suppression of tonic TRH secretion or by release of a specific thyrotropin-inhibiting factor (TIF). Attempts to purify hypothalamic extracts for releasing factor activity have not produced any conclusive evidence in the mammal, of a dual regulatory system for TSH control such as exists for prolactin and growth hormone (see Chapter 2). It has been suggested that stress-induced TSH suppression is in part due to inhibitory feed-back effects of adrenal cortical hormones (see p. 78) although detailed time course studies to prove this fact are still lacking. Lomax and associates[31] have studied the effects of morphine-induced TSH suppression in the rat. Both systemic administration and local intrahypothalamic injection of morphine were shown to depress the release of radioiodine from the thyroid gland of rats. Effective hypothalamic sites for such inhibition included the suprachiasmatic region and supramammillary and posterior hypothalamic regions within 1 mm of the midline. The latter placements were similar in location to the sites which were found to be effective in blocking the inhibitory effects of systemically-administered morphine. The possibility that the posterior hypothalamus contains an inhibitory regulatory region for thyroid control was also suggested by the electrical stimulation studies of Vertes et al.[32]. It is possible that such lesions block inputs from inhibitory regions such as the brain stem or habenula (see p. 74).

Evidence derived from experiments in the goldfish have indicated that hypothalamic inhibition of TSH secretion is the primary regulatory mechanism in this species. Stalk section in the goldfish causes increased TSH secretion and pituitaries from this species incubated in vitro show increased secretory activity resembling that observed in prolactin producing cells of the mammalian pituitary explant[33, 34]. Peter[34] has postulated that the hypothalamic inhibition is mediated by a TIF although to date there has been no elaboration of its chemical or physical properties. These phylogenetic differences in TSH control are of interest because they may provide insights into the potential inter-relationships between TSH and prolactin regulation in the mammal.

3.3.1.4 Summary

In summary, it appears that basal TSH secretion is dependent upon the tonic release of TRH by the hypothalamus. A disturbance in this relationship by hypothalamic–pituitary disconnection, intrahypothalamic deafferentation or by focal hypothalamic lesions results in pituitary TSH deficiency and subsequent hypothyroidism. This relationship appears to hold true in man as well. Secondary hypopituitarism due to TRH deficiency has now been documented to be the underlying disturbance in many cases of idiopathic hypopituitarism[6, 35]. The severity of the hypothyroidism in such cases, often resulting in virtually unmeasurable plasma thyroid hormone levels, argues strongly that TRH secretion in man is also required for maintenance of basal pituitary–thyroid function. On the other hand, acute increases in plasma TSH levels can be induced by hypothalamic electrical stimulation, with a time course similar to that which occurs after TRH administration or acute cold exposure (see p. 80).

3.3.2   Extrahypothalmic control of TSH secretion

Considering the number of observations which have been made concerning the role of extrahypothalamic structures in ACTH and gonadotropin regulation, it is somewhat surprising that so little information is available with respect to the function of these structures in TSH control. Although the medial basal hypothalamus appears capable of maintaining basal TSH secretion, phasic release of TSH, such as occurs in diurnal or circadian rhythms, stress-induced inhibition or cold-induced release are probably mediated via extrahypothalamic structures and inputs. These particular responses will be considered in detail later. In this section, evidence suggesting a role of extrahypothalamic structures in TSH secretion will be considered.

3.3.2.1   *Habenula and pineal*

Of extrahypothalamic structures, the function of the habenula in thyroid control has received the most attention, particularly by Szentagothai and colleagues[36]. Based on the effects of habenular lesions on thyroid responses to cold exposure (utilising a TSH bioassay in which TSH effects were assessed by changes in karyometrics of thyroid follicle cells), these workers postulated that the habenula functions in an indirect and primarily inhibitory manner, outside the primary TH feed-back loop, to integrate neural homeostatic responses with hormonal needs. They proposed that these effects are mediated via the anterior hypothalamic thyrotropic area since lesions of this region of the hypothalamus blocked supranormal thyroid responses which occurred in habenular-lesioned rats. Unfortunately, these observations were based upon disputable bioassay determinations of TSH and do not entirely exclude the possibility of non-TSH mediated effects. Earlier reports also implicated inhibitory effects of the habenula in thyroid control but there have been no recent reports to either confirm or deny the relevance of these observations. It is of interest that the major efferent pathway from the habenula is the fasciculus retroflexus which terminates in the medial mesencephalic region (interpeduncular nucleus), an area which forms part of the midbrain limbic system as defined by Nauta[37], and which has important relays to the hypothalamus via the medial forebrain bundle. Thus, significant anatomical inputs do exist to connect the habenula with the hypothalamus.

   Of equal uncertainty is the role of the pineal in TSH and thyroid control. Observations which have employed various parameters of thyroid secretion have suggested a pineal influence, predominantly inhibitory, and perhaps mediated by melatonin[38, 39]. Thus melatonin decreases thyroid weight and ^{131}I uptake and causes a reduction in thyroid secretory rate. On the other hand, pinealectomy is reported to cause thyroid hyperactivity in the tadpole[40] and an enhanced thyroid secretory rate in the rat[41]. The question as to whether these effects are mediated by changes in TSH secretion has been recently examined. Rowe et al.[42] found no differences in plasma TSH levels, as measured by radioimmunoassay, 27–28 days after pinealectomy. Relkin[43], however, has recently shown that pinealectomy in 21-day-old rats results in a transient period of increased TSH secretion which is detectable on the 4th but not the 8th day after pinealectomy. The mechanism of this transient elevation in TSH levels has not been demonstrated but it would appear to be of minimal physiological significance.

3.3.2.2 Extrapyramidal and limbic structures

In 1962, Lupulescu and his co-workers[44] reported that bilateral lesions of the globus pallidus and septal area cause increased thyroid activity as indicated by increased thyroid weight, ^{131}I uptake and enhanced goitrogenic response to propylthiouracil. Cheifetz[45] recently confirmed this finding and suggested that tonic inhibitory influences may arise from extrapyramidal structures.

The role of the 'limbic system' in TSH control has not been adequately defined. Shizumi et al.[46] reported that electrical stimulation of the hippo-campal formation in thiopental-anaesthetised dogs caused thyroid activation and increased TSH blood levels (within 30 min) as measured by the McKenzie bioassay. Stimulation of the orbital frontal cortex or the amygdaloid nuclear complex did not result in a significant change in thyroid secretion. Eleftheriou and Zolovick[47] found that corticomedial amygdaloid lesions in the deermouse caused thyroid atrophy and increased bioassayable TSH levels in the pituitary and decreased levels in plasma. These effects, which were interpreted to indicate a decrease in TSH secretion, persisted for as long as 16 days. Kovacs et al.[48] failed to detect changes in thyroid activity in rats with amygdaloid lesions, but reported that low frequency stimulation (15 Hz) produced an elevation in ^{131}I uptake.

The hippocampus has also been implicated in inhibition of ACTH. Because of the reciprocal effects of stress on ACTH and TSH (causing release of the former and inhibition of the latter), Dupont et al.[49] assessed the effects of hippocampal stimulation on TSH and ACTH responses to simultaneous cold exposure and mild psychic stress. Their observations are interesting. Control rats exposed to cold showed an increase in both plasma cortico-sterone and TSH levels (McKenzie bioassay). The presence of an observer in the room during exposure to cold caused an enhanced corticosterone response but prevented TSH release. Stimulation of the hippocampus in unanaesthetised rats was shown to inhibit corticosterone responses and to reinstate the TSH response to cold. It was concluded from these experiments that hippocampal activation may induce these reciprocal responses, causing inhibition of ACTH secretion and activation of TSH release.

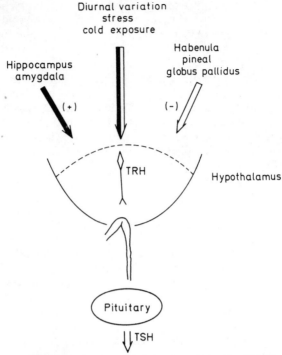

Figure 3.3 Diagrammatic representation of extrahypo-thalamic regions implicated in TSH control. These regions may contribute to phasic changes in TSH secretion such as those associated with diurnal rhythms, stress or cold exposure

In summary, it is evident at this point that data on the role of extrahypo-thalamic structures in TSH control are fragmentary and inconclusive (Figure 3.3). It is interesting that both inhibitory and excitatory inputs have been suggested. However, until the precise role of these structures in pituitary-thyroid control has been more adequately defined and until it has been clearly shown that none of the effects are secondary to changes in adrenal or other hormonal alterations, definitive conclusions concerning the role of these structures must remain tentative.

3.3.3 Mechanisms of phasic TSH secretion

The pituitary–thyroid axis has been traditionally viewed as a sluggishly reactive, steady-state system which is not readily responsive to acute perturb-ations. This concept has been derived in part from observations of the pro-gressive increase in time course of the metabolic effects induced by each successive component of the system. TRH-induced release of TSH occurs rapidly and is of short duration. The effects of TSH on the thyroid are more prolonged, leading to an early preferential release of T_3, with the total effects on thyroid secretion lasting for several hours. The biological half-life and metabolic actions of TH, in particular T_4, extend over several days. The kinetics of such a system thus has the effect of smoothing out over a prolonged period of time any acute perturbation of the neural regulatory component.

Despite this characteristic, it is now known that small acute changes in TRH or T_3 and T_4 feed-back do influence TSH secretion very rapidly, and such influences appear to comprise a significant component of the factors which regulate the system. It appears justified, therefore, to examine the factors which cause abrupt or acute changes in TSH levels, effects which may be broadly referred to as phasic changes in TSH secretion.

3.3.3.1 Diurnal variation in TSH secretion

The factors which determine circadian variation in plasma hormone levels and the association of hormone release with wake and sleep cycles are of considerable current interest in neuroendocrine research. The question of whether a diurnal variation occurs with respect to TSH levels remains controversial. Circadian plasma TSH variations in the rat have been reported and, in general, seem to indicate a small variation which is opposite in phase to that of corticosterone[50-52]. Studies of this question in man have been inconclusive and conflicting, in a large part due to the lack of sufficiently sensitive and precise radioimmunoassay methods to document the relatively small changes which occur[6]. Nicoloff and his associates showed that diurnal variations in serum TSH could be demonstrated in man, as indicated both by changes in thyroid iodine release[53] and by direct measurement of serum TSH by radioimmunoassay[54]. It was their conclusion that TSH diurnal rhythm was inverse to, and probably affected by, the ACTH–cortisol rhythm. Most other observers have failed to note any significant variation in TSH levels in man as studied during a 24 h period[6, 55, 56]. An exception to this is a recent preliminary report by Vanhaelst et al.[57] in which both a circadian TSH rhythm (characterised by an increased level of TSH during the latter part of the sleep cycle) and an episodic (phasic) release of TSH was described in eight subjects. Episodic TSH release (with a periodicity of 1–3 h) occurred throughout the day and night. This observation, if confirmed, will add TSH secretion to a growing list of anterior pituitary trophic hormones which appear to be secreted in a pulsatile manner. Vanhaelst et al.[57] concluded that the plasma TSH rise during the latter part of sleep coincides with the ACTH–cortisol increase and is not, therefore, likely to be due to an inhibitory effect of adrenal steroids on TSH secretion. The mechanism of this nocturnal rise is not clear at present. Lemarchand-Beraud and Vannotti[55] have reported that circadian variations of blood T_3 and T_4 levels can be demonstrated in man with a nadir at 4 a.m. Vanhaelst and his co-workers[57] postulate that the increased TSH levels in the plasma during this period of the night may be secondary to decreased negative feed-back effects of TH. On the other hand, this period of the sleep–wake cycle has also been shown to be characterised by pulsatile cortisol secretion and it is conceivable that the TSH episodes are entrained to similar neural stimuli as those inducing ACTH–cortisol release. Alternatively, secretory bursts of cortisol may have acute negative feed-back effects on TSH secretion. A critical analysis of this problem will necessitate concomitant measurement of T_4, T_3, TSH and cortisol levels at sufficiently frequent intervals to indicate whether there is a precise inter-relationship between these hormones. A recent report that prolactin release also occurs during this period of sleep[58] is of interest since TRH is reported to stimulate both TSH and prolactin release. The physiological significance of such diurnal rhythms and of episodic release of anterior pituitary hormones, in general, remains to be elucidated.

3.3.3.2 Effects of stress on TSH secretion

There have been numerous investigations of the effects of psychic or physical stress on pituitary–thyroid function. In general, these studies have indicated that TSH secretion is inhibited by stress in several species, including the rabbit, rat, guinea-pig and man (see Refs. 59 and 60 for reviews). These conclusions have been based, almost without exception, on indirect measurements of TSH release as inferred from alterations of TH secretion. A few studies have indicated abrupt increases in TH secretion after acute stress such as emotional stimuli (in the sheep)[59] or shock avoidance tests (in the Rhesus monkey)[60]. However, none of these studies entirely exclude the possibility that changes in haemoconcentration, thyroid hormone binding or thyroid gland blood flow may have been related to the alterations noted. In addition, effects secondary to the release of other hormones may have been involved in these responses.

There have been very few studies on the effects of stress in which plasma TSH levels have been measured directly. The recent studies of Fortier et al.[61] are particularly valuable in this regard. These investigators demonstrated that a number of stresses, including systemic trauma (tibial fracture), repeated electric shock and ether administration caused significant decreases in plasma TSH levels within 30 min in the rat. Similar rapid falls in bio-assayable TSH levels have also been reported following stress in the rabbit[62]. It has not been shown that stress acutely inhibits TSH in man; the stress of surgery had no effect on TSH levels in one report[63].

Since stress is associated with activation of the pituitary-adrenal axis, the question arises whether inhibition of TSH secretion which accompanies stress is: (a) a manifestation of neural inhibition of TRH secretion, (b) due to a concomitant reciprocal effect of ACTH release and TSH inhibition or (c) secondary to feed-back inhibition imposed by ACTH or adrenal steroids on hypothalamic or pituitary mechanisms for TSH control. A number of studies in both the rat and man have attempted to resolve this issue. Fortier and his co-workers[61, 64] showed that stress-induced TSH inhibition (as induced by a combination of ether anaesthetic plus intra-venous saline), caused a reduction in plasma TSH levels in the rat and a sixfold rise in plasma corticosterone. Intravenous injection of TRF (in a dose of 200 ng) instead of saline, resulted in a twofold rise in TSH levels over that of non-stressed controls, with no change in the plasma corticosterone response. ACTH suppression by dexamethasone pre-treatment in a dose sufficient to block the corticosterone rise (500 µg subcutaneously 5 h before the experiment) did not affect the TSH response to TRH[64]. These studies fail to indicate any inherent competition between TSH and ACTH secretion at the pituitary level and suggest that neuroendocrine mechanisms at a hypothalamic or extrahypothalamic level mediate these reciprocal responses. In support of this contention is the observation that stress-induced inhibition of TSH secretion is comparable in both normal and dexamethasone-treated rats[61]. From these results it was concluded that the inhibition of TSH secretion in response to stress is coincident to, rather than a consequence of, ACTH release.

The subsequent observation of Dupont *et al.*[49] that stimulation of the hippocampus in cold-exposed rats will restore the TSH response at the same time that ACTH release is inhibited suggests that extrahypothalamic regulatory mechanisms are involved in the integration and co-ordination of these complex neuroendocrine interactions. This is of interest because it has also been demonstrated that electrical stimulation of the hippocampus in the rat releases growth hormone, a hormone which is also inhibited by stress in this species[191].

Wilber and Utiger[65] have studied the effects of large doses of glucocorticoids on TSH secretion in both man and the rat. Their data indicate that TSH suppression following glucocorticoid administration in man occurs within a few hours but they did not document the early time course of this response. Intravenous administration of 100 µg dexamethasone in the rat was followed by a significant reduction in plasma TSH levels within 30 min, with a maximum effect at 1 h and a continuing effect evident as long as 4 h. Significantly, treatment with dexamethasone did not affect the rise in plasma TSH levels induced by TRF (using partially-purified TRF). From these observations it was concluded that the suppressive actions of steroids are exerted at the hypothalamic level leading to an inhibition of the secretion of TRF. The alternative possibility that glucocorticoids might accelerate degradation of TSH or increase the TSH distribution space has not been examined, but as pointed out by Wilber and Utiger, it is difficult to see how such a mechanism could explain the rapid effect or the post-treatment TSH rebound which was observed. It is also unlikely that such acute effects could result from influences on plasma thyroxine binding globulins as have been reported with longer courses of adrenal steroid therapy.

In summary, it would appear that there is more than one mechanism by which stress may result in inhibition of TSH secretion. Although detailed time-course analyses on the responses are not available, the rapidity of TSH inhibition suggests that a primary neural event, perhaps mediated by extrahypothalamic structures, is involved in the response. In addition, however, corticosteroids and other hormones may well have secondary suppressive effects at the hypothalamic level. Although hypothalamic lesions have been shown to prevent the release of TSH to cold exposure, no studies have been reported on the effects of hypothalamic or extrahypothalamic lesions on TSH inhibition. It would be of interest to examine the effects on stress-induced TSH inhibition of lesions in those areas of the brain which have been identified to possibly mediate TSH inhibition, i.e. globus pallidus or habenula (Figure 3.3).

3.3.3.3 Effects of changes in ambient temperature

One of the recognised responses of the pituitary–thyroid system is the activation of secretion which occurs during exposure to a lowered ambient
temperature. Previous reviews dealing with the regulation of TSH secretion
have considered in detail the historical data and controversies concerning
the effects of both acute and chronic cold exposure[2-4, 7, 66, 67].

Although it has been clearly demonstrated that TH is essential for survival
at lowered environmental temperatures, it has not been established whether
changes in thyroid secretion form an important homeostatic mechanism for
regulation of metabolism during cold exposure. It is appropriate, for the
purposes of a consideration of this literature, to divide pituitary–thyroid

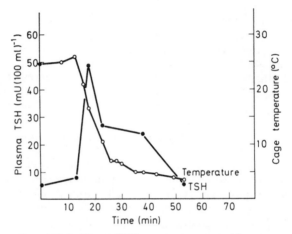

Figure 3.4   Plasma TSH response to acute cold exposure
in an unanaesthetised rat. This animal shows a marked
early TSH response with a fivefold rise less than 5 min after
onset of cold exposure. Plasma TSH returned to baseline
approximately 40 min after onset of cold. (From Reichlin
et al.[7], by courtesy of Academic Press)

responses into those which occur to acute (minutes to hours) versus chronic
(days to weeks) exposure to lowered environmental temperature.

(a) *Acute cold exposure*—There is now substantial evidence that acute
cold exposure in the rat causes a burst of TSH release which occurs sufficiently
rapidly to imply activation by a neuroendocrine reflex. Abrupt lowering of
the ambient temperature by sudden introduction of cold air into a closed
cage was shown to elicit a rise in immunoassayable plasma TSH levels
within 5–10 min in unanaesthetised rats bearing chronic indwelling jugular
cannulae (Figure 3.4)[7, 68]. This TSH surge proved to be short-lived with a
return to baseline within 40–60 min. A similar rapid increase in plasma TSH
levels, as measured by radioimmunoassay, was reported by Hershman and
Pittman[69] in rats transferred to a 2–4°C room. This time course is in agreement with that reported for bioassayable TSH levels by Itoh et al.[70] (TSH

increased at 15 min) and by Fortier *et al.*[61] (TSH increased at 30 min). The latter two groups also reported that the TSH rise was transient although the total duration of the response was somewhat longer.

Fortier *et al.*[61] have reported combined data on corticosterone, plasma T_4 and plasma and pituitary TSH responses to acute cold which are the most complete which have appeared to date. In a comprehensive analysis utilising pooled samples of blood assayed for TSH by the McKenzie bioassay, their results clearly show that in acute cold-exposed rats: (a) the rise in TSH levels is sufficient to cause a subsequent significant elevation of plasma T_4 levels; (b) neither adrenalectomy nor dexamethasone administration significantly affect the TSH response to cold; (c) thyroidectomised rats with elevated TSH levels show a further rise in TSH on exposure to cold. The rapidity of the time course and the large response in thyroidectomised rats are both consistent with the hypothesis that acute TSH release is mediated by hypothalamic discharge of TRH.

TSH responses to acute cold exposure have also been studied in man. Transient cold-induced TSH release occurs in the infant[71,72], but minimal, if any, effect has been noted in the adult[73,74].

That acute cold-exposure induced TSH release is probably triggered by peripheral cold receptors is suggested by the finding that during acute cold exposure, hypothalamic core temperature either shows no change or a slight rise[7,68]. On the other hand, TSH release can also be induced by lowering of core temperature (by ganglionic blockade) in animals kept at constant ambient temperature, indicating that either peripheral or central thermoreceptor inputs may trigger TSH secretion[7]. These observations confirm that experiments showing activation of TH secretion following hypothalamic cooling in the goat[75], rat[76] and baboon[77] are probably mediated by enhanced pituitary TSH secretion, although one recent report failed to document this effect in the rat[78].

Only one recent report has appeared on the effects of TH feed-back on cold-induced thyroid activation, in which it was reported that L-T_4 (12 µg $(100 \text{ g})^{-1}$ body wt. administered 2 h before cold exposure prevented thyroid activation as determined by an increase in plasma $[^{125}I]$PBI levels[79].

Additional evidence of thyroid secretion during acute cold exposure and a study of the central pathways involved in this response was reported by Kajihara *et al.*[80]. In these experiments, thyroid colloid droplet formation was utilised as the endpoint in assessing thyroid activation. The authors provide convincing evidence that this technique is a reliable index of thyroid activation by showing that the number of droplets formed has a log (dose) relationship to the amount of TSH administered. TRH was also effective in inducing thyroid colloid-droplet formation. Acute exposure of either rats or guinea-pigs to 5°C caused a detectable increase in droplet formation within 10 min, with a peak response at 30 min followed by a subsequent decline over the next 1.5 h. Measurement of $[^{131}I]$PBI release in guinea-pigs showed a peak increase at 4 h after cold exposure. These effects were not induced by administration of hydrocortisone, norepinephrine or epinephrine, all agents which are known to be released during acute cold exposure.

Thyroid activation to cold exposure in the guinea-pig was completely prevented by midbrain decerebration, although the thyroid was still shown to be responsive to TRH. This was interpreted to mean that peripheral cold receptors activate hypothalamic centres via ascending pathways transmitted through the brain stem. The authors did not, however, measure core temperature in decerebrate animals following cold exposure. It is possible that the dysthermoregulation induced by decerebration may have caused such a rapid fall in core temperature that TRH secretion was suppressed secondary to the severe stress. This was observed to occur in ganglionic-blocked animals exposed to 6°C[7, 68].

These results suggest that an acute neuroendocrine reflex exists for TSH release in rodents and in human infants, which is probably mediated by peripheral cold receptors and relayed to hypothalamic centres where TRH release occurs. The TSH response is as rapid as that following electrical stimulation or TRH administration and is accompanied by significant thyroid activation as evidenced by morphological changes of increased secretory activity and by increases in plasma TH levels. The significance of this response in terms of acute homeostatic defence against cold is not entirely evident, but significant increases in plasma TH induced by acute cold exposure may mediate important, but as yet undefined responses, perhaps in association with concomitant increases in catecholamine and adrenocortical secretion.

(b) *Chronic cold exposure*—There is much less certainty concerning the role of the hypothalamic–pituitary–thyroid system in homeostatic responses to prolonged cold exposure[7, 67, 81]. The bulk of experiments performed in a number of species, including man, have, in general, failed to show any change in plasma T_4 levels (total or free) during chronic cold exposure and, in fact, a fall in plasma TH levels has been noted in some studies[67]. The observation that TSH and TH secretion are increased, however, during prolonged cold exposure has been demonstrated repeatedly in the rat. This response has been largely attributed to increased utilisation, excretion and/or degradation of T_4. In this species, increased faecal excretion of T_4 secondary to enhanced food intake is an important component of the response to cold exposure. Activation of the pituitary–thyroid axis may thus not involve hypothalamic mechanisms and may be entirely secondary to a decrease in negative feedback effects on TSH secretion resulting from falling plasma TH levels.

Fortier *et al.*[61] have reported data concerning the metabolic clearance rates and secretory rates of TSH and T_4 during cold exposure. Exposure of rats to 5°C for 32 days was shown to result in no detectable change in plasma TSH levels and a 50% reduction in plasma T_4 levels. Calculations of the TSH secretory rate showed an increase in cold-exposed animals from 236 ± 25 to 452 ± 95 μU min^{-1} accompanied by an increased metabolic clearance rate. On the contrary, the secretory rate of T_4, calculated from disappearance rates of labelled T_4 from blood, showed no change. The metabolic clearance rate of T_4 was, however, increased. The authors reconstruct these data in the following manner. During cold exposure, increased TSH release is stimulated initially by hypothalamic mechanisms but this is not reflected by an elevation of plasma TSH levels because of increased metabolic clearance of TSH. During prolonged cold exposure, enhanced clearance of T_4 from the blood leads to an increased secretion of TSH which, because of its more rapid clearance from the blood, is not reflected by any absolute increase in plasma TSH levels. These data do not support the hypothesis that continued hypothalamic activation of the pituitary–thyroid axis is an important component of the response.

A variation in experimental method was employed by the author in an attempt to answer this question[7, 81]. It was reasoned that if the hypothalamus integrates autonomic and endocrine temperature homeostatic mechanisms, a deficit in autonomic mechanisms might be expected to elicit a compensatory increase in the pituitary–thyroid component. The sympathetic nervous system is known to play a major role in the process of cold adaptation[81, 82] with increased secretion of catecholamines, both from sympathetic nerve endings and from the adrenal medulla, comprising an essential component of the response. Important interactions between catecholamines and TH have been previously demonstrated which support the existence of compensatory interactions between thyroid and sympathetic nervous system activity for the maintenance of body temperature. In the thyroid-blocked (methimazole-treated) rat, cold exposure is associated with increased urinary excretion of catecholamines[83]; in the thyroidectomised baboon, urinary catecholamines are also increased[84]. These findings suggest that thyroid deficiency is accompanied by compensatory sympathetic nervous system activity.

In an attempt to assess the role of the hypothalamic–pituitary–thyroid axis in homeostatic responses to chronic cold exposure, the converse question was asked. Are rats with defective temperature regulation capable of developing compensatory pituitary–thyroid activity? To test this hypothesis, pituitary –thyroid responses were assessed in immunosympathectomised–adrenodemedullated rats exposed to $6\,°C$ for 2 weeks. Such animals were shown to have a chronic core hypothermia of *ca.* $1\,°C$[7, 81]. Although evidence of enhanced TSH secretion was derived by increased thyroid weight and plasma TSH levels (as measured by radioimmunoassay), there were no changes in either total or free (diffusible) T_4 levels in plasma. These experiments thus also failed to show any change in setpoint of regulation as far as T_4 levels were concerned.

A new wrinkle to this question has been suggested recently by the observations of Nejad *et al.*[85], which indicate that plasma T_3 levels are increased in cold-exposed rats (4 weeks at $6\,°C$). Whether the rise in plasma T_3 levels is due to increased T_3 secretion by the thyroid, to increased peripheral deiodination of T_4 to T_3 or to reduced plasma clearance of T_3 is unknown. Whatever the mechanism, if these observations are confirmed, they will provide an interesting alternative explanation for the numerous experimental failures to demonstrate a change in hypothalamic–pituitary–thyroid setpoint during cold exposure. This may indicate that neural drive (via TRH–TSH release, sympathetic control or a combination of both) may cause preferential secretion of the more biologically potent T_3. In unpublished experiments, we have found that immunosympathectomised–adrenodemedullated rats show reduced plasma T_3 levels at room temperature and fail to increase T_3 levels on cold exposure. This raises the possibility that enhanced T_3 secretion during cold exposure may be dependent in part upon sympathetic innervation of the thyroid, circulating catecholamines or both. Further studies will be required to elucidate this relationship.

Final proof of hypothalamic-activated TSH release during chronic cold exposure requires demonstration that TRH synthesis and secretion are enhanced. Redding and Schally[86] have reported increased TRH levels as measured by an *in vitro* bioassay for TRH in the peripheral plasma of hypophysectomised cold-exposed rats. Increased hypothalamic TRF levels were also reported by Fukatsu[87] in cold-exposed rats. Direct evidence of a hypothalamic role in chronic cold exposure has been provided by the experiments of Reichlin *et al.*[7], in which it was shown that TRH synthesis by hypothalamic extracts *in vitro* is enhanced by prior exposure of the rat to cold.

3.3.4 Thyrotropin-releasing hormone

3.3.4.1 *Hypothalamic localisation and synthesis of TRH*

In 1969, Burgus *et al.*[88] and Böler *et al.*[89] and their respective collaborators simultaneously reported the structure of TRH isolated from hypothalamic tissue of ovine and porcine origin[90]. This substance, a cyclic tripeptide, pyroglutamyl-histidyl-proline-amide (mol. wt. 362) (Figure 3.5) has since been shown to have all the biological and chemical characteristics of the native material. Synthetic TRH is now widely available for both experimental and clinical use. TRH has been shown to be active in every mammalian species to which it has been administered, although a recent report suggests that it may not be active in the fowl[91].

In an elegant series of experiments, Mitnick and Reichlin[92, 93] have shown conclusively that hypothalamic fragments cultured *in vitro* are capable of

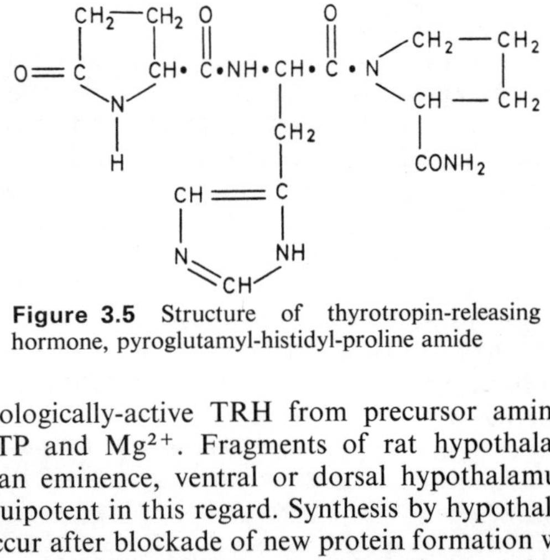

Figure 3.5 Structure of thyrotropin-releasing hormone, pyroglutamyl-histidyl-proline amide

synthesising biologically-active TRH from precursor amino acids in the presence of ATP and Mg^{2+}. Fragments of rat hypothalamus, including the stalk median eminence, ventral or dorsal hypothalamus, but not the cortex, were equipotent in this regard. Synthesis by hypothalamic fragments continued to occur after blockade of new protein formation with puromycin. Proof that the synthesising system was enzymatic was obtained from the demonstration that a soluble particulate-free extract of porcine hypothalamic tissue was capable of synthesising TRH in the presence of the appropriate co-factors.

In further studies, the authors have reported that the rate of incorporation of labelled precursor amino acids into TRH is influenced by the prior thyroid state of the animal[7]. Hypothalami from T_4-treated animals showed an increase in TRH synthesis, whereas in thyroidectomised animals synthesis was retarded markedly. However, in these experiments dose–response relationships were not established and only the extremes of thyroid function were assessed.

The question of whether TRH acts via CSF pathways has been considered by two investigators. These studies are important because morphological observations of the structure of the infundibular recess of the 3rd ventricle have raised the possibility that secretory processes arising from ependymal cells in this portion of the ventricular system may actively imbibe materials from the CSF and discharge them into the portal capillaries of the median eminence. Bioassayable TRF is reported to be detectable in the CSF of the rabbit[94]. Kendall *et al.*[95] reported that injection of TRH into the lateral ventricle of the rat, was not more effective in releasing TSH (as determined by an increase in thyroidal ^{131}I release from the pre-labelled gland) than intravenous administration. Gordon *et al.*[96] showed that immunoassayable TSH release occurs following injection of small quantities of TRH which were thought to be confined to the 3rd ventricular space. However, the TRH administered in this manner was much less effective than equivalent doses administered either parenterally or directly into the median eminence. These observations argue against there being an important transport mechanism for TRH from CSF to the median eminence. In a recent report it was shown that polypeptide substances such as LH and ACTH appear in the portal blood after intraventricular administration[97]. A similar experiment with labelled TRH has not been reported. TRH has been shown to be effective in causing TSH release when injected directly into a portal capillary[98].

3.3.4.2 Assay of TRH in peripheral blood

A limiting factor in the analysis of the role of TRH has been the difficulty in measuring the small quantities of the substance present in the hypothalamus or portal plasma. The existing *in vitro* and *in vivo* assay methods for TRH have been reviewed by Guillemin[90]. Given the limitations of assays for TRH, there are now several reports in which changes in TRH activity have been measured in hypothalamic tissues[68, 115] or portal blood[30, 116]. TRF activity has also been found in peripheral plasma of hypophysectomised rats[86], supporting the contention that residual pituitary TSH secretory capacity in stalk-sectioned or pituitary-transplanted rats is due to the continued secretion of TRH which reaches the pituitary in the systemic circulation. It is probable that in the near future, specific radioimmunoassay[99] or receptor binding radiostereoassays[100] will be developed which are sufficiently sensitive to measure TRH levels in blood and tissue.

TRH is rapidly inactivated in plasma[101-103] (but not CSF)[95] by an enzyme, the nature of which is not entirely clear at this time. Nair *et al.*[103] reported that 1 h of incubation at 37 °C results in a 72% decrease in the activity of both natural, synthetic and [^{14}C]proline labelled TRH. The recovered inactive material was shown to be a tripeptide which lacked the terminal proline amide group. Bassiri and Utiger[99] found that immunological activity of pharmacological doses of TRH was rapidly destroyed by incubation in plasma at 37 °C, a significant effect being evident within 2 min. Less than 50% of the immunological activity of the added TRH remained after 10 min incubation and only 1% after 2 h. Smaller amounts of TRH were inactivated even more rapidly. Dilutions of serum up to 1:64 were still active. It was concluded that serum contains a heat-, acid- and alkali-labile substance(s) which inactivates both immunological and biological TRH activity. It has been shown that the activity of this enzyme is related to thyroid state, it is enhanced in hyperthyroidism and decreased or absent following thyroidectomy or hypophysectomy.

The estimated half-life of TRH in the rat is 4.16 min with a volume of distribution of 18.5% of body wt. (*ca.* 2 × blood volume)[104]. A considerable proportion of labelled TRH is rapidly excreted in the urine in an unchanged form in both the rat and in man. Since excretion of TRH from plasma into urine is so rapid, the physiological significance of the inactivating plasma enzyme is unclear. Whatever the mechanism of TRH inactivation in plasma and its physiological significance, this effect represents a major practical obstacle which must be overcome if sensitive assay methods for TRH in biological fluids are to be achieved.

3.3.4.3   Structure–activity–relationships

It is beyond the scope of the present article to summarise the enormous strides which have been made in the structure–activity relationships for TRH. Hundreds of analogues have now been synthesised and with few exceptions have been shown to be inactive[90, 105-107]. The terminal proline-amide group is critical for the full activity of the molecule. Interestingly, one compound, p-Glu-N^{3im}-Me-His-Pro-amide has an activity 10 times that of the natural hormone[107]. It is probable that the structure of TRH is critical in terms of specific receptor binding sites on the thyrotrope cell.

3.3.4.4   Mechanisms of action

TRH is effective when administered either parenterally or orally and is active both *in vivo* and *in vitro*[90]. The effects of intravenous TRH are extremely rapid with measurable increases in plasma TSH levels occurring within 1–2 min in both man and animals[90]. This is in contrast to the negative feed-back effects of TH on pituitary TSH secretion which require at least 15 min to develop *in vitro* and an even longer period *in vivo*. The potency of TRH is indicated by the fact that estimations of the multiplication factor of TRH-induced TSH release, on a molar ratio, are of the order of 1:100 000; i.e. a single molecule of TRH induces release of more than 100 000 molecules of TSH[68].

TRH stimulatory effects appear to be the result of activation of cellular secretory processes initiated by attachment of the TRH molecule to specific membrane receptor sites on the thyrotrope cell. Labrie and his co-workers[100] have shown that *in vitro* binding of tritiated TRH to bovine pituitary cell membrane occurs very rapidly (within 5 min) and is dissociable by the addition of unlabelled hormone. The binding of TRH was not altered by administration of MSH-inhibiting hormone, lysine vasopressin, ACTH, GH, prolactin, luteinising hormone, insulin, glucagon, or significantly, the thyroid hormones T_4 and T_3. The remarkable sensitivity of the binding of labelled TRH to cell membrane and its displacement by cold TRH gives promise that this method may be a feasible technique for assay of small quantities of TRH. Other workers have confirmed these observations using thyrotrope tumour cells and whole mouse pituitary extracts[108].

The sequence of events which is set into motion by the attachment of TRH to the receptor site has not been entirely clarified but do appear to involve activation of an adenyl cyclase–cyclic AMP system. This effect was first reported by Wilber and Utiger in 1968[109], and has since been confirmed by others[5]. Prolonged pituitary stimulation by TRH apparently leads to increased TSH synthesis as well as release[110]. TSH release *in vitro* can also be stimulated by addition of excess K^+ and both TRF and excess K^+ require the presence of Ca^{2+}[111, 112]. Milligan and Kraicer[113] have shown that addition of K^+ results in a reversal of transmembrane potential in most rat anterior pituitary cells incubated *in vitro* accompanied by cellular ^{45}Ca uptake. The precise role of calcium in the secretory response to TRF remains unidentified. Recent evidence suggests that a protein kinase present in anterior pituitary tissue may be involved in the cyclic AMP activation of hormone secretion[114]. The action of TRH in inducing acute TSH release is not affected by pretreatment with protein synthesis inhibitors such as puromycin or cycloheximide. Further details of the effects of TRH are included in Chapter 2.

3.3.4.5 Specificity of TRH action

In early reports it was shown that TRH administration had no effect on plasma levels of GH, FSH, LH or cortisol[90]. Following the development of sensitive radioimmunoassays for prolactin, it was observed that intravenous TRH also causes *in vivo* prolactin release in man[117, 118], an effect not observed in the rat[119]. The TRH–prolactin response in man is quantitatively similar to the TSH response. The significance of this observation is still unclear, but it has been shown that TRH administration in lactating females is associated with sufficient prolactin release to enhance milk secretion[120]. The interesting possibility must be considered that this is a phylogenetic holdover of a more primitive thyroid regulatory system in premammalian species. In the goldfish, for example, hypothalamic control of TSH appears to be predominantly inhibitory (as for prolactin in the mammal). Perhaps other functional interrelationships between prolactin and TSH control will be demonstrated in the future.

It has also been reported that TRH administration induces GH release in acromegaly[121] and in some normal subjects following oral TRH administration[122].

3.3.4.6 Effects of TRH on brain

Several recent reports have suggested the possibility that TRH may have direct effects on brain metabolism. Intravenous TRH is reported to produce apparent acute relief of symptoms of depression[123, 124]. Plotnikoff and associates[124] observed that TRH enhanced the behavioural effects of L-DOPA in rats pretreated with pargyline (a monoamine oxidase inhibitor). Since this potentiation persisted after hypophysectomy, the phenomenon was interpreted to be independent of thyroid activation. Although these studies are preliminary, they suggest that TRH may soon join the growing list of polypeptide hormones which have direct effects on brain metabolism.

3.3.5   Role of monoamines in regulation of TRH secretion

Despite extensive experimental observations which support the hypothesis that central monoamines (in particular norepinephrine, dopamine, and serotonin) have important modulating effects on hypothalamic secretion of hypophysiotrophic hormones for regulation of LH, FSH, prolactin and GH (see Chapter 2); the effects of these substances on TRH release have been seldom studied. Fuxe and Hökfelt[125] found no alteration in dopamine fluorescence of the median eminence or arcuate nucleus following thiouracil or T_4 administration. On the other hand, Lichtensteiger[126] reported an increase in fluorescent intensity of tuberoinfundibular neurones in response to acute cold exposure, an effect which was prevented by prior T_4 administration. Brown and his co-workers[127] found a significant decrease in dopamine levels in the anterior and middle hypothalamus after daily T_4 administration in a dose sufficient to elevate plasma PBI levels (50 μg T_4 day^{-1} orally). There were no effects on norepinephrine levels, however.

A more direct approach to the problem of the role of monoamines in hypothalamic TRH synthesis and release has been provided by Reichlin and co-workers[7, 192]. In these experiments, the capacity of hypothalamic extracts to synthesise TRH *in vitro* was examined in rats pretreated with reserpine in a dose which was shown to cause significant reduction in plasma TSH levels (1 mg kg^{-1}, administered on five occasions over a 17 day period). Hypothalamic tissue from such rats showed a decreased rate of incorporation of [^{14}C]proline into chromatographically identified TRH. However, the rats appeared chronically ill and it was not possible to exclude the non-specific effects of chronic stress on TRH synthesis. In subsequent experiments, the effects of monoamines was assessed on TRH release from incubated hypothalamic tissue[192]. Pulse-labelled hypothalamic fragments from reserpine-treated rats showed a much slower spontaneous release of labelled TRH than controls. Norepinephrine (10^{-4} M) consistently and repeatedly caused increased TRH release from incubated hypothalamic tissue. Dopamine also had a stimulatory effect but this appeared to result from conversion of dopamine to norepinephrine since pharmacological blockade of this enzymatic step prevented dopamine-induced TRH release. Conversely, serotonin consistently inhibited TRH release, whereas acetylcholine had no effect. It was concluded from these experiments that catecholaminergic neurones may function in a regulatory manner to control synthesis and/or release of TRH in a manner analogous to the role of norepinephrine in induction of pineal synthesis of melatonin. It would be worth while to assess the possible role of neurotransmitters on TSH release induced by acute cold exposure by determining the effects of catecholamine-depleting agents. This is particularly pertinent since catecholamines have clearly been implicated in hypothalamic thermoregulatory mechanisms.

L-DOPA[128] administration, which in man causes acute GH release, is not associated with any change in plasma TSH levels; on the contrary, chronic L-DOPA administration is reported to interfere with TSH release induced by TRH, suggesting an effect of L-DOPA at the pituitary level. This is of interest because L-DOPA causes inhibition of prolactin secretion *in vitro* in the rat by direct effects on pituitary prolactin-producing cells[129]. In man, neither the administration of phentolamine (an α-adrenergic blocking agent) nor propranolol (a β-adrenergic blocker) has any effect on TRH-induced TSH secretion[130].

3.3.6 Thyroid hormone feed-back effects on brain for TRH–TSH control

As summarised by Reichlin *et al.*[7], it is currently believed that the primary site of negative feed-back control of TSH secretion is exerted by TH at the level of the pituitary. With the characterisation of TRH, it became possible to define this interaction in more precise terms (see p. 91). Despite indication that the setpoint for regulation of TSH secretion is determined by interactions at the pituitary thyrotrope level, the possibility that TH may also have an effect upon brain mechanisms for TRH synthesis or release has continued to receive considerable attention.

Experiments which have utilised application of TH directly into hypothalamic sites have been subject to criticism in the past because they did not distinguish effects mediated at the brain level from those secondary to diffusion of the substances to the pituitary via the portal vessels[2]. Kajihara and Kendall[131] attempted to resolve this problem by the use of multiple pituitary transplants to the kidney capsule in hypophysectomised rats. They observed that residual pituitary–thyroid function, as indicated by thyroidal ^{131}I uptake and thyroidal radioactive hormone release rates, was obliterated in transplanted rats by bilateral lesions in the region of the paraventricular nuclei, an effect presumed due to decreased TRH reaching the transplanted pituitary via systemic blood. T_4 implants (0.5 and 1.5 µg) into the anterior hypothalamus, but not the cerebral cortex, were also effective in causing thyroid depression due presumably to inhibition of TRH release. The crux of their argument was dependent on the fact that residual radioactivity in brain sites was similar in implantations made in cortex and hypothalamus, consisting of *ca.* 46% of the administered dose 24 h after implantation.

These studies are inconclusive because they do not exclude entirely the possibility that peripheral circulating T_4 may have suppressed pituitary transplants in a renal capsule site since such transplanted pituitaries have been shown to be extraordinarily sensitive to parenteral T_4[132]. A simple determination of residual radioactivity in the brain at one time interval does not exclude the possibility that the time course of diffusion of the remaining dose away from the anterior hypothalamus may have been different than from the cortex. In a subsequent study, Averill[132] demonstrated that the quantities of radioactive T_4 released from the hypothalamus in transplanted animals were much greater than Kajihara and Kendall[131] observed; at 24 h, less than 1 % remained at the site of implantation.

A series of interesting observations has been made by Joseph and Knigge[15, 133] concerning the site of feed-back effects of T_4 on TSH secretion in the cat. In these experiments, they circumvented the diffusion problem by using hypothalamic deafferentation and by using implants in the preoptic region of the hypothalamus. They studied responses to hemithyroidectomy and T_4 treatment in normal and hypothalamic-deafferented cats. Both deafferented and intact cats showed compensatory thyroid enlargement following hemithyroidectomy. However, T_4 in a dose of 2.5 µg kg^{-1} day^{-1} for 2 weeks caused inhibition of thyroid function in normal cats but not in deafferented animals. Implantation of T_4 pellets into the preoptic region was shown to be effective in inhibiting thyroidectomy responses in intact cats but not in deafferented animals. The authors conclude that an inhibitory neural pathway extends from the preoptic area to the medial basal hypothalamus and that this region is sensitive to feed-back actions of T_4. In a subsequent study[133], responses to hemithyroidectomy and T_4 treatment were examined in normal and deafferented kittens (5–21 days old). Hemithyroidectomy in 5-day-old kittens did not induce a compensatory increase in thyroid weight or ^{131}I uptake. On the other hand, deafferentation resulted in a marked increase in gland weight, as did T_4 implants into the preoptic area of the hypothalamus. They concluded that the preoptic area of the hypothalamus contains an inhibitory neural pathway in the kitten as well as in the adult, but that the neurones in the kitten respond differently to T_4 than do those of the adult, indicating positive feed-back effects in the kitten.

These studies are of interest in view of the demonstrated effects of systemic TH administration in the perinatal period on subsequent thyroid activity in the rat. Bakke and Lawrence[193] reported that such administration causes permanent hypothyroidism. They have recently shown that hypothalamic T_4 implants (in systemically ineffective doses) in neonatal rats also cause a permanent hypothyroid state characterised by growth failure, thyroid atrophy and reduced pituitary and plasma TSH levels[134]. The authors argue that neonatal administration of T_4, like androgen treatment of the female, can lead to a permanent alteration in hypothalamic–pituitary regulation. The amounts of T_4 implanted into the hypothalamus in these experiments were very large (smallest dose 20 µg) and may well have had non-specific local toxic effects. The experiments do not exclude, as the authors note, the possibility of diffusion of T_4 to the pituitary where the effects may have been mediated.

Several attempts have been made to estimate changes in TRH content or synthesis in response to different thyroid states. Sinha and Meites[115] reported that TRH levels in the hypothalamus were increased in thyroidecto-mised rats, but were not altered by T_4 treatment. A different approach to the problem of the effects of T_4 on hypothalamic TRH regulation has been reported by Reichlin et al.[7]. In these studies, the effects of prior thyroid state on the rate of incorporation of labelled amino acid precursors into TRH was examined in vitro. It was demonstrated that hypothalamic tissue from

T_4-treated animals (dose of $4\,\mu g$ $(100\,g)^{-1}$ body wt. day^{-1}) showed an increased capacity to synthesise TRH. On the other hand, thyroidectomised animals showed minimal TRH synthesis. From these observations it was postulated that T_4 has a positive feed-back effect upon hypothalamic synthesising mechanisms for TRH. In a formulation of the regulatory mechanism of the hypothalamic–pituitary–thyroid system by these authors, it was proposed that the T_4 feed-back effect upon the system is inherent to the genetic control system which establishes the functional long-term level of activity (or the setpoint of control) of the entire system. This allows for the primary site of acute feed-back regulation to occur at the pituitary level through the interaction between TRH and TH and to result in minute to minute changes in TSH secretion. The effects of microiontophoretic application of TH on single neurones have been reported[137]. The results indicate that most central neurones, in widely distributed regions of the hypothalamus, spinal cord and cortex are activated by local TH.

Interpretation of the effects of TH on neural feed-back regulatory mechanisms must remain cautious. In most experiments, large amounts of TH have been used. The possibility must be considered that the effects of such large quantities of TH may be reflected in generalised changes in cerebral protein synthesis[135] or be secondary to alteration in monamine synthesis or release[127, 136]. These effects might in themselves produce profound disturbances of neural mechanisms which are not necessarily physiologically important in feed-back regulation.

In conclusion, the possibility that feed-back effects of TH may be mediated at the hypothalamic level has been reconsidered by several investigators in the past few years. In spite of new approaches and of evidence suggesting that TH does have effects on hypothalamic mechanisms, it has not been clearly shown that these effects are physiological and not pharmacological. In addition, in future studies it will be necessary to examine the effects of T_3 as well as T_4.

3.4 PITUITARY TSH SECRETION

3.4.1 Interactions of TRH and TH in control of TSH secretion

TSH is synthesised and secreted by specific cells of the anterior pituitary which can be identified positively by histochemical, electron microscopic and immunofluorescent techniques. The structures of both human and bovine pituitary TSH are similar; the amino acid sequence of the latter has now been elucidated by Pierce and his co-workers[138] and shown to consist of two subunits, a and β; the former is identical to and interchangeable with the same subunit of LH. The immunological and biological determinants of the intact hormone appear to reside in the β subunit.

TSH secretion by the pituitary thyrotrope appears to be under the precise control of the levels of TH. Several analyses of TH and TSH feed-back interactions in man have been reported[139, 140]. Administration of increasing doses of T_4 or T_3 to hypothyroid patients produces a graded depression of plasma TSH levels. When data relating TSH to T_4 concentration were plotted to show TSH as a function of plasma T_4, a curvilinear relationship between these two variables was evident. Similar findings have been demonstrated in the rat[141]. Pituitary–thyroid feed-back regulation can thus be defined in terms of a specific plasma TSH level which is determined by a specific plasma TH concentration. In terms of servosystems analysis, the TH level in blood can be looked upon as the controlled variable. The normal 'setpoint' of pituitary–thyroid function is the resting level of plasma TH for the maintenance of which a specific level of TSH is required. Secretion of TSH is regulated inversely by the level of TH so that deviations from the setpoint of control lead to appropriate changes in the rate of TSH secretion.

The actual 'setpoint' of regulation of TSH–TH feed-back appears to be determined by the levels of TRH secreted by the hypothalamus. The mechanism of this interaction at the pituitary level has received considerable attention in recent years[142-145]. The TSH-releasing effects of hypothalamic TRH are immediate; increases in plasma TSH levels are detectable within minutes following i.v. administration of TRH in both the rat and man. On the other hand, inhibition of TSH secretion following T_4 or T_3 administration requires 15–45 min to develop. The effects of TRH administration can be blocked by prior treatment with either T_4 or T_3 both *in vivo* and *in vitro*. Such inhibition can, however, be overcome by administration of larger doses of TRH. These studies indicate that a competitive inhibition interaction exists between TRH and TH. It has been further shown that TH inhibition, but not TRH stimulation, is dependent upon new protein synthesis since the former, but not the latter, can be inhibited by a variety of protein synthesis inhibitors including actinomycin D, puromycin and cycloheximide[143, 145]. These findings have led to the postulation that TH acts on the thyrotrope by stimulating the production of an inhibitory protein which subsequently interferes with the TSH-releasing effects of TRH.

The remarkable sensitivity of the system to small changes in plasma levels of TH has been well documented. Snyder and Utiger[146] showed that the daily administration to normal human volunteers of small doses of TH (15 µg T_3 and 60 µg T_4 daily for 3–4 weeks), which were insufficient to produce measurable increases in plasma T_3 or T_4 levels, were effective in substantially reducing plasma TSH responses to intravenous TRH. These data suggest that the setpoint of control between TRH and TH is extremely sensitive to alterations in hormonal feed-back effects within the physiological range. The effects of TH feed-back inhibition can be overcome, however, by exogenous administration of TRH or by endogenous release such as occurs in acute cold exposure. On the other hand, increased plasma TH levels, such as occur in hyperthyroidism, result in the pituitary being relatively refractory to TRH administration.

The question of the relative importance of T_4 versus T_3 in producing the feed-back effects of TH on pituitary TSH secretion has been considered. Reichlin *et al.*[147] showed that pituitary tissue has a potent mechanism for deiodination of T_4[147]. More recently, Schadlow *et al.*[148] have described high affinity, T_3 binding sites in cell homogenates of rat pituitary. The specific binding of T_3 (which was 9.8 times as strong as T_4) led them to suggest that T_3 may be the primary agent in feed-back control. They postulated, moreover, that at the physiological level, T_3 sites are almost entirely saturated, indicating that feed-back inhibition is close to complete. Proof of the latter will require physiological studies of the feed-back effects of T_3 on TSH secretion, which have not been critically assessed to date, although the data of Snyder and Utiger[146] are consistent with this interpretation.

3.4.2 Mechanisms of action of TSH

Several excellent reviews have appeared in the past few years which discuss in detail the mechanisms of TSH action on the thyroid gland[8-11]. There is now conclusive evidence that circulating TSH binds to a hormone receptor site on thyroid follicle cells to initiate a wide range of effects, ultimately resulting in stimulation of iodide uptake, TH synthesis and release and, after a delay, an increase in thyroid tissue mass. Extensive evidence supports the hypothesis that binding of TSH to the follicle cell activates adenyl cyclase, resulting in the generation of cyclic-3'5'AMP[8, 9, 11]. The effects of TSH are rapid, both as observed biochemically and morphologically. Increases in adenylcyclase activity are detectable *in vitro* within 1 min after the addition of TSH to bovine and canine thyroid cells[149, 150]. Administration of TSH *in vivo* is followed within 5 min by evidence of the formation of pseudopods at the apical end of the follicle cell and by ingestion of colloid droplets with the peak increase in intracellular colloid droplet formation occurring *ca.* 1 h after TSH administration[151]. Most of the criteria described by Sutherland[152] for the hypothesis of cyclic AMP-mediated hormone release have been met in the case of TSH. This subject has been reviewed extensively by Dumont[8] and the questions which remain to be answered are clearly outlined by him. There is evidence that cyclic-AMP acts by stimulation of a specific protein kinase within thyroid cells[153, 154] in a manner similar to that which has been previously described in adrenal cortex, muscle and brain tissue.

Of current interest is the role of prostaglandins in activation of adenylcyclase. Both prostaglandin PGE_1 and PGE_2 activate thyroid adenyl cyclase and increase cyclic AMP content in the thyroid cell[150, 155]. Conversely, prostaglandin antagonists block the effects of both TSH and PGE_1 on the thyroid adenyl cyclase–cyclic AMP system[156]. In a recent paper, TSH administration was shown to increase tissue prostaglandin levels, as measured by radioimmunoassay[157]. Both PGE_1 and $PGF_{2\alpha}$ were increased by 30–80% within 5–15 min after addition of TSH *in vitro* to bovine thyroid-cell preparations. This rapid rise in cell prostaglandins following TSH administration closely paralleled the temporal character of TSH-induced activation of adenylcyclase. The stimulatory effect was shown to be specific for TSH with no change in prostaglandin levels following equivalent doses of LH, GH, ACTH or glucagon. These results suggest a possible role of prostaglandins in mediation of TSH effects on the thyroid.

Following the endocytosis of colloid, intracellular colloid droplets are approached by lysosomes which migrate from the basal portion of the cell and which function to remove enzymatically iodinated thyronines from thyroglobulin. This is followed by the secretion of TH from the basal portion of the cell into the blood. This stimulation of radioiodine release in the mouse, *in vivo*, is mimicked by theophylline (phosphodiesterase inhibitor) and by cyclic-AMP, but not by other nucleotides[8]. The process of secretion appears to involve microtubules, since both intracellular colloid droplet formation and TH secretion in thyroid slices are inhibited by colchicine, vincristine and other agents which share the common property of interfering with the function of microtubules[158]. Cytocholasin, an inhibitor of the microfilament system, also interferes with TH secretion in incubated thyroid slices[8].

The demonstration by Douglas[159] of Ca^{2+} dependent stimulus-secretion coupling in a number of endocrine glands has raised the question of whether Ca^{2+} has any role in triggering TH release. Willems and Dumont[160] found no stimulation of colloid droplet formation *in vitro* by the addition of Ca^{2+} or Ba^{2+}. Protein kinase activity in isolated bovine thyroid glands is enhanced by Mg^{2+} but markedly inhibited by Ca^{2+} [153]. A similar divalent cation requirement of protein kinases isolated from other tissues has been reported.

In conclusion, the effects of TSH are rapid and multiple and a complete characterisation of all the steps in stimulation of the thyroid is still not possible. It is clear that TSH is membrane bound and that activation of adenyl cyclase initiates most of the cellular events which follow both acute and chronic TSH administration. The action of cyclic-AMP is mediated through a protein kinase which does not appear to require Ca^{2+} for activation. Interestingly, the process of endocytosis itself appears to stimulate several of the subsequent metabolic events within the thyroid cell and it is possible that endocytosis secondarily increases cyclic-AMP levels[161]. Evidence of a role for prostaglandins in activation of thyroid secretion is convincing but the physiological importance of this mechanism has not been defined entirely.

3.4.3 Interaction of TSH and monoamines in thyroid secretion

Although TSH is the primary regulator of TH secretion, the possibility that circulating catecholamines or direct sympathetic innervation of the thyroid also exert a physiological effect on TH secretion has been investigated extensively (see Refs. 1, 4, 66 and 162–164 for reviews). A renewed interest in this subject has been evidenced by the appearance of several recent reports which have re-assessed these interactions both *in vivo* and *in vitro*.

The physiological role, if any, of these agents *in vivo* has been difficult to define. Melander and his co-workers[165-170] have published a series of significant studies which indicate that catecholamines and sympathetic terminations in the thyroid do influence thyroid hormone secretion in mice and rats. These investigators have shown that in the T_4-blocked mouse, L-epinephrine, L-norepinephrine, L-isoproterenol, and 5-HT, like TSH, induce formation of intracellular colloid droplets in the thyroid[165, 167], accompanied by release of ^{131}I-labelled TH. In contrast, these same agents administered to non-T_4 blocked mice caused a decrease in blood ^{131}I levels. In T_4-blocked animals, the stimulating effects of epinephrine and 5-HT were prevented by the prior administration of the *a*-adrenergic blocking agent, phentolamine, but were unchanged by propranolol. The critical point emphasised by these studies is that the effects of monoamine administration are dependent on the level of thyroid activity and sensitivity, both of which are in turn dependent on TSH secretion. In the T_4-blocked mouse, the effects of monoamines and TSH were found to be additive when administered simultaneously. That the source of the catecholamines may include sympathetic nerve terminals ending in the thyroid gland was suggested by experiments in which electrical stimulation of the cervical sympathetic trunk also caused an increase in intracellular colloid droplet formation and ^{131}I release[168]. This effect was also blocked by phentolamine administered 1.5 h before stimulation. The authors argue convincingly that these effects cannot be explained simply on the basis of changes in blood flow.

The same workers have extensively investigated the role of thyroid mast cells in thyroid regulation[166, 169]. The thyroid gland of the rodent contains numerous mast cells, the number of which correlates directly with TSH levels in plasma. In the rat, mast cells contain histamine and serotonin and both agents are released rapidly after a single intravenous dose of TSH (in T_4 treated rats). Mast cell histamine release (as assessed by histochemical fluorescence) occurred within 1 min after TSH administration with a return of histamine levels to normal by 2 h. Serotonin fluorescence, on the other hand, showed a progressive decline over this time interval. Release of these monoamines following TSH administration provides an explanation for observed acute TSH-induced changes in thyroid blood flow. Release of mast cell contents may, however, have a function beyond simple regulation of blood flow. Mast cell stimulation with 48/80 resulted in acute formation of intracellular colloid droplets and an increase in blood ^{131}I TH levels in the mouse. Species differences were noted, however, as in rats, the administration of 48/80 resulted in a decrease in ^{131}I release.

Because of the inherent difficulties in interpretation of studies on the effects of monoamines *in vivo* (due mainly to the problem of effects on gland blood flow), Ingbar and associates[171-172] have examined the effects of these agents *in vitro* using a bovine thyroid incubation technique. Epinephrine in concentrations of 1 and 10 µg ml^{-1} was shown to markedly stimulate the formation of iodothyronines. Equipotent in this respect was adrenochrome, the oxidative product of epinephrine; both agents stimulated adenylcyclase activity and their actions were blocked by phentolamine but not by propranolol. These effects resembled in several, but not all respects, those induced by TSH. Similar concentrations of serotonin were also effective in generation of cyclic AMP and these effects, like those of epinephrine, were prevented by phentolamine. These data argue in favour of a direct effect of serotonin and epinephrine on thyroid cell metabolism.

A precise characterisation of the role of (a) circulating catecholamines and (b) sympathetic thyroid innervation of TH secretion is still not possible from the available evidence. The fact that thyroid denervation does not noticeably affect pituitary–thyroid control does not exclude the possibility that under certain circumstances, catecholamines (and serotonin) might serve to modulate or alter TH secretion (as for example in favour of T_3 as opposed to T_4 release). Of interest in this respect is the recent observation of Nejad *et al.*[85] that chronic cold exposure (with its attendant activation of the sympathetic nervous system) is accompanied by enhanced TSH secretion and elevation in plasma T_3 but not T_4 levels. In the future, it will be important to assess critically the interaction between TSH and monoamines in terms of the differential effect on T_4 v. T_3 secretion.

3.5 CIRCULATION AND METABOLIC EFFECTS OF THYROID HORMONES

3.5.1 Role of T_4 v. T_3

Although it is beyond the scope of the present review to consider in detail the circulation, plasma binding, and metabolic effects of TH, advances in methodology within the last 3–5 years have re-opened the issue of the relative importance of T_4 v. T_3 in TH regulation of metabolism. Tri-iodothyronine was first identified in human plasma in 1952 by Gross and Pitt-Rivers[173] and early experiments indicated that T_3 was formed and secreted by the thyroid. Since that time, controversy has continued over the relative importance of this form of TH, particularly with the recognition that T_3 (a) has higher biological potency that T_4, accompanied by a shorter biological half-life; (b) circulates in plasma less tightly bound to plasma proteins; and (c) is more widely distributed in tissues than T_4. However, problems in measuring the plasma levels of T_3 made it difficult to accurately assess the role of this hormone. With the recent development of reliable chromatographic[174] and radioimmunoassay techniques[175-179], renewed interest in the function of T_3 developed and it is now apparent that, in man, at least 50–75% of TH metabolic effects are attributable to T_3.

There is still debate concerning the absolute levels of T_3 in plasma. Sterling and his co-workers[174], using chromatographic separation techniques, reported normal human serum levels of 2.2 ng ml^{-1}, a value which is ca. 1/40th that of serum T_4 levels. Subsequent radioimmunoassay determinations of T_3 suggest that T_3 levels are slightly lower than those initially reported by Sterling, ranging between 1 and 1.8 ng ml^{-1}[175-178]. Radioimmunoassay determinations of plasma T_3 levels in the rat have shown considerably lower levels (160 pg ml^{-1})[85] whereas those in the sheep are ca. one-half those reported in man (0.55 ng ml^{-1})[179].

Both T_4 and T_3 circulate in the plasma bound to specific binding proteins. The binding of T_4 is considerably more complete than that of T_3. If it is assumed that the free (diffusible or non-protein bound) portion of TH is the physiologically-active component, then the free T_3 concentration in man is ca. 4.3 pg ml^{-1} which amounts to 1/5 of the absolute concentration of free T_4 in human serum[178]. Using the calculated metabolic activity of T_3 of ca. four times that of T_4, it is apparent that the contributions of free T_4 and free T_3 are approximately equal in terms of biological activity.

Studies in several species have now clearly shown that a significant proportion (as much as $\frac{1}{2}$–$\frac{2}{3}$) of circulating T_3 is derived from extrathyroidal de-iodination of T_4[180-182]. Conversely, it is estimated that of circulating T_4, ca. one-third is eventually de-iodinated to T_3[181-182]. Extrathyroidal conversion of T_4 to T_3 has also been demonstrated in other species. In the sheep, it has been calculated that ca. 91% of daily T_3 turnover is derived from peripheral monodeiodination of T_4[179].

The possibility must again be considered as suggested by Galton and Ingbar[183] that the metabolic effect of T_4 is totally dependent upon its deiodination to T_3. Oppenheimer and co-workers[184-186] have extensively investigated tissue and cellular binding sites for T_4 and T_3. They have demonstrated recently specific T_3 nuclear membrane binding sites in liver cell homogenates[185]. Calculations of the concentration of T_3 in rat plasma and of the specific activity of injected T_3 led to the conclusion that a small increment in the plasma T_3 was accompanied by significant displacement of nuclear T_3. These studies show a clear difference between tissue distribution of T_3 as opposed to T_4. T_4 is distributed in the same ratio throughout all sub-cellular components, whereas T_3 appears to have specific binding sites. The authors relate this finding to the suggestion of Tata[187], that an early step in the cellular action of TH is nuclear stimulation of RNA-polymerase activity. They suggest that this indicates that conversion of T_4 to T_3 may be a necessary prerequisite for metabolic activity of T_4[188].

A critical question which arises is: what are the effects of physiological thyroid stimulation on T_3 v. T_4 release? Hollander and his co-workers[189] have shown that significant elevations in plasma T_3 levels are measurable in man following a single intravenous injection of TRH (100 µg)[189]. The rise in T_3 levels was detected as early as 10 min after TRH administration and the level was still increasing at the end of 1 h. In contrast, changes in plasma T_4 levels following a single injection of TRH were negligible and occurred much later. These authors speculate that this indicates that the acute effects of a pharmacological dose of TRH may be a preferential secretion of T_3. Administration of TSH is also followed by a more rapid and greater fractional rise in plasma T_3 than in T_4 levels[177, 178]. Shimoda and Greer[190] reported that following TSH stimulation, incorporation of iodide into T_3 occurred preferentially to that of T_4 *in vitro*.

Nejad and co-workers[85] have shown that many of the factors which influence T_3 levels in man also operate in the rat. Extrathyroid conversion of T_4 and T_3 has also been demonstrated to occur in this species[188]. These observations are important because they indicate the usefulness of the rat as a model for further studies of T_4, T_3 interrelationships.

3.6 CONCLUSION

Regulation of the pituitary–thyroid axis is achieved by both closed-loop and open-loop components (Figure 3.6). The primary site of acute regulatory control is the pituitary thyrotrope cell; the secretion of TSH is exquisitely controlled by the interaction of the stimulatory effects of TRH and the negative feed-back effects of TH. Basal TSH secretion, which is dependent upon continuing or tonic TRH secretion, can be increased acutely by TRH or decreased, after a modest delay, by administration of T_4 or T_3. Elevated levels of TH cause attenuation of or completely prevent TRH-mediated acute TSH release.

The medial basal hypothalamus is capable of maintaining near normal pituitary–thyroid function. Extrahypothalamic inputs, although not clearly defined as yet, probably determine diurnal variations, stress-induced inhibition and cold-induced release of TSH by effects mediated via TRH releasing neurones of the medial basal hypothalamus. The role of monoaminergic neurones in control of TRH secretion is still not clearly defined. Preliminary evidence has implicated noradrenergic neurones as active in stimulating release and synthesis of TRH.

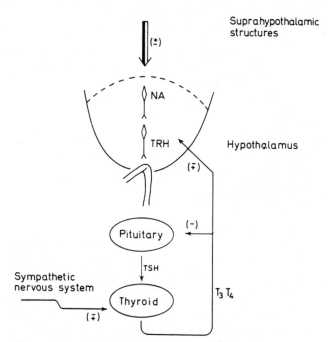

Figure 3.6 Hypothalamic–pituitary–thyroid system for control of thyroid hormone secretion. The principal site of acute feed-back regulation is at the level of the thyrotrope. Tonic TRH release establishes the sensitivity of T_3 and T_4 feed-back effects. Peptidergic (TRH producing neurones) are influenced by several extrahypothalamic inputs and some of these effects may be mediated via noradrenergic neurones. The function of negative *v*. positive feed-back effects of TH on the hypothalamus remains unresolved.

The feed-back effects of thyroid hormones on the brain have been difficult to assess due, in large part, to the profound effects of thyroid hormone deficiency or excess on neural metabolic function in general. Arguments have been made for both negative and positive feed-back effects. Whatever the case, it is likely that these effects cause only long-term adjustments in the system and do not acutely affect hypothalamic–pituitary–thyroid responses.

There is a renewed need for further assessment of the effects of the sympathetic nervous system on thyroid control and an analysis of the interaction which occurs between TSH, circulating catecholamines, sympathetic innervation and monoamine containing mast cells of the thyroid gland. There are undoubtedly important species differences in these mechanisms.

Current evidence supports the concept that T_3 is the primary, and perhaps only, metabolically-active thyroid hormone. The resolution of this problem will also require further study.

References

1. Hoskins, R. G. (1949). The thyroid-pituitary apparatus as a servo (feedback) mechanism. *J. Clin. Endocrinol.*, **9**, 1429
2. Reichlin, S. (1966). Control of thyrotropin hormone secretion. *Neuroendocrinology*, vol. 1, 445 (L. Martini and W. Ganong, editors) (New York: Academic Press)
3. Brown-Grant, K. (1966). The control of TSH secretion. *The Pituitary Gland*, vol. 2, 235 (G. W. Harris and B. T. Donovan, editors) (London: Butterworth)
4. Harris, G. W. and George, R. (1969). Neurohumoral control of the adenohypophysis and the regulation of the secretion of TSH, ACTH and growth hormone. *The Hypothalamus*, 326 (W. Haymaker, E. Anderson and W. J. H. Nauta, editors) (Springfield: Thomas)
5. McKenzie, J. M., Adiga, P. R. and Solomon, S. H. (1970). Hypothalamic control of thyrotropin. *The Hypothalamus*, 335 (L. Martini, M. Motta and F. Fraschini, editors) (New York: Academic Press)
6. Hershman, J. M. and Pittmann, J. A. Jr. (1971). Control of thyrotropin secretion in man. *N. Engl. J. Med.*, **285**, 997
7. Reichlin, S., Martin, J. B., Mitnick, M. A., Boshans, R. L., Grimm, Y., Bollinger, J., Gordon, J. and Malacara, J. (1972). The hypothalamus in pituitary-thyroid regulation. *Rec. Progr. Horm. Res.*, **28**, 229
8. Dumont, J. E. (1971). The action of thyrotropin on thyroid metabolism. *Vitam. Horm.*, **29**, 287
9. Field, J. B. (1970). Mechanism of action of thyroid-stimulating hormone. *Proc. 6th Midwest Conf. on the Thyroid*, 89 (A. D. Kenny and R. R. Anderson, editors) (Columbia, Mo.: Columbia Press)
10. Liberti, P. and Stanbury, J. B. (1971). The pharmacology of substances affecting the thyroid gland. *Ann. Rev. Pharmacol.*, **11**, 113
11. Burke, G. (1971). Thyroid stimulators and thyroid stimulation. *Acta Endocrinol.*, **66**, 558
12. Larsen, P. R. (1972) Triiodothyronine: Review of recent studies of its physiology and pathophysiology in man. *Metabolism*, **21**, 1073
13. Halasz, B., Florsheim, W. H., Corcorran, N. I. and Gorski, R. S. (1967). Thyrotrophic hormone secretion in rats after partial or total interruption of neural afferents to the median basal hypothalamus. *Endocrinology*, **80**, 1075
14. Voloschin, L., Joseph, S. A. and Knigge, K. M. (1968). Endocrine function in male rats following complete and partial isolations of the hypothalamopituitary unit. *Neuroendocrinology*, **3**, 387
15. Knigge, K. M. and Joseph, S. A. (1971). Neural regulation of TSH secretion: sites of thyroxine feedback. *Neuroendocrinology*, **8**, 273
16. Van Rees, G. P. and Moll, J. (1968). Influence of thyroidectomy with and without thyroxine treatment on thyrotrophin secretion in gonadectomised rats with anterior hypothalamic lesions. *Neuroendocrinology*, **3**, 115
17. Martin, J. B., Boshans, R. and Reichlin, S. (1970). Feedback regulation of TSH secretion in rats with hypothalamic lesions. *Endocrinology*, **87**, 1032
18. Guillemin, R. (1970). Discussion: Unsolved problems in the portal vessel-chemotransmitter hypothesis. *Hypophysiotropic Hormones of the Hypothalamus Assay and Chemistry*, 14 (J. Meites, editor) (Baltimore: Williams and Wilkins)
19. Jonsson, G., Fuxe, K. and Hökfelt, T. (1971). On the catecholamine innervation of the hypothalamus, with special reference to the median eminence. *Brain Res.*, **40**, 271
20. Makara, G. B., Harris, M. D. and Spyer, K. M. (1972). Identification and distribution of tuberoinfundibular neurones. *Brain Res.*, **40**, 283
21. Martini, L., Fraschini, F. and Motta, M. (1968). Neural control of anterior pituitary functions. *Rec. Progr. Horm. Res.*, **24**, 439

22. Flament-Durand, J. (1971). Tentative localisation of the structures responsible for the synthesis of the thyrotropin releasing hormone. Autoradiographic study of ^{3}H proline incorporation in the nervous system of the normal rat. *Arch. Biol. (Liege)*, **82**, 245

23. D'Angelo, S. A., Snyder, J. and Grodin, J. M. (1964). Electrical stimulation of the hypothalamus; simultaneous effects on the pituitary-adrenal and thyroid systems of the rat. *Endocrinology*, **75**, 417

24. Martin, J. B. and Reichlin, S. (1970). Thyrotropin secretion in the rat following hypothalamic stimulation or injection of synthetic TSH releasing factor. *Science*, **168**, 1366

25. Martin, J. B. and Reichlin, S. (1972). Plasma thyrotropin (TSH) response to hypothalamic electrical stimulation and to injection of synthetic thyrotropin-releasing hormone (TRH). *Endocrinology*, **90**, 1079

26. Ohsawa, K. (1972). Experimental studies on neurohumoral control of TSH secretion. I. Effect of electrical stimulation of the hypothalamus on the pituitary-thyroid function in dogs. *Med. J. Kobe Univ.*, **32**, 1

27. Averill, R. L. W. and Salaman, D. F. (1967). Elevation of plasma thyrotropin (TSH) during electrical stimulation in the rabbit hypothalamus. *Endocrinology*, **81**, 173

28. Martin, J. B. and Reichlin, S. (1971). Anatomical specificity of hypothalamic sites for release of thyrotropin and growth hormone. *Neurology*, **21**, 436

29. Krulich, L., Illner, P., Fawcett, C. P., Quijada, M. and McCann, S. M. (1972). Dual hypothalamic regulation of growth hormone secretion. *Growth and Growth Hormone* 306. (A. Peale and E. E. Müller, editors) (Amsterdam: Excerpta Medica)

30. Wilber, J. F. and Porter, J. C. (1970). Thyrotropin and growth hormone releasing activity in hypophysial portal blood. *Endocrinology*, **87**, 807

31. Lomax, P., Kokka, N. and George, R. (1970). Thyroid activity following intracerebral injection of morphine in the rat. *Neuroendocrinology*, **6**, 146

32. Vertes, M., Vertes, T. and Kovacs, S. (1965). Effect of hypothalamic stimulation on pituitary thyroid function. *Acta Physiol. Acad. Sci. Hung.*, **27**, 229

33. Peter, R. E. (1970). Hypothalamic control of thyroid gland activity and gonadal activity in the goldfish, *Carassius auratus*, *J. Endocrinol.*, **51**, 31

34. Peter, R. E. (1971). Feedback effects of thyroxine on the hypothalamus and pituitary of goldfish, *Carassius auratus*. *J. Endocrinol.*, **51**, 31

35. Martin, L. G., Martul, P., Connor, T. B. and Wiswell, J. G. (1972). Hypothalamic origin of idiopathic hypopituitarism, *Metabolism*, **21**, 143

36. Szentagothai, J., Flerko, B., Mess, B. and Halasz, B. (1968). *Hypothalamic Control of the Anterior Pituitary*, 184 (Budapest: Akademiai Kiado)

37. Nauta, W. J. H. (1963). Central nervous organisation and the endocrine motor system. *Advances in Neuroendocrinology*, 5 (A. V. Nalbandov, editor) (Urbana, Ill.: Univ. Illinois Press)

38. Singh, D. V. and Turner, C. W. (1972). Effect of melatonin upon thyroid hormone secretion rate in female hamsters and male rats. *Acta Endocrinol.*, **69**, 35

39. Defronzo, R. A. and Roth, W. D. (1972). Evidence for the existence of a pineal-adrenal and a pineal-thyroid axis. *Acta Endocrinol.*, **70**, 31

40. Remy, C. and Disclos, P. (1970). Influence de l'epiphysectomie sur le dévelopment de la thyroide et des gonads chez les têtrads d'Alytes obstetricians. *Compt. Rend. Soc. Biol.*, **164**, 1989

41. Singh, D. V., Narang, C. D. and Turner, C. W. (1969). Effect of melatonin and its withdrawal on thyroid hormone secretion rate of female rats. *J. Endocrinol.*, **43**, 489

42. Rowe, J. W., Richert, J. R., Klein, D. C. and Reichlin, S. (1970). Relation of the pineal gland and environmental lighting to thyroid function in the rat. *Neuroendocrinology*, **6**, 247

43. Relkin, R. (1972). Effects of pinealectomy and constant light and darkness on thyrotropin levels in pituitary and plasma of rat. *Neuroendocrinology*, **10**, 46

44. Lupulescu, A., Nicolescu, A., Gheorghiescu, B., Merculiev, E. and Lungu, M. (1962). Neural control of the thyroid gland: studies on the role of extrapyramidal and rhinencephalon areas in the development of the goiter. *Endocrinology*, **70**, 517

45. Cheifetz, P. N. (1969). Effect of lesions in the globus pallidus upon thyroid function. *J. Endocrinol.*, **43**, 36

46. Shizumi, K., Matsuzaki, F., Iino, S., Matsuda, K., Nagataki, S. and Okinaka, S.

(1962). Effect of electrical stimulation of the limbic system on pituitary-thyroid function. *Endocrinology*, **71,** 456

47. Eleftheriou, B. E. and Zolovick, A. J. (1968). Effect of amygdaloid lesions on plasma and pituitary thyrotropin levels in the deermouse. *Proc. Soc. Exp. Biol. Med.*, **127,** 671

48. Kovacs, S., Sandor, A., Vertes, Z. and Vertes, M. (1965). The effect of lesions and stimulation of the amygdala on pituitary-thyroid function. *Acta Physiol. Acad. Sci. Hung.*, **27,** 221

49. Dupont, A., Bastarache, E., Endröczi, E. and Fortier, C. (1972). Effect of hippcampal stimulation on the plasma thyrotropin (TSH) and corticosterone responses to acute cold exposure in the rat. *Can. J. Physiol. Pharm.*, **50,** 364

50. Retiene, K., Zimmerman, E., Schindler, W. J., Neuenschwander, J. and Lipscombe, H. S. (1968). A correlation study of endocrine rhythms in rats. *Acta Endocrinol.*, **57,** 1

51. Bakke, J. L. and Lawrence, N. (1965). Circadian periodicity in thyroid stimulating hormone titer in the rat hypophysis and serum. *Metabolism*, **14,** 841

52. Singh, D. V., Panda, J. N. and Anderson, R. R. (1967). Diurnal variation of plasma and pituitary thyrotropin (TSH) of rats. *Proc. Soc. Exp. Biol. Med.*, **126,** 553

53. Nicoloff, J. T. (1970). A new method for the measurement of thyroidal iodine release in man. *J. Clin. Invest.*, **49,** 1912

54. Nicoloff, J. T., Fisher, D. A. and Applean, M. D. Jr. (1970). The role of glucocorticoids in the regulation of thyroid function in man. *J. Clin. Invest.*, **49,** 1922

55. Lemarchand-Beraud, T. and Vannotti, A. (1969). Relationships between blood thyrotropin level, protein bound iodine and free thyroxine concentration in man under normal physiological conditions. *Acta Endocrinol.*, **60,** 315

56. Webster, B. R., Guansing, A. R. and Paice, J. C. (1972). Absence of diurnal variation of serum TSH. *J. Clin. Endocrinol.*, **34,** 899

57. Vanhaelst, L., Van Cauter, E., Degaute, J. P. and Goldstein, J. (1972). Circadian variations of serum thyrotropin levels in man. *J. Clin. Endocrinol.*, **35,** 479

58. Sassin, J. F., Frantz, A. G., Weitzman, E. D. and Kapen, S. (1972). Human prolactin: 24-hour pattern with increased release during sleep. *Science*, **177,** 1205

59. Dewhurst, K. E., elKabir, D. J. and Harris, G. W. (1968). A review of the effect of stress on the activity of the central nervous-pituitary–thyroid axis in animals and man. *Confin. Neurol.*, **30,** 161

60. Mason, J. W. (1968). A Review of psychoendocrine research on the pituitary–thyroid system. *Psychosom. Med.*, **30,** 666

61. Fortier, C., Delgado, A., Ducommon, P., Ducommun, S., Dupont, A., Jobin, M., Kraicer, J., MacIntosh-Hardt, B., Marceau, H., Miathe, P., Miathe-Voloss, C., Rerup, C. and Van Rees, G. P. (1970). Functional interrelationships between the adenohypophysis, thyroid, adrenal cortex and gonads. *Can. Med. Assoc. J.*, **103,** 864

62. Leppaluoto, J. (1972). Blood bioassayable thyrotrophin and corticosteroid levels during various physiological and stress conditions in the rabbit. *Acta Endocrinol.*, Suppl. 165, 1

63. Charters, A. C., Odell, W. D. and Thompson, J. C. (1969). Anterior pituitary function during surgical stress and convalescence. Radioimmunassay measurement of blood TSH, LH, FSH and growth hormone. *J. Clin. Endocrinol.*, **29,** 63

64. Koch, B., Jobin, M., Dulac, S. and Fortier, C. (1972). Thyrotropin (TSH) response to synthetic TSH-releasing factor following pharmacological blockade of adrenocorticotropin (ACTH) secretion. *Can. J. Physiol. Pharm.*, **50,** 360

65. Wilber, J. F. and Utiger, R. D. (1969). The effect of glucocorticoids on thyrotropin secretion. *J. Clin. Invest.*, **48,** 2096

66. D'Angelo, S. A. (1963). Central nervous regulation of the secretion and release of thyroid stimulating hormone. *Advances in Neuroendocrinology*, 158, (A. V. Nalbandov, editor) (Urbana, Ill.: Univ. Illinois Press)

67. Galton, V. A. and Nisula, B C. (1969). Thyroxine metabolism and thyroid function in the cold-adapted rat. *Endocrinology*, **85,** 79

68. Martin, J. B. and Reichlin, S. (1970). Neural regulation of the pituitary-thyroid axis. *Proc. 6th Midwest Conf. on the Thyroid* 1. (A. D. Kenny and R. R. Anderson, editors) (Columbia, Mo.: Univ. Columbia Press)

69. Hershman, J. M. and Pittman, J. A. (1971). Utility of the radioimmunassay of serum thyrotrophin in man. *Ann. Int. Med.*, **74,** 481

70. Itoh, S., Hiroshige, T., Koseki, T. and Nakatsugawa, T. (1966). Release of thyro-
    tropin in relation to cold exposure. *Fed. Proc.* (*Fed. Amer. Soc. Exp. Biol.*), **25**, 1187
71. Fisher, D. A. and Odell, W. D. (1971). Effect of cold on TSH secretion in man.
    J. Clin. Endocrinol., **33**, 859
72. Wilber, J. F. and Baum, D. (1970). Elevation of plasma TSH during surgical hypo-
    thermia. *J. Clin. Endocrinol.*, **31**, 372
73. Berg, G. R., Utiger, R. D., Schalch, D. S. and Reichlin, S. (1966). Effect of central
    cooling in man on pituitary-thyroid function and growth hormone secretion. *J. Appl.
    Physiol.*, **21**, 1791
74. Hershman, J. M., Read, D. G., Bailey, A. L. Norman, V. D. and Gibson, T. B. (1970).
    Effect of cold exposure on serum thyrotropin. *J. Clin. Endocrinol.*, **30**, 430
75. Andersson, B., Ekman, L., Gale, C. C. and Sundsten, J. W. (1962). Activation of the
    thyroid gland by cooling of the pre-optic area in the goat. *Acta Physiol. Scand.*, **54**, 191
76. Reichlin, S. (1964). Function of the hypothalamus in regulation of pituitary-thyroid
    activity. *Brain-Thyroid Relationships*, Ciba Foundation Study Group No. **18**, 13
77. Gale, C. C., Jobin, M., Proppe, D. W., Notter, D. and Fox, H. (1970). Endocrine
    thermoregulatory responses to local hypothalamic cooling in unanesthetized baboons.
    Amer. J. Physiol., **219**, 193
78. Jobin, M., Endröczi, E., Hontela, S. and Fortier, C. (1970). Effect of hypothalamic
    cooling on the behaviour and the pituitary–thyroid activity in the rat. *J. Physiol.*
    (Lyon), **63**, 309
79. Brown, M. R. and Hedge, C. A. (1972). Thyroid secretion in the unanesthetised,
    stress-free rat and its suppression by pentobarbital. *Neuroendocrinology*, **9**, 158
80. Kajihara, A., Onaya, T., Yamada, T., Takemura, Y. and Kotani, M. (1972). Further
    studies on the acute stimulatory effect of cold on thyroid activity and its mechanism.
    Endocrinology, **90**, 538
81. Martin, J. B. (1972). Immunosympathectomy as a tool in endocrinologic studies,
    Immunosympathectomy, 177. (G. Steiner and E. Schönbaum, editors) (Amsterdam:
    Elsevier)
82. Himms-Hagen, J. (1967). Sympathetic regulation of metabolism. *Pharmacol. Rev.*, **19**,
    367
83. Johnson, G. E., Flattery, K. V. and Schönbaum, E. (1965). The influence of methi-
    mazole on the catecholamine excretion of cold-stressed rats. *Can. J. Physiol.
    Pharmacol.* **45**, 415
84. Gale, C. C., Toivola, P., Schonbaum, M. L. D. (1969). Thyroid-sympathetic nervous
    interactions in thermo-regulation. *Program 51st Meeting of the Endocrine Society*,
    New York, p. 114
85. Nejad, I. F., Bollinger, J. A., Mitnick, M. and Reichlin, S. (1972). Importance of
    T_3 (triiodothyronine) secretion in altered states of thyroid function in the rat: cold
    exposure, subtotal thyroidectomy, and hypophysectomy. *Trans. Ass. Amer. Phys.*,
    85, 295
86. Redding, T. W. and Schally, A. V. (1969). Studies of the thyrotropin-releasing
    hormone (TRH) activity in peripheral blood. *Proc. Soc. Exp. Biol. Med.*, **131**, 420
87. Fukatsu, H. (1971). Experimental studies on regulating mechanism of TSH secretion
    by TRH and thyroxine in rats. *Folia Endocrinol. Jap.*, **47**, 236
88. Burgus, R., Dunn, T. F., Desidiero, D. and Guilleman, R. (1969). Molecular structure
    of the hypothalamic hypophysiotropic TRF factor of ovine origin: mass spectrometry
    demonstration of the PCA-His-Pro-NH_2 sequence. *CR Acad. Sci.* (*Paris*), **269**, 1870
89. Böler, J., Enzman, F., Folkers, K., Bowers, C. Y. and Sehally, A. V. (1969). The iden-
    tity of chemical and hormonal properties of the thyrotropin releasing hormone and
    pyroglutamyl-histidyl-proline amide. *Biochem. Biophys. Res. Commun.*, **37**, 705
90. Guillemin, R., Burgus, R. and Vale, W. (1971). The hypothalamic hypophysiotropic
    thyrotropin-releasing factor. *Vitam. Horm.*, **29**, 1
91. Ochi, Y., Shiomi, K., Hachiya, T., Yoshimura, M. and Miyazaki, T. (1972). Failure
    of TRH (thyrotropin-releasing hormone) to stimulate thyroid function in the chick.
    Endocrinology, **91**, 832
92. Mitnick, M. and Reichlin, S. (1971). Thyrotropin-releasing hormone: biosynthesis
    by rat hypothalamic fragments *in vitro*. *Science*, **172**, 1241
93. Mitnick, M. and Reichlin, S. (1972). Enzymatic synthesis of thyrotropin-releasing
    hormone (TRH) by hypothalamic 'TRH synthetase'. *Endocrinology*, **91**, 1145

94. Averill, R. L. W. and Kennedy, T. H. (1967). Elevation of thyrotropin release by intrapituitary infusion of crude hypothalamic extracts. *Endocrinology*, **81**, 113

95. Kendall, J. W., Rees, L. H. and Kramer, R. (1971). Thyrotropin releasing hormone stimulation of thyroidal radioiodine release in the rat: comparison between intravenous and intraventricular administration. *Endocrinology*, **88**, 1503

96. Gordon, J. H., Bollinger, J. and Reichlin, S. (1972). Plasma thyrotropin responses to thyrotropin-releasing hormone after injection into the third ventricle, systemic circulation, median eminence and anterior pituitary. *Endocrinology*, **91**, 696

97. Ondo, J. G., Mical, R. S. and Porter, J. C. (1972). Passage of radioactive substances from CSF to hypophysial portal blood. *Endocrinology*, **91**, 1239

98. Porter, J. C., Vale, W., Burgus, R., Mical, R. S. and Guillemin, R. (1971). Release of TSH by TRF infused directly into a pituitary stalk portal vessel. *Endocrinology*, **89**, 1054

99. Bassiri, R. M. and Utiger, R. D. (1972). The preparation and specificity of antibody to thyrotropin releasing hormone. *Endocrinology*, **90**, 722

100. Labrie, F., Barden, N., Poirier, G. and McLean, A. (1972). Binding of thyrotropin-releasing hormone to plasma membranes of bovine anterior pituitary gland. *Proc. Nat. Acad. Sci. USA*, **69**, 283

101. Vale, W. W., Burgus, R., Dunn, T. F. and Guillemin, R. (1971). *In vitro* plasma inactivation of thyrotropin releasing factor (TRF) and related peptides: its inhibition by various means and by the synthetic dipeptide PCA-his-pro-O-me. *Hormones*, **2**, 193

102. Bassiri, R. and Utiger, R. D. (1972). Serum inactivation of the immunological and biological activity of thyrotropin-releasing hormone (TRH). *Endocrinology*, **91**, 657

103. Nair, R. M. G., Redding, T. W. and Schally, A. V. (1971). Site of inactivation of thyrotropin-releasing hormone by human plasma. *Biochemistry*, **10**, 3621

104. Redding, T. W. and Schally, A. V. (1972). On the half-life of thyrotropin-releasing hormone in rats. *Neuroendocrinology*, **9**, 250

105. Rivier, J., Vale, W., Monahan, M., Ling, N. and Burgus, R. (1972). Synthetic thyrotropin-releasing factor analogues. 3 Effect of replacement or modification of histidine residue on biological activity. *J. Med. Chem.*, **15**, 479

106. Sievertsson, H., Chang, J. K., Folkers, K. and Bowers, C. T. (1972). Synthesis of di- and tripeptides and assay *in vivo* for activity in the thyrotropin-releasing hormone and luteinising releasing hormone systems. *J. Med. Chem.*, **15**, 8

107. Vale, W., Rivier, J. and Burgus, R. (1971). Synthetic TRF (thyrotropin-releasing factor) analogues: II. p-Glu-N^{3im} Me-His.ProNH$_2$: A synthetic analogue with specific activity greater than that of TRF. *Endocrinology*, **89**, 1485

108. Grant, G., Vale, W. and Guillemin, R. (1972). Interaction of thyrotropin-releasing factor with membrane receptors of pituitary cells. *Biochem. Biophys. Res. Commun.*, **46**, 28

109. Wilber, J. F. and Utiger, R. D. (1968). *In vitro* studies on mechanism of action of thyrotropin releasing factor. *Proc. Soc. Exp. Biol. Med.*, **127**, 488

110. Wilber, J. F. (1971). Stimulation of [^{14}C]-glucosamine and [^{14}C]-alanine incorporation into thyrotropin by synthetic thyrotropin-releasing hormone. *Endocrinology*, **89**, 873

111. Vale, W. and Guillemin, R. (1967). Potassium-induced stimulation of thyrotropin release *in vitro*. Requirement for presence of calcium and inhibition by thyroxine. *Experientia*, **23**, 855

112. Vale, W., Burgus, R. and Guillemin, R. (1967). Presence of calcium ions as a requisite for the *in vitro* stimulation of TSH-release by hypothalamic TRF. *Experientia*, **23**, 853

113. Milligan, J. V. and Kraicer, J. (1971). ^{45}Ca uptake during the *in vitro* release of hormones from the rat adenohypophysis. *Endocrinology*, **89**, 766

114. Labrie, F., Lemaire, S. and Courte, C. (1971). Adenosine 3′,5′-monophosphate-dependent protein kinase from bovine anterior pituitary gland. *J. Biol. Chem.*, **246**, 7293

115. Sinha, D. and Meites, J. (1965). Effects of thyroidectomy and thyroxine on hypothalamic control of 'thyrotropin releasing factor' and pituitary content of thyrotropin in rats. *Neuroendocrinology*, **1**, 4

116. Averill, R. L. W., Salaman, D. F. and Worrhington, W. C. Jr., (1966). Thyrotropin releasing factor in hypophyseal portal blood. *Nature (London)*, **211**, 144

117. Jacobs, L. S., Snyder, P. J., Wilber, J. F., Utiger, R. D. and Daughaday, W. H. (1971).

Increased serum prolactin after administration of synthetic TRH in man. *J. Clin. Endocrinol.*, **33**, 996

118. Foley, T. P. Jr., Jacobs, K. S., Hoffman, W., Daughaday, W. H. and Blizzard, R. M. (1972). Human prolactin and thyrotropin concentrations in the serums of normal and hypopituitary children before and after the administration of synthetic thyrotropin-releasing hormone. *J. Clin. Invest.*, **51**, 2143

119. Lu, K-H, Shaar, C. J., Kortright, K. H. and Meites, J. (1972). Effects of synthetic TRH on *in vitro* and *in vivo* prolactin release in the rat. *Endocrinology*, **91**, 1540

120. Tyson, J. E., Friesen, H. G. and Anderson, M. S. (1972). Human lactational and ovarian response to endogenous prolactin release. *Science*, **177**, 897

121. Irie, M. and Tsushima, T. (1972). Increase of serum growth hormone concentration following thyrotropin releasing hormone injection in patients with acromegaly and gigantism. *J. Clin. Endocrinol.*, **35**, 97

122. Eastman, V. J. and Lazarus, L. (1972). The effect of orally administered synthetic thyrotropin-releasing factor on adenohypophyseal function. *Horm. Metab. Res.*, **4**, 158

123. Kastin, A. J., Ehrensing, R. H., Schalch, D. S. and Anderson, M. S. (1972). Improvement in mental depression with decreased thyrotropin response after administration of thyrotropin-releasing hormone. *Lancet*, **2**, 740

124. Plotnikoff, N. P., Prange, A. J. Jr., Breese, G. R., Anderson, M. S. and Wilson, I. C. (1972). Thyrotropin releasing hormone: Enhancement of Dopa activity by a hypothalamic hormone. *Science*, **178**, 417

125. Fuxe, K. and Hokfelt, T. (1969). Catecholamines in the hypothalamus and pituitary gland; *Frontiers in Neuroendocrinology*, 47 (W. Ganong and L. Martini, editors) (New York: Oxford University Press)

126. Lichtensteiger, W. (1969). The catecholamine content of hypothalamic nerve cells after acute exposure to cold and thyroxine administration. *J. Physiol. (London)*, **203**, 675

127. Brown, G. M., Krigstein, E., Dankova, J. and Hornykiewiez, O. (1972). Relationship between hypothalamic and median eminence catechalamines and thyroid function. *Neuroendocrinology*, **10**, 207

128. Spaulding, S. W, Burrow, G. N., Donabedian, R. and Van, M. (1972). L-Dopa suppression of thyrotropin releasing hormone response in man. *J. Clin. Endocr.*, **35**, 182

129. Malarkey, W. B. and Daughaday, W. H. (1972). The influence of Levodopa and adrenergic blockade on growth hormone and prolactin secretion in the MSt TW15 tumor-bearing rat. *Endocrinology*, **91**, 1314

130. Woolf, P. D., Lee, L. A. and Schalch, D. S. (1972). Adrenergic manipulation and thyrotropin-releasing hormone (TRH)-induced thyrotropin (TSH) release. *J. Clin. Endocrinol.*, **35**, 616

131. Khajchara, A. and Kendall, J. W. (1969). Studies on the hypothalamic control of TSH secretion. *Neuroendocrinology*, **5**, 53

132. Averill, R. L. W. (1970). Disappearance of ^{131}I-labelled thyroxin (^{131}I-T_4) from agar pellets implanted in the hypothalamus of rats. *Endocrinology*, **87**, 176

133. Joseph, S. A. and Knigge, K. M. (1972). Neural regulation of TSH secretion: Thyroxine feedback in the newborn. *Neuroendocrinology*, **10**, 197

134. Bakke, J. L., Lawrence, N. and Robinson, S. (1972). Late effects of thyroxine injected into the hypothalamus of the neonatal rat. *Neuroendocrinology*, **10**, 183

135. Kohl, H. H. (1972). Depressed RNA synthesis in the brains and livers of thyroidectomised, normal and hormone injected rats. *Brain Res.*, **40**, 445

136. Emlen, W., Segal, D. S. and Mandell, A. J. (1972). Thyroid state: Effects on pre- and post-synaptic central noradrenergic mechanisms. *Science*, **175**, 79

137. Davidoff, R. A. and Ruskin, H. M. (1972). The effects of microelectrophoretically applied thyroid hormone on single cat central nervous system neurons. *Neurology*, **22**, 467

138. Pierce, J. G. (1971). The subunits of pituitary thyrotropin: their relationship to other glycoprotein hormones. *Endocrinology*, **89**, 1331

139. Reichlin, S. and Utiger, R. D. (1967). Regulation of the pituitary thyroid axis in man: The relationship of TSH concentration to free and total thyroxine level in plasma. *J. Clin. Endocrinol.*, **27**, 251

140. Cotton, G. E., Gorman, C. A. and Mayberry, W. E. (1971). Suppression of thyrotropin

(L-TSH) in serums of patients with myxedema of varying etiology treated with thyroid hormones. *N. Engl., J. Med.* **285**, 529

141. Reichlin, S., Martin, J. B., Boshans, R. L., Schalch, D. S., Pierce, J. G. and Bollinger, J. (1970). Measurement of TSH in plasma and pituitary of the rat by a radioimmuno-assay utilizing bovine TSH: effect of thyroidectomy or thyroxine administration on plasma TSH levels. *Endocrinology*, **87**, 1022

142. Bowers, C. Y., Schally, A. V., Reynolds, G. A. and Hawley, W. D. (1967). Interactions of l-thyroxine or l-tri-iodothyronine and thyrotropin releasing factor on the release and synthesis of thyrotropin from the anterior pituitary gland of mice. *Endocrinology*, **81**, 741

143. Bowers, C. Y., Lee, K. L. and Schally, A. V. (1968). A study on the interaction of the thyrotropin-releasing factor and l-tri-iodothyronine: Effects of puromycin and cycloheximide. *Endocrinology*, **82**, 75

144. Vale, W., Burgus, R. and Guillemin, R. (1967). Competition between thyroxine and TRF at the pituitary level in the release of TSH. *Proc. Soc. Exp. Biol. Med.*, **125**, 210

145. Vale, W., Burgus, R. and Guillemin, R. (1968). On the mechanism of action of TRF: Effects of cycloheximide and actinomycin on the release of TSH stimulated *in vitro* by TRF and its inhibition by thyroxine. *Neuroendocrinology*, **3**, 34

146. Snyder, P. J. and Utiger, R. D. (1972). Inhibition of thyrotropin response to thyro-tropin-releasing hormone by small quantities of thyroid hormones. *J. Clin. Invest.*, **51**, 2077

147. Reichlin, S., Volpert, E. M. and Werner, S. C. (1966). Hypothalamic infiuence on thyroxine monodeiodination by rat anterior pituitary gland. *Endocrinology*, **78**, 302

148. Schadlow, A. R., Surks, M. I., Schwartz, H. I. and Oppenheimer, J. H. (1972). Specific tri-iodothyronine binding sites in the anterior pituitary of the rat. *Science*, **176**, 1252

149. Pastan, I. and Katzen, R. (1967). Activation of adenyl cyclase in thyroid homogenates by thyroid stimulating hormone. *Biochem. Biophys. Res. Commun.*, **29**, 792

150. Zor, U., Kaneko, T., Lowe, I. P., Bloom, G. and Field J. B. (1969). Effect of thyroid stimulating hormone and prostaglandins on thyroid adenyl cyclase activation and cyclic adenosine 3′,5′-monophosphate. *J. Biol. Chem.*, **244**, 5189

151. Wollman, S. H. (1965). Heterogeneity of the thyroid gland. *Current Topics in Thyroid Research* (C. Cassano and M. Andreoli, editors) (New York: Academic Press)

152. Sutherland, E. W. (1972). Studies on the mechanism of hormone action. *Science*, **177**, 401

153. Yamashita, K. and Field, J. B. (1972). Cyclic AMP-stimulated protein kinase pre-pared from bovine thyroid glands. *Metabolism*, **21**, 150

154. Kuo, J. F., Krueger, B. K., Sane, J. R. and Greengard, P. (1970). Cyclic nucleotide-dependent protein kinases. V. Preparation and properties of adenosine 3′,5′-mono-phosphate-dependent protein kinase from various bovine tissues. *Biochim. Biophys. Acta*, **212**, 79

155. Ahn, C. S. and Rosenberg, I. N. (1970). Proteolysis in thyroid slices: Effects of TSH, dibutyryl cyclic 3′,5′-AMP and prostaglandin E. *Endocrinology*, **86**, 870

156. Sato, S., Szabo, M., Kowalski, K. and Burke, G. (1972). Role of prostaglandin in thyrotropin action on thyroid. *Endocrinology*, **90**, 343

157. Yu, S. C., Chang, L. and Burke, G. (1972). Thyrotropin increases prostaglandin levels in isolated thyroid cells. *J. Clin. Invest.*, **51**, 1038

158. Nève, P., Willems, C. and Dumont, J. (1970). Involvement of the microtubule-micro filament system in thyroid secretion. *Exp. Cell Res.*, **63**, 457

159. Douglas, W. W. (1968). Stimulus secretion coupling: the concept and clues from chromaffin and other cells. *Brit. J. Pharmacol.*, **34**, 451

160. Willems, C., Roemans, P. A. and Dumont, J. E. (1971). Stimulation *in vitro* by thyro-tropin, cyclic 3′,5′-AMP, dibutyryl cyclic 3′,5′-AMP and prostaglandin E_1 of secretion by thyroid dog slices. *Biochim. Biophys. Acta*, **222**, 474

161. Kowalski, K., Babiarz, D., Sato, S. and Burke, G. (1972). Stimulatory effects of induced phagocytosis on the function of isolated thyroid cells. *J. Clin. Invest.*, **51**, 2808

162. Chuprinova, S. I. (1967). Effect of the sympathetic nervous system on hormone formation in the thyroid. *Bull. Exp. Biol. Med. (USSR)*, **64**, 937

163. Chuprinova, S. I. (1968). The influence of sympathetic impulses on the secretion of the thyroid hormones. *Dokl. Akad. Sci. USSR*, **179**, 155

164. Kraemer, H. (1968). The consequences of right cervical sympathectomy on thyroid and adrenals in castrated rats. *J. Physiol. (Paris)*, **60**, Suppl. 2, 478

165. Ericson, L. E., Melander, A., Owman, C. and Sundler, F. (1970). Endocytosis of thyroglobulin and release of thyroid hormone in mice by catecholamines and 5-hydroxy tryptamine. *Endocrinology*, **87**, 915

166. Melander, A., Owman, C. and Sundler, F. (1971). TSH-induced appearance and stimulation of amine-containing mast cells in the mouse thyroid. *Endocrinology*, **89**, 528

167. Melander, A. and Sundler, F. (1972). Interactions between catecholamines, 5-hydroxytryptamine and TSH on the secretion of thyroid hormone. *Endocrinology*, **90**, 188

168. Melander, A., Nilsson, E. and Sundler, F. (1972). Sympathetic activation of thyroid hormone secretion in mice. *Endocrinology*, **90**, 194

169. Ericson, L. E., Hakanson, R., Melander, A., Owman, C. and Sundler, F. (1972). TSH-induced release of 5-hydroxytryptamine and histamine from rat thyroid mast cells. *Endocrinology*, **90**, 795

170. Melander, A. and Sundler, F. (1972). Significance of thyroid mast cells in thyroid hormone secretion. *Endocrinology*, **90**, 802

171. Maayan, M. L. and Ingbar, S. H. (1970). Effects of epinephrine on iodide and intermediary metabolism in isolated thyroid cells. *Endocrinology*, **87**, 588

172. Maayan, M. L., Miller, S. L. and Ingbar, S. H. (1971). Effects of serotonin on iodine and intermediary metabolism in isolated thyroid cells. *Endocrinology*, **88**, 620

173. Gross, J. and Pitt-Rivers, R. (1952). The identification of 3:5′,3′-L-tri-iodothyronine in human plasma. *Lancet*, **1**, 439

174. Sterling, K., Bellabarba, D., Newman, E. S. and Brenner, M. A. (1969). Determination of tri-iodothyronine concentration in human serum. *J. Clin. Invest.*, **48**, 1150

175. Chopra, I. J., Solomon, D. H. and Beall, G. N. (1971). Radioimmunoassay for measurement of triiodothyronine in human serum. *J. Clin. Invest.*, **50**, 2033

176. Mitsuma, T., Nihei, N., Gershengorn, M. C. and Hollander, C. S. (1971). Serum triiodothyronine: measurements in human serum by radioimmunoassay with corroboration by gas–liquid chromatography. *J. Clin. Invest.*, **50**, 2679

177. Lieblich, J. and Utiger, R. D. (1972). Triiodothyronine radioimmunoassay. *J. Clin. Invest.*, **51**, 157

178. Larsen, P. R. (1972). Direct immunoassay of triiodothyronine in human serum. *J. Clin. Invest.*, **51**, 1939

179. Fisher, D. A., Chopra, I. J. and Dussault, J. H. (1972). Extrathyroidal conversion of thyroxine to triiodothyronine in sheep. *Endocrinology*, **91**, 1141

180. Braverman, L. E., Ingbar, S. H. and Sterling, K. (1970). Conversion of thyroxine (T_4) to triiodothyronine (T_3) in athyreotic subjects. *J. Clin. Invest.*, **49**, 855

181. Pittman, C. S., Chambers, J. B., Jr. and Read, V. H. (1971). The extrathyroidal conversion rate of thyroxine to triiodothyronine in normal male. *J. Clin. Invest.*, **50**, 1187

182. Sterling, K., Brenner, M. A. and Newman, E. S. (1970). Conversion of thyroxine to triiodothyronine in normal human subjects. *Science*, **169**, 1099

183. Galton, V. A. and Ingbar, S. H. (1966). Observations on the nature of the heat resistant thyroxine deiodinating system of rat liver. *Endocrinology*, **78**, 855

184. Oppenheimer, J. H., Schwartz, H. L., Shapiro, H. C., Bernstein, G. and Surks, M. I. (1970). Differences in primary cellular factors influencing the metabolism and distribution of 3,5,3′-L-tri-iodothyronine and L-thyroxine. *J. Clin. Invest.*, **49**, 1016

185. Oppenheimer, J. H., Koerner, D., Schwartz, H. L. and Surks, M. I. (1972). Specific nuclear triiodothyronine binding sites in rat liver and kidney. *J. Clin. Endocrinol.*, **35**, 330

186. Oppenheimer, J. H. (1972). Thyroid hormones in liver. *Mayo Clin. Proc.*, **47**, 854

187. Tata, J. R. and Windell, C. C. (1966). Ribonucleic acid synthesis during the early action of thyroid hormones. *Biochem. J.*, **98**, 604

188. Schwartz, H. L., Surks, M. I. and Oppenheimer, J. H. (1971). Quantitation of extrathyroidal conversion of L-thyroxine to 3′5,3′-triiodo-L-thyronine in the rat. *J. Clin. Invest.*, **50**, 1124

189. Hollander, C. S., Mitsuma, T., Shenkman, L., Woolf, P. and Gershengorn, M. C. (1972). Thyrotropin releasing hormone: evidence for thyroid response to intravenous injection in man. *Science*, **175**, 209

190. Shimoda, S. and Greer, M. A. (1966). Stimulation of *in vitro* iodothyronine synthesis in thyroid lobes from rats given a low iodine diet, propylthiouracil or TSH *in vivo*. *Endocrinology*, **78**, 715

191. Martin, J. B. (1972). Plasma growth hormone (GH) response to hypothalamic or extrahypothalamic electrical stimulation. *Endocrinology*, **91**, 107

192. Grimm, Y. and Reichlin, S. (1973). Thyrotropin-releasing hormone (TRH): Neurotransmitter regulation of secretion by mouse hypothalamic tissue *in vitro*. *Endocrinology*, **93**, 626

193. Bakke, J. L. and Lawrence, N. (1966). Persistent thyrotropin insufficiency following neonatal thyroxine administration. *J. Lab. Clin. Med.*, **67**, 477

4
The Pituitary Adrenal Cortical System: Stimulation and Inhibition of Secretion of Corticotrophin

F. E. YATES
University of Southern California

J. W. MARAN
Stanford University

G. L. CRYER and D. S. GANN
Johns Hopkins University

4.1 INTRODUCTION

4.1.1 History of interrelations among the brain, pituitary and adrenal

Recognition that the pituitary exerts an influence on adrenal cortical structure and function can be traced to the observation of *Ascoli* and *Legnani* in 1912, who found that the inner zones of the adrenal cortex atrophied following hypophysectomy in dogs[1]. This conclusion was subsequently confirmed by the elegant work of *Smith*[2]. *MacKay* and *MacKay* found that removal of one adrenal was followed by an enlargement (compensatory hypertrophy) of the remaining gland[3], and *Shumacker* and *Firor* demonstrated that this pheno-menon did not occur in hypophysectomised animals[4].

An adrenocorticotrophic hormone (ACTH) was obtained from pituitary extracts during the 1940s, and by 1954 the structure of ACTH had been established[5]. In 1963 the first complete synthesis of the full ACTH molecule was reported[6].

During the 1960s many lines of evidence converged to establish that the anterior, medial, basal hypothalamus stores a substance, still unidentified, that is secreted into the hypothalamic–pituitary portal vascular system, and that stimulates ACTH release (see Ref. 7 for review). This hypothalamic hormone has been designated corticotrophin-releasing hormone (CRH). More generally, any substance that acts on the pituitary to cause ACTH release is referred to as a corticotrophin-releasing factor (CRF). There are many CRFs experimentally demonstrable.

The problem of the identification of CRH is discussed elsewhere in this volume (Chapter 2). Two recent reviews provide more detailed descriptions of the system and extensive bibliographies covering early as well as recent work on the control of ACTH release[8, 9].

4.2 OVERVIEW OF THE PHYSIOLOGICAL CONTROL OF RELEASE OF ACTH

The control of ACTH release has three aspects: (a) the modulation at the pituitary of stimulation of release of ACTH by CRH (see Section 4.3); (b) stimulation of release of ACTH by agents other than CRH (see Section 4.4); and (c) the control of secretion of CRH (see Sections 4.7, 4.8 and 4.9).

Figure 4.1 shows the causal chain between the brain and the target cells for cortisol or corticosterone, and some of the influences that have been thought to modulate the performance of the chain. These influences are discussed in subsequent sections of this review.

Before turning to a consideration of the control of release of ACTH, we wish to consider several properties of ACTH itself, and the corticotropes that synthesise and store it.

4.2.1 Potency of ACTH

A 24 amino acid fragment of ACTH, beginning with the *N*-terminal end of the molecule, has the full potency of the 39 amino acid, natural peptide. The

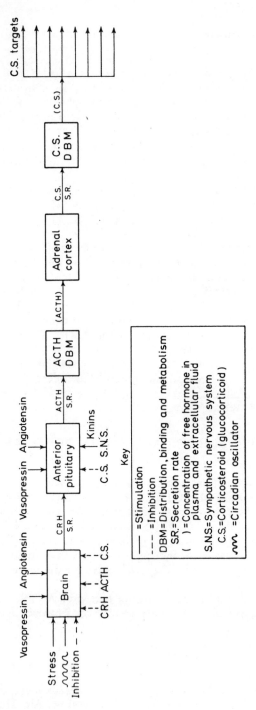

Figure 4.1 The adrenocortical glucocorticoid system. Not all stimulatory and inhibitory influences indicated are known with certainty to be physiologically significant. All can be demonstrated experimentally.

bioassayable potency of natural ACTH, or of the fully-active fragment, varies with the route of administration, but is approximately 100 U mg^{-1}*. The full dynamic range of ACTH concentrations in plasma appears to be approximately the same in all mammals so far studied: 0–100 µU ml^{-1} (0–1 ng ml^{-1}). The concentrations are affected by many variables and show a marked circadian rhythm, as will be discussed later. The usual level reported in unstimulated, normal animals, at the nadir of their circadian rhythm, is *ca.* 0–5 µU ml^{-1} (0–50 pg ml^{-1}).

ACTH may be bound to plasma proteins[11, 12]. If so, the concentration of the unbound, active fraction will have a physiological dynamic range smaller than that for the total concentration in plasma given above.

4.2.2 Localisation of stores of ACTH

The corticotropes of the pituitary that synthesise and store ACTH are present in both the pars distalis and pars intermedia of the adenohypophysis[13-18]. In the rat, injections of exogenous partially-purified ovine hypothalamic CRH are most potent in provoking release of ACTH when given at the junction of the intermedia, or into the pars intermedia itself[19]. The significance of the presence of ACTH in the pars intermedia (or, for that matter, in the basal hypothalamus itself, where it has also been reported) is not clear. *In vitro* corticotropic cells of the pars distalis appear to have most of the responses to stimuli that are associated with physiological release of ACTH *in vivo*.

4.3 MODULATION BY CORTICOSTEROIDS OF THE ACTH-RELEASING RESPONSE TO CRH

4.3.1 Failure to demonstrate corticosteroid inhibition, of release of ACTH at the pituitary

Since it has long been known that exogenous corticosteroids can inhibit release of ACTH[20-22], it was reasonable to consider the possibility that in so doing they acted directly upon the corticotropes of the pituitary. In some studies, however, neither infusions[23, 24], nor crystalline implants[25-28] of corticosteroids directly into the pituitary caused any significant impairment of ACTH release. Furthermore, Egdahl[29] found that dexamethasone (a potent synthetic corticosteroid) could not inhibit hypersecretion of ACTH from isolated pituitaries in dogs with brain tissue removed (to be discussed later).

Hedge and Smelik demonstrated indirectly that the pituitary retains some responsiveness to endogenous CRH in rats 2 h after pretreatment systemically with dexamethasone in doses sufficient to prevent stimulation of endogenous CRH release by certain stimuli which ordinarily provoke it[30]. At first glance, these results seem to suggest that the dexamethasone did not act at the pituitary level to inhibit the system, even though the conditions of the study appear to be similar to those described below in which an impaired response to CRH

---

* The potency of ACTH was defined in bioassay units (U), before the structure and molecular weight of the hormone were known[10].

following dexamethasone can be demonstrated[31]. However, the pituitary may have been inhibited in the studies of Hedge and Smelik. In the absence of comparative tests with and without dexamethasone it is impossible to tell.

4.3.2 Demonstration of corticosteroid inhibition of release of ACTH by an action at the pituitary

Many studies have demonstrated clearly that corticosteroids can act at the pituitary under experimental conditions to diminish or abolish secretion of ACTH. Rose and Nelson infused cortisol into the hypophysial area of unilaterally adrenalectomised rats, and inhibited the ACTH-dependent compensatory adrenal hypertrophy that ordinarily occurs in such animals[32]. Dexamethasone implants in the pituitary have also been reported to decrease adenohypophysial ACTH content[33]. Direct injection of dexamethasone into the anterior pituitary of the rat *in vivo* inhibits ACTH release[31]. In unanaesthetised dogs, dexamethasone given subcutaneously 2 h before stimulation of release of ACTH by micro-injection of exogenous CRH directly into the pituitary, abolishes the ACTH-releasing action of CRH[34]. deWied showed that dexamethasone impaired the release of ACTH provoked by vasopressin, or crude hypothalamic extracts, in rats with lesions of the hypothalamic median eminence[35]. He concluded that corticosteroids can inhibit release of ACTH by an action on the pituitary.

Other data also support the view that corticosteroids act at the pituitary to inhibit release of ACTH. Both pituitary cells in monolayer culture[36], and incubated pituitary glands show corticosteroid inhibition of ACTH release ordinarily provoked by various CRFs and ions[37-42]. Vernikos-Danellis showed that exogenous steroid could suppress the effectiveness of CRFs on the release of ACTH from the pituitary[43]. Furthermore, systemic injections of corticosteroids diminish release of ACTH following CRH, or other CRFs, in animals with parts of the brain damaged or removed so that the source of endogenous CRH is presumably abolished[35, 44, 45]. In such animals, corticosteroids can still cause adrenal atrophy[46, 47], an effect known to require diminution of ACTH secretion. Finally, Kendall and Allen have found that dexamethasone decreased plasma corticosteroid concentrations in hypophysectomised rats with anterior pituitaries transplanted under their renal capsules[48].

The wide variety of data reviewed above definitely establishes that release of ACTH induced by either exogenous or endogenous CRFs or by CRH can be inhibited locally at the pituitary by corticosteroids under some experimental conditions. These results and conclusions raise the possibility that the anterior pituitary may be the site of physiological feed-back inhibition in the adrenal cortical system. Henkin *et al.* found that the anterior pituitary of the cat contained both cortisol and corticosterone at tissue concentrations 800 times higher than those present in plasma[49].

The possibility that corticosteroids may also inhibit the adrenal cortical system by an action on the brain is discussed in Section 4.7.

4.4 STIMULATION OF ACTH RELEASE BY MEANS OTHER THAN CRH

4.4.1 Vasopressin

Some substance present in the neurohypophysis has long been known to result in release of ACTH when it is given systemically[50, 51]. Synthetic vasopressins and their analogues have similar effects[52-55]. Such studies do not localise the point of action of vasopressin in causing stimulation of the adrenal cortical system, and more specific studies have involved direct presentation of vasopressin to pituitary tissue *in vivo* or *in vitro*. Release of ACTH from rat pituitaries incubated *in vitro* is readily stimulated by vasopressin[39]. The peptide hormone also stimulates release of ACTH when it is micro-injected into the pituitaries of unanaesthetised dogs in doses that are ineffective when given intravenously[34]. (However, in anaesthetised rats pretreated with dexamethasone, vasopressin is not effective in provoking release of ACTH when it is injected directly into the anterior pituitary[52, 56-59] except at very high doses[60], presumably because for moderate stimulation by CRFs dexamethasone suppresses release of ACTH by an action at the pituitary, as discussed in the previous section.) Vasopressin is also effective in causing ACTH release in animals with hypothalamic lesions[35, 61] in whom endogenous CRH sources are presumably absent. We conclude that vasopressin is a CRF.

In rats with a genetic defect that prevents synthesis of vasopressin, release of ACTH is only slightly impaired, if at all[62-64]. Neurohypophysectomy also fails to prevent release of ACTH, although its magnitude may be diminished[65-70]. Therefore, it is apparent that vasopressin cannot be CRH, even though it is an experimentally-effective CRF.

Vasopressin appears to potentiate the ACTH-releasing action of CRH itself. When a subthreshold dose (with respect to ACTH release) of vasopressin is placed into the anterior pituitary of rats, it fails to release ACTH itself, but increases 2.5 times the response to exogenous CRH given intravenously[64]. The same study demonstrated that in the mildly dehydrated animal the apparent potency of exogenous CRH is increased, and therefore it is possible that the potentiation is a physiological effect of antidiuretic hormone (vasopressin). Vasopressin also can act at the median eminence to release endogenous CRH (see Section 4.8.1).

4.4.2 Other CRFs

In principle, any number of substances could cause release of ACTH by direct action on the pituitary under experimental conditions, if they damaged corticotropes and caused them to leak stored ACTH. A more interesting group of substances to consider as CRFs are those that might be presented to the pituitary under physiological conditions. In the rat pretreated with pentobarbital and dexamethasone, injections in the pituitary region revealed that 10 ng of histamine caused release of ACTH (but 100 ng did not); 100 ng of spermidine were effective also, and so was angiotensin II at 75 ng. or vasopressin at doses greater than 100 ng[60]. Numerous other substances were shown to be ineffective: e.g. epinephrine, oxytocin, serotonin, norepinephrine, L-Dopa, dopamine, acetylcholine, carbachol, putrescine and bradykinin[60]. Various prostaglandins are also ineffective[71]. The doses of the effective substances are relatively high, either because the dexamethasone pretreatment suppresses the sensitivity of the ACTH-releasing process at the pituitary, as discussed above, or because some of the substances have no physiological action at the site.

Release of ACTH can be provoked by changes in the ionic composition of the medium bathing pituitary tissue *in vitro*. In the presence of ionised calcium increased external potassium ion concentrations are associated with enhanced release of ACTH[72].

4.4.3 Sympathetic innervation of the pituitary, and release of ACTH

In 1959, Story *et al.* made the remarkable discovery that removal of all brain tissues rostral to the mesencephalon in the dog led to sustained hypersecretion of cortisol[73]. The phenomenon has been confirmed in dogs[74-76], in rats[77], and in monkeys with complete removal of the forebrain[78]. In the dog, steroid hypersecretion is not inhibited by barbiturates, but in the rat treated approximately in the same manner, the anaesthetic does inhibit the hypersecretion[77].

In the rat, hypersecretion is also present following isolation of the medial, basal hypothalamus–pituitary complex from the rest of the brain by surgical deafferentation, without brain removal. This preparation can increase the already elevated corticosteroid secretion rate following a variety of stimuli including ether, trauma, immobilisation or application of a tourniquet to the leg[79-83]. Compensatory adrenal hypertrophy can also occur[79]. Similarly, in the dog the hypersecretion following brain removal often can be increased by burn, constriction of the thoracic inferior vena cava, nerve stimulation or haemorrhage[74, 75, 84].

The hypersecretion will continue even in the absence of hindbrain and spinal cord, posterior pituitary, kidneys or abdominal viscera[74, 85]. Apparently, it is provoked by some stimulus acting directly on the pituitary. The failure of dexamethasone to inhibit the hypersecretion in some preparations may mean merely that the hypersecretion results from a very strong stimulus, because it is already known that powerful CRF stimuli can override dexamethasone inhibition of the ACTH releasing process at the pituitary[31, 56, 64]. Alternatively, the stimulus may act distal to the site of action of dexamethasone, or perhaps normal suppression by corticosteroids requires an action at the brain, even though experimentally an action at the pituitary is demonstrable. In any case, the inhibitory effect of dexamethasone at the pituitary saturates before the stimulatory effect of CRH does[64].

A possible explanation of the phenomenon of hypersecretion of corticosteroids in animals with the hypothalamus isolated or removed has been advanced by Gann and Cryer[86]. They showed that the hypersecretion of cortisol which usually follows brain removal in the dog can be prevented by prior extirpation of the cervical sympathetic and nodose ganglia. They also found that expansion of the blood volume prevented or reversed the hypersecretion in 50% of the experiments. They proposed that brain removal releases tonic inhibition of the sympathetic nervous system, which then stimulates pituitary release of ACTH. The sympathetic projection must be directly to the pituitary since hypersecretion does not depend on the presence of any tissue containing CRH. Expansion of the blood volume might inhibit the release of ACTH by increasing inhibition of sympathetic efferents through baroreceptor afferents. The finding that steroid hypersecretion persists even in the absence of the brain and spinal cord does not necessarily exclude a role for the sympathetic nervous system, since the post ganglionic cervical sympathetic nerves may be stimulated by circulating kinins, whose levels may be increased by haemorrhage. Redgate showed that release of ACTH provoked by severe haemorrhage persists after pre-ganglionic section of the cervical sympathetic pathways, and that infusion of bradykinin can induce release of ACTH. He concluded that post-ganglionic sympathetic fibres might be stimulated by circulating kinins under certain circumstances[87], but such an action has never been demonstrated directly.

Allen *et al.* have found that afferent pathways which leave the spinal cord in the thoracic segments mediate the release of ACTH after application of a tourniquet to the legs[88]. They suggested that the pathway might be sympathetic nerves reaching the pituitary. It is remarkable that cervical sympathetic ganglionectomy even prevents the compensatory hypersecretion following unilateral adrenalectomy[89], although it does not prevent the compensatory hypertrophy later.

The above experiments indicate that the sympathetic nervous system might under certain circumstances modulate release of ACTH from the anterior pituitary. Whether it does so through a secretomotor or a vasomotor action is not known. In 1955, Harris summarised the projections of the sympathetic nervous system to the anterior pituitary[90], but he thought they had no secretomotor action. However, in 1959, Smelik emphasised that even a vasomotor action of sympathetics on the pituitary might participate in variations in the release of ACTH[91].

4.5 OVERVIEW OF STIMULATION AND INHIBITION OF RELEASE OF CRH

The only certain physiological stimulus for release of ACTH is hypothalamic CRH and the coupling between input and output at the pituitary is tight, and almost instantaneous. Release of CRH from neurones of the medial basal hypothalamus is a final common pathway for neural control of ACTH release (with the possible exception of the sympathetic pathway to the pituitary discussed previously). The CRH containing neurones can be stimulated or inhibited by neural pathways and transmitters, but hormones (and other chemical agents) acting on the brain can also modulate release of CRH.

Neural and chemical stimulation and inhibition of CRH release will be discussed in detail in Section 4.7.

4.5.1 Localisation of hypothalamic CRH

CRH is stored in synaptosome granules of the hypothalamic median eminence[92]. Almost all hypothalamic extracts reported to be rich in CRH have included the median eminence. Nevertheless, CRH could be synthesised elsewhere, and transported through axon channels to synaptic terminals located in the median eminence. It could even arise from different neurones elsewhere in the brain which discharge CRH into cerebrospinal fluid. Such a discharge has never been proved, but if it occurred, the CRH might be transferred across the ependymal cells lining the floor of the third ventricle, and there be taken up by neurones in the median eminence, or even be transferred directly to the pituitary–portal vascular system[93, 94].

The above conjectures are made very implausible by the experiments of Rethelyi and Halasz[95], who showed that neurones in the surface zone (zona palisadica) of the median eminence do not show terminal axon degeneration after separation of this layer from the rest of the hypothalamus. Apparently the cell bodies and axons of neurones that synthesise and store CRH may be confined to the limited region of the medial basal hypothalamus isolated in these studies in the rat. If so, then many of the chemical and neural influences on release of CRH may take place elsewhere on secondary neurones that synapse with the CRH-containing cells. The dendritic field of the CRH-containing neurone is not known, but it could be extensive. In any case, nerve cells lying outside the zona palisadica in the rat have no axon terminals within it.

Before turning to the details of neural and hormonal or chemical stimulation and inhibition of release of CRH, we wish to consider the general classes of inputs that can activate the adrenocortical system, to aid in the interpretation of the material presented in Sections 4.7–4.9.

4.6 PHENOMENOLOGICAL STIMULATORY INPUTS TO THE ADRENAL CORTICAL SYSTEM: STRESSES AND RHYTHMS

4.6.1 Stresses

We have defined a 'stressor' as any stimulus, internal or external, that ultimately causes increases in secretion rates of CRH, ACTH and corticosteroids to produce a rise in plasma corticosteroid concentrations above the levels found at that time of day in unperturbed subjects on the same sleep/wakefulness cycle. This definition specifically excludes from consideration as stress responses those increases in secretion rate of ACTH that result either from the normal rhythmic inputs to the system (to be described later), or from decreases in the concentration of unbound (free) plasma corticosteroids. Under our definition, the increase in plasma corticosteroid levels observed in pregnancy would be considered a stress response, since both the bound and unbound fractions then increase in absolute magnitude. Therefore, the enhanced production of transcortin, the corticosteroid-binding globulin, known to occur in pregnancy cannot act on the system only by absorbing free corticosteroids in plasma and thereby releasing feed-back inhibition of the system. Under such circumstances the concentration of unbound corticosteroids would be normal or low—contrary to the facts.

In both the basal and stressed states, secretion rates of CRH, ACTH and corticosteroids, and plasma corticosteroid levels are all tightly coupled. The four variables change in the same direction: in the stressed states they all increase together and in the basal states, they vary periodically together.

Stresses which activate the various stimulatory pathways to the CRH-releasing neurones are so numerous that they almost defy listing.

Most stresses studied have been experimental contrivances. However, certain ACTH-releasing stimuli may occur in the lives of free-ranging animals. These include: haemorrhage, pain, hypoglycaemia, cold exposure, fear, overwhelming general sensation of any modality, and pregnancy. The physiological significance of stimulation of the adrenal cortical system in each of these cases remains unknown.

4.6.2 Adrenocortical rhythms

For the past 20 years it has been known that in man the plasma concentration of cortisol rises in the morning and declines subsequently in the afternoon and evening[96, 97]. An adrenocortical rhythm is present in many mammalian species, and is presumably associated with 24 h variations in secretion rates of ACTH and CRH. Plasma concentration of ACTH[98-100] and hypothalamic content of CRH[52, 101, 102] have been shown to exhibit circadian rhythms.

With rapid sampling of blood, it can be shown that the 24 h period in the adrenal cortical system is created by intermittent discharges of CRH and ACTH, and therefore of cortisol and/or corticosterone. Hume was the first to note, in the dog, intermittent bursts of secretion of cortisol, which appeared in the absence of any known stimulus to release ACTH, but which were dependent on ACTH released by the pituitary[103]. He suggested that these 'puffs' of ACTH might serve to maintain the sensitivity of the adrenal cortex to ACTH. Gann[104] has shown that the maintenance of this sensitivity depends upon the integrity of the carotid baroreceptors. Thus, the adrenal cortical system may be coupled to the circulation through this pathway, as well as through some dependence of adrenocortical function on its own local blood flow[105, 106].

In man, also, it is clear that ACTH (and presumably CRH) is released intermittently, in about eight bursts every 24 h[107-109]. These bursts are more frequent during the circadian rise in plasma corticosteroid levels than at other times, when the bursts may be spaced so widely that much of the time adrenal secretion rate is zero. The protein-binding of cortisol in plasma acts as a low-pass filter and smoothes the episodic variations in secretion rates of CRH–ACTH–cortisol–corticosterone into continuous corticosteroid concentration functions possessing a 24 h periodicity. It is not yet clear whether the faster, episodic variations are themselves near-periodic, with a period of *ca.* 3 h, or whether they are truly aperiodic, and merely constitute the mechanism whereby the 24 h rhythm in plasma concentration of corticosteroids is achieved.

4.6.3 Origin of the periodicities in the basal adrenocortical state

The periodic performance of the adrenal cortical system could arise from periodic inputs at the hypothalamic median eminence, or by the action of autonomous oscillators in one of the components of the system (hypothalamic median eminence, pituitary, adrenal cortex, cardiac output or regional blood flows, or metabolic processes for ACTH and cortisol).

Periodic variations in cortisol inactivation or in adrenal sensitivity to ACTH have been reported. Hamster adrenal glands *in vitro* (organ culture) show spontaneous variations in conversion of acetate to corticosterone, without any ACTH input, and these variations constitute a circadian rhythm lasting at least 2 days[110]. However, since it is well known that the adrenal *in vivo* fails to secrete significant amounts of cortisol or corticosterone following hypophysectomy, it is obvious that the reported spontaneous circadian rhythm of the isolated adrenal cortex does not account for the observed circadian rhythm in the intact system. Furthermore, the adrenal secretory response to submaximal doses of ACTH given intravenously in unanaesthetised dogs is nearly the same in the morning as it is in the afternoon (R. E. Miller, J. W. Maran and F. E. Yates, unpublished observations). If a constant infusion of ACTH is given to people, sufficient to elevate plasma corticosteroid levels to the expected peak circadian value, and then is sustained for 4 days, relatively constant plasma glucocorticoid levels result[111] (when sampled four times per day). If the blood flow, metabolism, binding or distribution parameters of the adrenocortical system were varying significantly, it is doubtful that this constancy would be obtained.

We conclude that the intermittent and the 24 h periodic variations in cortisol output levels in man arise from neural input signals to the median eminence, and that the adrenal cortical system is not intrinsically oscillatory.

4.6.4 Circadian variation in magnitude of stress responses

We have emphasised that the circadian variations occur in the basal state of the adrenal cortical system, and that this state is distinct from the stressed state. Nevertheless, the possibility exists that the basal oscillations will affect, in a periodic fashion, the magnitude of responses to random, stress inputs. To determine whether or not the stress-induced increment in plasma corticosteroid levels is of constant value, Gibbs attempted to suppress the circadian variation in basal corticosteroid levels in rats by small doses of dexamethasone, insufficient to prevent the response to the chosen stress (ether anaesthesia)[112]. After the basal circadian rhythm was suppressed, the standard stress produced a larger effect in the afternoon, at the time of the expected circadian peak in basal corticosterone levels. (Being a nocturnal animal, the rat has a rhythm shifted 180 degrees out of phase with that of man.) Gibbs concluded that more ACTH was released following the stress in the afternoon than in the morning. Unfortunately, he used the same dose of dexamethasone in the morning as in the afternoon to inhibit the basal state of the adrenocortical system. Since the basal circadian drive of the system is minimal in the morning, in rats, he should have used less dexamethasone to inhibit the system at that time. The excessive dose in the morning could have contributed to inhibition of the response to stress at that time, and led to the erroneous conclusion that more ACTH was released following stress in the afternoon.

In the morning the basal levels are nearly zero, and little or no dexamethasone would be needed to reduce them.

In man, stresses have been reported to cause more ACTH release when they are applied at the nadir of the basal circadian rhythm[113, 114]. It should be noted, however, that stress responses superimposed upon peak basal levels may saturate the adrenal response to ACTH, so that the magnitude of the stress increment in ACTH may then be under-estimated at the time of the circadian zenith.

We conclude that the question of whether responses to a given stress show circadian variations remains open.

4.7 HORMONAL INHIBITION OF RELEASE OF CRH

4.7.1 Inhibition of release of CRH by CRH

Motta et al. have suggested that hypothalamic-releasing factors may in some fashion inhibit their own release[115]. The suggestion was based upon a study of gonadotrophin secretion. The possibility of inhibition of release of endogenous CRH by CRH itself has never been tested.

4.7.2 Inhibition of release of CRH by ACTH

The possibility that ACTH might in some way lead to inhibition of its own release has often been suggested[116-123]. This action of ACTH does not depend upon increased corticosteroid secretion following stimulation of the adrenal: the effect can be demonstrated in adrenalectomised rats[117]. It could indicate that ACTH inhibits its own release by action at the pituitary itself, as has been suggested, on slender evidence, for the case of melanocyte-stimulating hormone[124]. However, hypothalamic implants of ACTH decrease corticosteroids levels in plasma[119], so ACTH may act at the brain to inhibit release of CRH. (Although the authors initially claimed that they were studying an inhibition of the basal release of CRH, it appears that the conditions were those of a mild stress.)

Most experiments purporting to demonstrate an inhibitory effect of ACTH upon ACTH release have required large doses and long periods of treatment. We know of no evidence that ACTH acts physiologically to adjust the secretion rates of either CRH or ACTH, except through its stimulation of corticosteroid output from the adrenal. Corticosteroids may then modulate releases of both CRH and ACTH, as will be described below.

4.7.3 Inhibition of release of CRH by corticosteroids

Labelled corticosteroids administered systemically are taken up by various regions of the brain, including the hypothalamus, hippocampus and septum[125-130]. Although the uptake could be by glial cells rather than by neurones, McEwen and his co-workers have shown by radioautography that the uptake appears to be in neurones, at least in the hippocampus. Furthermore, since corticosteroids affect brain excitability[131-134] and morphology[135], and can either increase or decrease neuronal firing rates, particularly in the hypothalamus and midbrain[136-140], it seems certain that uptake does occur into neurones. Therefore, corticosteroids might affect adrenocortical function by varying rates of synthesis or release of CRH.

Care must be taken in the evaluation of reports allegedly demonstrating corticosteroid effects on the adrenal cortical system following injections or implantations of dissolved or crystalline corticosteroids into various regions of the brain. Spread of the corticosteroids from brain to the pituitary through cerebrospinal fluid and the pituitary portal system could give misleading results, but such a phenomenon cannot explain all the published results. We will summarise the data obtained from such experiments on the assumption that spread to the pituitary was not responsible for the observations in all of the cases.

Corticosteroids introduced into the midbrain, hypothalamus or septum have repeatedly been shown to inhibit the adrenal cortical system[25,28,31,33,116,141-150] but in two cases implantation of corticosteroids increased basal plasma corticosterone levels in the rat after the steroids were placed in the hippocampus[142,151]. Corticosteroids can increase, have no effect, or decrease firing rates of various neurones in the brain[136-140]. All these findings suggest that corticosteroids might act in several ways on the brain components of the CRH-releasing system. They could inhibit the system either by inhibiting neurones that lead to stimulation of release of CRH, or by stimulating neurones that lead to inhibition.

The following six lines of additional evidence also suggest that corticosteroid inhibition of release of CRH occurs in the brain. McHugh and Smith showed that systemic administration of cortisol in monkeys was more effective in inhibiting release of ACTH following stimulation of the amygdala than following stimulation of the hypothalamus[152]. These results could indicate the existence of a corticosteroid negative feed-back point somewhere in a pathway between the amygdala and the hypothalamus. Hedge and Smelik[30] found that resynthesis of CRH after stimulation of release of CRH by mechanical perturbation of the hypothalamus, prior handling of the animals, or by vasopressin, was inhibited by dexamethasone. Leeman et al. administered corticosteroids systemically and tested responses to a crude hypothalamic CRH preparation. It was equally effective with and without steroid pretreatment[50]. They concluded that the data provided evidence for a central nervous system site for inhibition of the adrenal cortical system by corticosteroids. Yates et al.[64] demonstrated that in experiments with graded doses of dexamethasone, progressive increases in dexamethasone levels will continue to cause progressive inhibition of the response of the adrenal cortical system to a CRH-releasing stimulus, without further affecting the response to CRH itself at the pituitary, after an initial decrease. These results were interpreted as indicating that separate central nervous system and pituitary sites for inhibition of the adrenal cortical system by corticosteroids exist, and that the pituitary sites saturate at lower doses of corticosteroids than do the brain sites. Earlier, Vernikos-Danellis reported results that we believe can be interpreted in the same manner[43]. Takebe et al. showed that administration of steroid led to a decrease in hypothalamic content of CRH[153]. Chowers *et al.* also found decreases in hypothalamic CRH after hypothalamic implantation of dexamethasone and increases in CRH after implantation in the anterior pituitary[33]. These workers concluded that steroids can suppress synthesis of CRH by an action on nervous tissue. If the only effect of the steroids had been at the pituitary, an increased CRH content would have been expected after hypothalamic implantation of dexamethasone.

We believe that all the evidence taken together points to the existence of sites for corticosteroid inhibition of release of ACTH at the pituitary, and for corticosteroid inhibition of synthesis of CRH through actions at several different points in the brain. How many such locations are present in the brain is not known at this time, nor do we know which of the two tissues, brain or pituitary, is the more important site for corticosteroid modulation of the activity of the adrenal cortical system under physiological conditions.

4.8 STIMULATION OF RELEASE OF CRH BY ENDOGENOUS CHEMICAL AGENTS

Makara *et al.* studied the responses of the adrenal cortical system in the rat to various chemical stimuli after antero-lateral or complete deafferentation of the medial basal hypothalamus[154, 155]. They found that even complete neural isolation of the medial basal hypothalamus failed to eliminate the ACTH release provoked by intraperitoneal administration of *E. coli* endotoxin, histamine $(5 \text{ mg} (100 \text{ g body wt.})^{-1})$, insulin, or large subcutaneous doses of formaldehyde. Ether will also stimulate ACTH release in animals with median eminence–pituitary islands[77, 79, 81]. These experiments do not establish the site of action of the stressors, because of the possible existence of a sympathetic neural pathway to the pituitary, discussed earlier.

4.8.1 Vasopressin and release of CRH

Hedge *et al.* showed that in animals pretreated with dexamethasone and morphine, it was possible to abolish the CRF-action of vasopressin, and that then vasopressin placed in the median eminence could activate the adrenal cortical system through stimulation of endogenous CRH release[57]. It is possible that vasopressin is a physiological transmitter activating the CRH-releasing neurone, because it has been shown that the neuronal systems that synthesise vasopressin also send branches into the medial basal hypothalamus[156]. Hedge and Smelik[30] further demonstrated that vasopressin was effective in releasing previously synthesised and stored CRH, but did not stimulate production of new CRH.

4.8.2 Angiotensin and release of CRH

Gann and Egdahl[157] showed that the kidney was not necessary for maximal adrenocortical response to a large haemorrhage, but that constriction of the descending aorta led to increased secretion of cortisol which was prevented by prior nephrectomy. Since this manoeuvre increases blood pressure in the carotid sinuses and aortic arch, it is surprising that it did not inhibit ACTH release, as pressor agents often do[158].

Gann and his associates[86, 159] subsequently showed that although nephrectomy does not change the static gain characteristics of the adrenocortical response to haemorrhage of various magnitudes ranging from 2–30 ml (kg body wt.)$^{-1}$ in anaesthetised dogs, it will do so after dexamethasone pretreatment. In the absence of the kidney, dexamethasone treatment increased both the threshold for the response to haemorrhage and the level at which the maximal response was obtained. The apparent paradox in which the kidney appeared to play no role in the system in the absence of inhibition by steroid, but a very large role in the presence of such inhibition, could be resolved by the hypothesis that angiotensin acts directly on the median eminence to induce release of CRH, but not by the alternative hypotheses that angiotensin acts on the pituitary or on the adrenal.

The hypothesis that angiotensin acts on the median eminence to release CRH, was subjected to experimental tests in dogs in which the anterior pituitary was either isolated, or left with the median eminence, in animals with the rest of the brain removed[160]. Angiotensin was then infused at rates equivalent to its rate of formation in dogs after haemorrhage. The presence of the median eminence was required for angiotensin to activate the adrenal cortical system. However, it is possible that the presence of the median eminence may merely have been necessary to maintain responsiveness of the pituitary to the agent. Earlier it had been suggested that angiotensin acts directly on the pituitary[161, 162], but the experiments did not distinguish between action at the two proposed sites. Hiroshige[60] showed that angiotensin placed into the pituitary of the rat, in very large doses, caused ACTH release but again the site of action is not certain.

The mathematical analyses performed by Gann and his associates[86, 159] have been employed to identify the structure of the adrenal cortical system at its most inaccessible regions. The analysis requires use of the locus of action of angiotensin in activating the system as a marker. Therefore, it is not a trivial matter to find that locus by direct experimentation, and particularly, its relation to the locus of action of dexamethasone.

4.9 NEURAL STIMULATION AND INHIBITION OF RELEASE OF CRH

In Figure 4.2 we present a summary of the stimulatory and inhibitory pathways which are described later.

4.9.1 Techniques for demonstration of neural pathways

Four techniques have been widely used in the identification of possible stimulatory and inhibitory pathways modulating release of CRH. These are: (a) stimulation of the nervous system; (b) lesions of the nervous system; (c) fluorescence studies of the localisation of norepinephrine, dopamine or sero-tonin in the brain; and (d) micro-injection of chemical substances into the brain, including both neural transmitters and blockers of synaptic trans-mission.

4.9.2 Pathways for stimulation of release of CRH

Stimulatory (and inhibitory) pathways for release of CRH have been postu-lated by numerous investigators who have measured changes in blood levels of ACTH or corticosteroids following electrical stimulation at various brain sites. Redgate[163] has reviewed much of this work and pointed out potential problems in interpretation of results. He found prompt increases in levels of ACTH following electrical stimulation of the amygdaloid–septal complex as have other investigators[163-168]. Redgate[163] also found a delayed (5–10 min) stimulatory response following electrical stimulation in a number of sites extending from the medulla to the posterior hypothalamus. There is some evidence for cholinergic mediation of these effects. Shute and Lewis[169] have described an ascending cholinergic neuronal system, partly arising from the substantia nigra and the ventral tegmental area of the midbrain (part of Nauta's[170, 171] 'limbic mid-brain area') and projecting through the hypo-thalamus and subthalamus to the basal fore-brain areas. Some of these fibres appear to enter the hypothalamus anteriorly. Hedge and Smelik[172] blocked the adrenocortical response to surgical and ether stresses by implan-tation of atropine in the anterior hypothalamus, and proposed an excitatory cholinergic pathway. Also, Steiner et al.[137, 139] found that steroid-sensitive neurones in hypothalamus and midbrain are stimulated by acetylcholine and inhibited by norepinephrine and dopamine.

4.9.3 Pathways for inhibition of release of CRH

Electrical stimulation of a number of brain locations leads to inhibition of release of CRH. The best known pathway involves the hippocampus[164-168, 173]. The amygdala[166] and the septum[174] may also inhibit release of CRH; and lesions of the septum lead to either a decrease or an increase, depending on location[175]. Another pathway has been reported, arising from the rostral, basal pre-optic region and entering the medial basal hypothalamus and leading to inhibition of release of CRH[176].

Nauta[170, 171] has traced the extensive interconnections between the limbic structures (which include the above-mentioned inhibitory sites) the hypo-thalamus and the midbrain. There are extensive reciprocal interconnections among the above limbic structures, lateral, medial, posterior and anterior hypothalamus and the 'limbic midbrain area' of Nauta. These connections are mediated principally by the medial forebrain bundle, stria terminalis and medullaris, dorsal longitudinal fasciculus and mammillary peduncle. Nauta and Kuypers have also outlined pathways by which cardiovascular afferents, which have known inhibitory effects on release of CRH, can project to this same 'limbic midbrain area'[171]. Recent evidence from Gann's laboratory[177] has demonstrated a part of a neural link from the cardiovascular system to CRH releasing neurones. Electrical stimulation of neurones in the posterior hypothalamus, which are connected to cardiovascular receptors sensitive to changes in blood volume, causes prompt inhibition of moderately elevated ACTH release. It is possible that this pathway may coincide with the ascending noradrenergic pathway of Fuxe and Hökfelt. Van Loon and his associates[178-181] have produced direct evidence for a noradrenergic inhibitory pathway. Whether or not these three pathways are the same remains to be seen.

4.9.4 Interconnectivity and redundancy of input pathways

The medial basal hypothalamus, anterior hypothalamus, pre-optic area, amygdala, septum and hippocampus are highly interconnected. Through the medial forebrain bundle, and the fornix, the limbic forebrain structures are connected posteriorly to the mammillary bodies, midbrain tegmentum, and to the posterior hypothalamus. Therefore, pathways arising from the forebrain limbic structures may enter the medial basal hypothalamus posteriorly, instead of anteriorly. The map we present in Figure 4.2 is an attempt to provide a compact summary of the connections that we believe influence release of CRH. Obviously, the map conceals the degree of interconnectivity that is present.

It has been reported that anterior pathways leading to CRH release act rapidly, whereas posterior pathways act much more slowly[163]. However, the

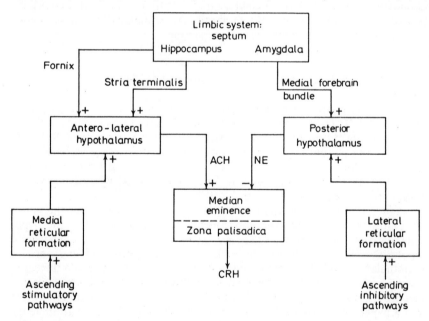

Figure 4.2 Neural input pathways of the adrenocortical system ACH = acetylcholine; NE = norepinephrine

apparent slowness of activation of the system following prolonged stimulation in the midbrain could be the result of a rapid overshoot following cessation of prolonged inhibitory stimulation[177]. At the present time, it is not known how the 'slow' response is processed.

Excellent summaries of the relationships between the limbic system and the medial basal hypothalamus can be found elsewhere[170, 182, 188].

We have found review of studies involving stimulation and lesions of the brain, with respect to effects on release of CRH, very discouraging. The techniques used have not been as refined as those now standard in neurophysiology proper. It is our hope that in the future the neural aspects of neuroendocrinology will be treated with the respect and care that have characterised approaches in modern neurophysiology.

4.9.5 Neurotransmitters in release of CRH

In describing the various stimulatory and inhibitory pathways, we have noted that the stimulatory pathways· may be cholinergic, and inhibitory pathways may be noradrenergic. However, Krieger and Krieger[189] have claimed that carbachol (related to acetylcholine), norepinephrine, serotonin, or γ-aminobutyric acid (GABA), when injected in certain areas of the hypothalamus and limbic system, all can lead to acute rises in plasma corticosteroid levels in adult male cats. It is difficult to interpret such general signs of stimulation. The non-specificity is disturbing. However, other studies have also shown that norepinephrine may be involved in stimulation of CRH secretion[190]. It is of course possible that multisynaptic stimulatory and inhibitory pathways can both employ a particular transmitter at some stage. These somewhat divergent results are perhaps indicative of the complexity of the interactions among various neural 'systems' involved in control of release of CRH.

4.10 THE OSCILLATORY INPUT TO THE ADRENAL CORTICAL SYSTEM

It is now evident that the circadian rhythm of the adrenal cortical system is imposed partly through stimulatory neural pathways entering the anterior regions of the hypothalamus. Lesions in this region abolish the circadian rhythm[79, 82, 191], at least transiently, without abolishing all stress responses. Unfortunately, the location of the pacemaker that imposes the rhythmic input through the anterior hypothalamus is not known. Both anticholinergic and antiserotoninergic agents interfere with the circadian rhythm[189, 192]. It is also possible that the circadian rhythm involves modulations in the inhibitory pathways entering from the posterior hypothalamus, but we have found no direct evidence on the point.

4.10.1 Zeitgeber for the circadian input

Liddle has concluded that the major rhythms in adrenal steroid secretion appear to be related to habitual patterns of activity, and not related in any fixed way to the external environment[193]. He suggests that the sleep/wakefulness schedule confers the apparent circadian rhythmicity on ACTH secretion, though other influences may entrain the adrenal cortical system.

A free-running circadian rhythm in ACTH levels is present in adult, adrenalectomised female rats, living in constant light[194]. Thus the rhythm must arise at early stages of the system, and not at the adrenal gland itself. A free running circadian rhythm is present in plasma corticosterone levels in rats, or in plasma cortisol levels in man under conditions of constant light or constant dark, but alternating light/dark patterns strongly entrain the rhythms[195-197]. Studies in which the sleep/wakefulness cycle was reversed show that as long as constant light is present, cortisol follows the activity cycle regardless of geophysical time.

In blind subjects, cortisol rhythms are abnormal but some relation to sleep/wakefulness patterns still persists[198].

The results and conclusions described above can be summarised in the following propositions:

(a) In man the adrenal cortical system has an endogenous rhythm with a free-running period of *ca*. 24 h.

(b) The sleep/wakefulness activity cycle and the dark/light (but not the light/dark) transition entrain the endogenous rhythm, or may impose a new rhythm on the system without abolishing its endogenous periodicity. In some persons, the two Zeitgeber easily entrain the rhythm, but in others the endogenous rhythm is so strong, or the coupling to the exogenous rhythm so weak, that the exogenous rhythm is merely added to the endogenous rhythm.

(c) When the sleep/wakefulness Zeitgeber and the dark/light Zeitgeber are out of phase with each other, the actions of both are seen, and the cortisol peak will appear at the time of awakening in its normal relationship to the sleep/wakefulness cycle, and another peak will appear when the lights are turned on.

(d) Ordinarily these two Zeitgeber have the same phase relationship to geophysical time and therefore usually reinforce each other.

4.11 PROPERTIES OF THE CORTICOSTEROID MODULATION OF THE ADRENAL CORTICAL SYSTEM

4.11.1 Inhibition, modulation and negative feed-back

Up to this point, we have referred to the inhibitory effects of corticosteroids on release of CRH and ACTH either as 'modulation' or as 'negative feed-back'. However, almost all experiments demonstrating the capcity of corticosteroids to inhibit the adrenocortical responses to stressors have involved administration of pharmacological doses of corticosteroids before the stressors were applied. Obviously, in the natural state, animals cannot increase their corticosteroid levels until after the system has become activated by the stressor. It is not yet clear in a quantitative sense just how effective corticosteroids are in shaping the pattern of corticosteroid secretion rates during an initial stress response.

4.11.2   Delayed level-sensitive and rapid rate-sensitive inhibition by corticosteroids of releases of ACTH and CRH

At any point during an infusion of corticosterone in rats, an injection of ACTH will cause release of endogenous corticosterone. However, if instead of administering ACTH, one injects histamine while the plasma corticosterone levels are low but rising steeply from the infusion, the histamine fails to cause the usual release of CRH–ACTH[199]. The stressor is ineffective until the plasma corticosterone levels have stopped rising and are at their steady, elevated level. One to two hours after attainment of steady-state corticosterone levels, histamine will again activate the system, without inhibition. However, after 2 h, a new period of inhibition appears, and the histamine is once again ineffective.

From the above results it was concluded that the corticosteroid modulation of releases of CRH–ACTH involves a fast rate-sensitive component and a delayed sensitive component. It is not known whether the two components are both present in the brain and in the pituitary. Studies in animals with median eminence lesions have indicated that the pituitary may be one locus of the fast feed-back (M. Jones *et al.* personal communication). Of course, the brain could also possess an independent fast feed-back locus.

Although, in retrospect, it is clear that earlier studies had demonstrated both fast rate-sensitive feed-back and delayed level-sensitive feed-back[200, 201], the existence of these two separate feed-back components was not formally recognised until 1969[199]. The presence of a rapid corticosteroid inhibition of the adrenal cortical system (produced by corticosterone secreted from the rat adrenal in response to stress) has recently been confirmed by Dallman *et al.*[202]

The proposed rate-sensitive characteristic of the fast feed-back, as suggested by Dallman and Yates[199], has been confirmed by Jones *et al.*[203], who repeated, with interesting modifications, the original experiments that defined the rate-sensitive pathway. By means of intermittent infusions of corticosterone in rats, they demonstrated clearly the existence of rapid feed-back inhibition of the system, and its dependence on rates of rise of plasma corticosterone rather than on absolute levels. Their experiments also showed that the rapid feed-back action lasts longer than was estimated by Dallman and Yates. Thus the phenomenon seems firmly established for the anaesthetised rat, but it remains to be seen if it is present in unanaesthetised animals of any species. Because dexamethasone is extremely potent (*ca.* 200 × corticosterone and *ca.* 40 × cortisol), and because the rate-sensitive pathway accommodates rapidly in the presence of high levels of corticosteroids[203], experiments to test for rate sensitivity must be designed with care to ensure their physiological significance.

4.11.3   Relationship between strength of a stressor and the inhibitory effectiveness of corticosteroids in the delayed level-sensitive pathway

In Figure 4.3 we have shown diagrammatically the relationship between the response of the adrenal cortical system to a stressor, the strength of the

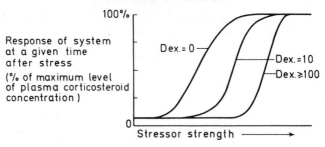

Figure 4.3 Relationships between strength of stressor and degree of negative feed-beck inhibition by corticosteroids. Dex = dexamethasone dose in arbitrary units. (If Dex is present more than 4 h, decreased adrenal sensitivity occurs from lack of stimulation by ACTH, and the maximum level of system output begins to drop.)

stressor, and the inhibitory potency of dexamethasone as a signal in the delayed level-sensitive pathway. It can be seen that the primary effect of dexamethasone is to shift the threshold for response of the system to higher stress levels. Eventually, however, a dose of dexamethasone is reached beyond which no further increase will enhance the inhibition.

Two possible explanations for the failure of dexamethasone to abolish all stress responses, at high doses, have been offered[116, 159, 204]: (a) the receptors for dexamethasone saturate at levels too low to inhibit strong CRH-releasing stimuli at the brain, or stimulation by CRH of release of ACTH at the pituitary; or (b) a corticosteroid-resistant pathway for activation of release of CRH, with a high threshold, might be present. An analysis by computer simulation[205] published in 1967 showed that either hypothesis could explain data of the type presented in Figure 4.3, although this result has been challenged[9].

Whatever the exact structure of the system responsible for data of the type shown in Figure 4.3, it appears that the delayed level-sensitive corticosteroid inhibitory pathway impinges upon both the brain and the pituitary, and that the dose of dexamethasone required to saturate the pathway at the pituitary is lower than that required to saturate its effects at the brain[64]. The effects of corticosteroids at the pituitary are probably important only during variations of corticosteroid concentrations in the lower ranges. In higher ranges, only the brain can still respond to variations in corticosteroid levels. Therefore it is possible that the brain and the pituitary together constitute multistage feedback loci for corticosteroids in the basal circadian rhythm range of operation of the system. However, during stress responses occurring at the circadian peak, only the brain elements might have sufficient, residual sensitivity to changes in corticosteroid levels, to modulate responses of the system. These conjectures require experimental validation.

Iproniazid (a monoamine oxidase inhibitor) increases the degree of inhibition of the adrenocortical system in the presence of dexamethasone and strong stresses, even when it fails to act as an inhibitor by itself[116, 159]. This result might mean that corticosteroids depress the system through stimulation of a noradrenergic inhibitory pathway that becomes more potent when inactivation of its transmitter is impaired.

4.12   MEMORY EFFECTS IN THE ADRENAL CORTICAL SYSTEM

4.12.1   Memory at the adrenal

Stimulation of the adrenal cortex by ACTH alters the responsiveness of the
adrenal cortex to subsequent ACTH stimulation. If a step input of ACTH is
presented from a zero-level baseline, sustained for *ca.* 1 h, and then removed,
the response to a subsequent similar step of ACTH will be less than the first,
if only 5 min is allowed for recovery, but it will be like the first if 40 min of
recovery is allowed[206-208]. Over longer time domains, the effect of a prior
stimulation by ACTH is to render the adrenal more responsive to subsequent
ACTH[111].

4.12.2   Memory effects from a previous stress

Recently, Dallman and Jones have shown that a prior stress response leaves a
trace effect on the response to a subsequent stress[209]. They noted that changes
in plasma corticosterone concentration in rats were as great (or greater)
during the second response to a stressor, as they were during the first response.
However, if the plasma corticosterone transient created during the first stress
response was mimicked by infusions of corticosterone in the absence of the
first stress, then the response to the stressor given subsequently was inhibited.
The authors concluded that the response to a first stress leaves the adrenal
cortical system in a hyperexcitable state, so that it would be hyper-responsive
to a subsequent stress were it not for the inhibitory effects of the increase in
corticosteroid levels associated with the first stress response. The corticosteroid inhibition approximately balances the hyperexcitability, so that a
second stress response appears to be about the same as the first. Further, in
adrenalectomised animals the release of ACTH following a second stress is
augmented[202]. The memory effects appear to involve the delayed level-
sensitive characteristics of the adrenal cortical system.

4.13   CONCLUSION

Combining the diagrams in Figures 4.1 and 4.2 provides a representation of
the complete adrenal cortical system. To achieve that synthesis, specific
assignment of the locations of corticosteroid feed-back sites in the brain to
elements shown in Figure 4.2 would be necessary, but we cannot make the
designations with assurance, for reasons that are obvious from the evidence
in Sections 4.7, 4.9, 4.11 and 4.12. The structure of the central parts of the
system remains uncertain, and the apparent structure can change in time.
   Whatever the extent of uncertainty about the central arrangements of the
adrenal cortical system, that confusion is not nearly as galling as is the failure,
after half a century of endeavour, to determine the physiological function of
the activation of the adrenal cortical system that can occur during or following
noxious stimuli such as haemorrhage, sensory overload, cold exposure, final
examinations, or the writing of a review article under a deadline.

Acknowledgements

We wish to thank Dr. Mary F. Dallman for helpful criticisms and comments during preparation of this manuscript.

References

1. Ascoli, G. and Legnani, T. (1912). Die Folgen der Existirpation der Hypophyse, *Münch med. Wschr.*, **59**, 518
2. Smith, P. E. (1930). Hypophysectomy and replacement therapy in the rat, *Amer. J. Anat.*, **45**, 205
3. MacKay, E. M. and MacKay, L. L. (1926). Compensatory hypertrophy of the adrenal cortex, *J. Expt. Med.*, **43**, 395
4. Shumacker, H. B. Jr. and Firor, W. M. (1934). The inter-relationship of the adrenal cortex and the anterior lobe of the hypophysis. *Endocrinology*, **18**, 676
5. Bell, P. H. (1954). Purification and structure of β-corticotrophin, *J. Amer. Chem. Soc.*, **76**, 5565
6. Schwyzer, R. and Siber, P. (1963). Total synthesis of adrenocortitrophic hormone, *Nature (London)*, **199**, 172
7. Yates, F. E. and Urquhart, J. (1962). Control of plasma concentrations of adreno-cortical hormones, *Physiol. Rev.*, **42**, 359
8. Yates, F. E. and Maran, J. W. (1974). Stimulation and inhibition of adrenocortico-tropin (ACTH) release. *Handbook of Physiology*, Vol. '*Hypothalamo-Hypophysial System*', (W. Sawyer and E. Knobil, editors) (Baltimore: Amer. Physiol. Soc.)
9. Gann, D. S. and Cryer, G. L. (1972). Models of adrenal cortical control, *Advan. Biomed. Engineer*, **2**, 1
10. Sayers, G. and Travis, R. H. (1970). Adrenocorticotropic hormone; adrenocortical steroids and their synthetic analogs, *The Pharmacological Basis of Therapeutics; a Textbook of Pharmacology, Toxicology and Therapeutics for Physicians and Medical Students*, 4th edn, 1610, (L. S. Goodman and A. Gilman, editors) (London: Macmillan)
11. Werder, K. V. von, Schwartz, K. and Scriba, P. C. (1968). Serumprotein-bindung von ACTH. I. Untersuchungen mit Dextrangelfiltration und ³H-ACTH, *Klin. Wochenschr.*, **46**, 940
12. Werder, K. V. von, Kluge, F., Schwartz, K. and Scriba, P. C. (1968). Serumprotein-bindung von ACTH. II. Untersuchungen mit Dichtegradientenzentrifugation und ³H-ACTH. *Klin. Wochenschr.*, **46**, 1028
13. Moriarty, G. C. (1972). Ultrastructural localization and study of adrenocorticotropin-producing cells with the use of immunocytochemical techniques (abstract), *Anat. Rec.*, **172**, 370
14. Baker, B. L., Pek, S., Midgley, A. R. Jr. and Gersten, B. E. (1970). Identification of the corticotropin cell in rat hypophyses with peroxidase-labelled antibody, *Anat. Rec.*, **166**, 557
15. Porte, A., Klein, J. M., Stoeckel, M. E. and Stutinsky, F. (1971). Sur l'existence de cellules de type corticotrope dans la pars intermedia de l'hypophyse du rat, *Z. Zellforsch*, **115**, 60
16. Phifer, R. F. and Spicer, S. S. (1970). Immunohistologic and immunopathologic demonstration of adrenocorticotropic hormone in the pars intermedia of the adeno-hypophysis, *Lab. Invest.*, **23**, 543
17. Gosbee, J. L., Kraicer, J., Kastin, A. J. and Schally, A. V. (1970). Functional relation-ship between the pars intermedia and ACTH secretion in the rat, *Endocrinology*, **86**, 560
18. Stoeckel, M. E., Dellmann, H.-D., Porte, A. and Gertner, C. (1971). The rostral zone of the intermediate lobe of the mouse hypophysis, a zone of particular concentration of corticotrophic cells, *Z. Zellforsch.*, **122**, 310
19. Wei, E., Maran, J. W., Dhariwal, A. P. S. and Yates, F. E. (1973). Regional responses

of the pituitary to corticotropin-releasing factor (CRF) and ammonium ions, *Endocrinology*, **92**, 710

20. Ingle, D. J. and Kendall, E. C. (1937). Atrophy of the adrenal cortex of the rat produced by the administration of large amounts of cortin, *Science*, **86**, 245

21. Ingle, D. J. and Higgens, G. M. (1938). Regeneration of the adrenal gland following enucleation. *Amer. J. Med. Sci.*, **196**, 232

22. Ingle, D. J., Higgens, G. M. and Kendall, E. C. (1938). Atrophy of the adrenal cortex in the rat produced by administration of large amounts of cortin. *Anat. Rec.*, **71**, 363

23. Kendall, J. W. (1962). Studies on inhibition of corticotropin and thyrotropin release utilizing microinjections into the pituitary, *Endocrinology*, **71**, 452

24. Stark, E., Gyévai, A., Acs, Zs., Szalay, K. Sz. and Varga, B. (1968). The site of the blocking action of dexamethasone on ACTH secretion: *In vivo* and *in vitro* studies, *Neuroendocrinology*, **3**, 275

25. Corbin, A., Mangili, G., Motta, M. and Martini, L. (1965). Effect of hypothalamic and mesencephalic steroid implantations on ACTH feedback mechanisms, *Endocrinology*, **76**, 811

26. Endröczi, E., Lissák, K. and Tekeres, M. (1961). Hormonal 'feed-back' regulation of pituitary-adrenocortical activity, *Acta. Physiol. Acad. Sci. Hung.*, **18**, 291

27. Feldman, S., Conforti, N. and Davidson, J. M. (1966). Adrenocortical responses in rats with corticosteroid and reserpine implants, *Neuroendocrinology*, **1**, 228

28. Smelik, P. G. and Sawyer, C. H. (1962). Effects of implantation of cortisol into the brain stem or pituitary gland on the adrenal response to stress in the rabbit. *Acta Endocrinologica*, **41**, 561

29. Egdahl, R. H. (1964). The acute effects of steroid administration on pituitary adrenal secretion in the dog, *J. Clin. Invest.*, **43**, 2178

30. Hedge, G. A. and Smelik, P. G. (1969). The action of dexamethasone and vasopressin on hypothalamic CRF production and release, *Neuroendocrinology*, **4**, 242

31. Russell, S. M., Dhariwal, A. P. S., McCann, S. M. and Yates, F. E. (1969). Inhibition by dexamethasone of the *in vivo* pituitary response to corticotropin-releasing factor (CRF), *Endocrinology*, **85**, 512

32. Rose, S. and Nelson, I. (1956). Hydrocortisone and ACTH release, *Aust. J. Exp. Biol. Med. Sci.*, **34**, 77

33. Chowers, I., Conforti, N. and Feldman, S. (1967). Effects of corticosteroids on hypothalamic corticotropin releasing factor and pituitary ACTH content, *Neuroendocrinology*, **2**, 193

34. Gonzalez-Luque, A., L'Age, M., Dhariwal, A. P. S. and Yates, F. E. (1970). Stimulation of corticotropin release by corticotropin-releasing factor (CRF) or by vasopressin following intrapituitary infusions in unanesthetized dogs: Inhibition of the responses by dexamethasone, *Endocrinology*, **86**, 1134

35. deWied, D. (1964). The site of the blocking action of dexamethasone on stress-induced pituitary ACTH release, *J. Endocrinology*, **29**, 29

36. Fleischer, N. and Rawls, W. E. (1970). ACTH synthesis and release in pituitary monolayer culture: effect of dexamethasone, *Amer. J. Physiol.*, **219**, 445

37. Arimura, A., Bowers, C. Y., Schally, A. V., Saito, M. and Miller, M. C. (1969). Effect of corticotropin-releasing factor, dexamethasone and actinomycin D on the release of ACTH from rat pituitaries *in vivo* and *in vitro*, *Endocrinology*, **85**, 300

38. Berthold, K., Arimura, A. and Schally, A. V. (1970). Effect of 6-dehydro-16-methylene hydrocortisone and dexamethasone on the release of ACTH from rat pituitary glands, *in vitro*, *Acta Endocrinologica*, **63**, 431

39. Fleischer, N. and Vale, W. (1968). Inhibition of vasopressin-induced ACTH release from the pituitary by glucocorticoids *in vitro*, *Endocrinology*, **83**, 1232

40. Kraicer, J., Milligan, J. V., Gosbee, J. L., Conrad, R. G. and Branson, C. M. (1969). Potassium, corticosterone, and adrenocorticotropic hormone release *in vitro*, *Science*, **164**, 426

41. Kraicer, J. and Milligan, J. V. (1970). Suppression of ACTH release from adenohypophysis by corticosterone: an *in vitro* study, *Endocrinology*, **87**, 371

42. Pollock, J. J. and La Bella, F. S. (1966). Inhibition by cortisol of ACTH release from anterior pituitary tissue *in vitro*, *Canad. J. Physiol.*, *Pharmacol.*, **44**, 549

43. Vernikos-Danellis, J. (1964). Estimation of corticotropin releasing activity of rat hypothalamus and neurohypophysis before and after stress, *Endocrinology*, **75**, 514

44. Dunn, J. and Critchlow, V. (1969). Feedback suppression of 'non-stress' pituitary adrenal function in rats with forebrain removed, *Neuroendocrinology*, **4**, 296

45. Dunn, J. and Critchlow, V. (1969). Feedback suppression of pituitary-adrenal function in rats with pituitary islands, *Life Sci.*, **8**, 9

46. Ganong, W. F. and Hume, D. M. (1955). Effect of hypothalamic lesions on steroid-induced atrophy of the adrenal cortex in the dog, *Proc. Soc. Exp. Biol. Med.*, **88**, 528

47. McCann, S. M., Fruit, A. and Fulford, B. D. (1958). Studies on the loci of action of cortical hormones in inhibiting the release of adrenocorticotrophin, *Endocrinology*, **63**, 29

48. Kendall, J. W. and Allen, C. (1968). Studies on the glucocorticoid feedback control of ACTH secretion, *Endocrinology*, **82**, 397

49. Henkin, R. I., Casper, A. G. T., Brown, R., Harlan, A. B. and Bartter, F. C. (1968). Presence of corticosterone and cortisol in the central and peripheral nervous system of the cat, *Endocrinology*, **82**, 1058

50. Leeman, S. E., Glenister, D. W. and Yates, F. E. (1962). Characterization of a calf hypothalamic extract with adrenocorticotropin-releasing properties: Evidence for a central nervous system site for corticosteroid inhibition of adrenocorticotropin release, *Endocrinology*, **70**, 249

51. Rumsfeld, H. W. and Porter, J. C. (1962). ACTH-releasing activity of bovine posterior pituitaries, *Endocrinology*, **70**, 62

52. Cheifetz, P. N., Gaffud, N. T. and Dingman, J. F. (1969). The effect of lysine vaso-pressin and hypothalamic extracts on the rate of corticosterone secretion in rats treated with dexamethasone and pentobarbitone, *J. Endocrinology*, **43**, 521

53. Arimura, A., Schally, A. V. and Bowers, C. Y. (1969). Corticotropin releasing activity of lysine vasopressin analogues, *Endocrinology*, **84**, 579

54. Doepfner, W., Stürmer, E. and Berde, B. (1963). On the corticotrophin-releasing activity of synthetic neurohypophysial hormones and some related peptides, *Endocrinology*, **72**, 897

55. Hilton, J. G., Scian, L. F., Westermann, C. D. and Kruése, O. R. (1959). Effect of synthetic lysine vasopressin on adrenocortical secretion, *Proc. Soc. Exp. Biol. Med.*, **100**, 523

56. Dhariwal, A. P. S., Russell, S. M., McCann, S. M. and Yates, F. E. (1969). Assay of corticotropin-releasing factors by injection into the anterior pituitary of intact rats, *Endocrinology*, **84**, 544

57. Hedge, G. A., Yates, M. B., Marcus, R. and Yates, F. E. (1966). Site of action of vasopressin in causing corticotropin release, *Endocrinology*, **79**, 328

58. Hiroshige, T., Kunita, H., Ogura, C. and Itoh, S. (1968). Effects on ACTH release of intrapituitary injections of posterior pituitary hormones and several amines in the hypothalamus, *Jap. J. Physiol.*, **18**, 609

59. Hiroshige, T. (1970). Role of vasopressin in the regulation of ACTH secretion: Studies with intrapituitary injection technique, *Med. J. Osaka University*, **21**, 161

60. Hiroshige, T. (1973). Assay of corticotropin releasing factor, *Brain–Pituitary Adrenal Interrelationships*, (A. Brodish and E. S. Redgate, editors) (Basle: Karger)

61. McCann, S. M. and Fruit, A. (1957). Effect of synthetic vasopressin on release of adrenocorticotrophin in rats with hypothalamic lesions, *Proc. Soc. Exp. Biol., Med.* **96**, 566

62. Arimura, A., Saito, T., Bowers, C. Y. and Schally, A. V. (1967). Pituitary-adrenal activation in rats with hereditary hypothalamic diabetes insipidus, *Acta Endocrinologica*, **54**, 155

63. McCann, S. M., Antunes-Rodrigues, J., Nallar, R. and Valtin, H. (1966). Pituitary-adrenal function in the absence of vasopressin, *Endocrinology*, **79**, 1058

64. Yates, F. E., Russell, S. M., Dallman, M. F., Hedge, G. A., McCann, S. M. and Dhari-wal, A. P. S. (1971). Potentiation by vasopressin of corticotropin release induced by corticotropin-releasing factor, *Endocrinology*, **88**, 3

65. Arimura, A., Yamaguchi, T., Yoshimura, K., Imazeki, T. and Itoh, S. (1965). Role of the neurohypophysis in the release of adrenocorticotrophic hormone in the rat, *Jap. J. Physiol.*, **15**, 278

66. deWied, D. (1961). The significance of the antidiuretic hormone in the release mechanism of corticotropin, *Endocrinology*, **68**, 956

67. deWied, D. (1968). Influence of vasopressin and of a crude CRF preparation on pituitary ACTH-release in posterior-lobectomized rats, *Neuroendocrinology*, **3**, 129
68. Itoh, S., Nishimura, Y., Yamamoto, M. and Takahashi, H. (1964). Adrenocortical response to epinephrine in neurohypophysectomized rats, *Jap. J. Physiol.*, **14**, 177
69. Nowell, N. W. (1959). Studies in the activation and inhibition of adrenocorticotrophin secretion. *Endocrinology*, **64**, 191
70. Smelik, P. G., Gaarenstroom, J. H., Konijnendijk, W., and deWied, D. (1962). Evaluation of the role of the posterior lobe of the hypophysis in the reflex secretion of corticotrophin, *Acta Physiol. Pharmacol. Neerl.*, **11**, 20
71. Hedge, G. A. (1972). The effects of prostaglandins on ACTH secretion, *Endocrinology*, **91**, 925
72. Kraicer, J., Milligan, J. V., Gosbee, J. L., Conrad, R. G. and Branson, C. M. (1969). *In vitro* release of ACTH: Effects of potassium, calcium and corticosterone, *Endocrinology*, **86**, 863
73. Story, J. L., Melby, J. C., Egdahl, R. H. and French, L. A. (1959). Adrenal cortical function following stepwise removal of the brain in the dog. *Amer. J. Physiol.*, **196**, 583
74. Egdahl, R. H. (1962). Further studies on adrenal cortical function in dogs with isolated pituitaries, *Endocrinology*, **71**, 926
75. Egdahl, R. H. (1960). Adrenal cortical and medullary responses to trauma in dogs with isolated pituitaries, *Endocrinology*, **66**, 200
76. Wise, B. L., Van Brunt, E. E. and Ganong, W. F. (1963). Effect of removal of various parts of the brain on ACTH secretion in dogs, *Proc. Soc. Exp. Biol. Med.*, **112**, 792
77. Greer, M. A. and Rockie, C. (1968). Inhibition of pentobarbital of ether-induced ACTH secretion in the rat, *Endocrinology*, **83**, 1247
78. Kendall, J. W. and Roth, J. G. (1969). Adrenocortical function in monkeys after forebrain removal or pituitary stalk section. *Endocrinology*, **84**, 686
79. Halász, B., Slusher, M. A. and Gorski, R. A. (1967). Adrenocorticotropic hormone secretion in rats after partial or total deafferentation of the medial basal hypothalamus, *Neuroendocrinology*, **2**, 43
80. Kendall, J. W. Jr., Matsuda, K., Duyck, C. and Greer, M. A. (1964). Studies of the location of the receptor site for negative feedback control of ACTH release, *Endocrinology*, **74**, 279
81. Dunn, J. and Critchlow, V. (1969). Pituitary–adrenal response to stress in rats with hypothalamic islands, *Brain Res.*, **16**, 395
82. Palka, Y., Coyer, D. and Critchlow, V. (1969). Effects of isolation of medial basal hypothalamus on pituitary–adrenal and pituitary–ovarian functions, *Neuroendocrinology*, **5**, 333
83. Greer, M. A., Allen, C. F., Gibbs, F. P. and Gullickson C. (1970). Pathways at the hypothalamic level through which traumatic stress activates ACTH secretion, *Endocrinology*, **86**, 1404
84. Egdahl, R. H. (1961). Corticosteroid secretion following caval constriction in dogs with isolated pituitaries, *Endocrinology*, **68**, 226
85. Ganong, W. F. (1963). The central nervous system and the synthesis and release of adrenocorticotropic hormone, *Advances in Neuroendocrinology*, pp. 92–157 (A. V. Nalbandov, editor) (Urbana: University of Illinois Press)
86. Gann, D. S. and Cryer, G. L. (1973). Feedback control of ACTH secretion by cortisol, *Brain-Pituitary Adrenal Interrelationships*, (A. Brodish and E. S. Redgate, editors) (Basel: Karger)
87. Redgate, E. S. (1968). Role of the baroreceptor reflexes and vasoactive polypeptides in the corticotropin release evoked by hypotension, *Endocrinology*, **82**, 704
88. Allen, J. P., Allen, C. F. and Greer, M. A. (1972). Demonstration of two discrete spinal cord pathways through which stress stimulates ACTH secretion, *Clin. Res.*, **20**, 215 (Abstract)
89. Fendler, K. and Endröczi, E. (1965). Changes of adrenal compensatory hypertrophy in the rat after removal of the sympathetic superior cervical ganglia, *Acta Physiol. Acad. Sci. Hung.*, **28**, 171
90. Harris, G. W. (1955). *Neural Control of the Pituitary Gland*, (London: Edward Arnold)
91. Smelik, P. G. (1959). Autonomic nervous involvement in stress-induced ACTH secretion, (PhD. dissertation), Rijksuniversiteit te Groningen, N. V. Drukkerij, V/H. H. Born, Assen.

92. Mulder, A. H., Gueze, J. J. and deWied, D. (1970). Studies on the subcellular localization of corticotrophin releasing factor (CRF) and vasopressin in the median eminence of the rat, *Endocrinology*, **87**, 61
93. Yates, F. E., Russell, S. M. and Maran, J. W. (1971). Brain adenohypophysial communication in mammals, *Ann. Rev. Physiol.*, **33**, 393
94. Ondo, J. G., Mical, R. S. and Porter, J. C. (1972). Passage of radioactive substances from CSF to hypophysial portal blood, *Endocrinology*, **91**, 1239
95. Réthelyi, M. and Halász, B. (1970). Origin of the nerve endings in the surface zone of the median eminence of the rat hypothalamus, *Exp. Brain Res.*, **11**, 145
96. Bliss, E. L., Sandberg, A. A., Nelson, D. H. and Eik-Nes, K. (1953). The normal levels of 17-hydroxycorticosteroids in the peripheral blood in man, *J. Clin. Invest.*, **32**, 818
97. Migeon, C. J., Tyler, F. H., Mahoney, J. P., Florentin, A. A., Castle, H., Bliss, E. L. and Samuels, L. T. (1956). The diurnal variation of plasma levels and urinary excretion of 17-hydroxycorticosteroids in normal subjects, night workers, and blind subjects, *J. Clin. Endocrinol., Metab.*, **17**, 1051
98. Berson, S. A. and Yalow, R. S. (1968). Radioimmunoassay of ACTH in plasma, *J. Clin. Invest.*, **47**, 2725
99. Demura, H., West, C. D., Nugent, C. A., Nakagawa, K. and Tyler, F. H. (1966). A sensitive radioimmunoassay for plasma ACTH levels, *J. Clin. Endocrinol. Metab.*, **26**, 1297
100. Conroy, R. T. W. L. and Mills, J. N. (1970). *Human Circadian Rhythms*, (London: J. & A. Churchill)
101. David-Nelson, M. A. and Brodish, A. (1969). Evidence for a diurnal rhythm of corticotrophin-releasing factor (CRF) in the hypothalamus, *Endocrinology*, **85**, 861
102. Hiroshige, T., Sakakura, M. and Itoh, S. (1969). Diurnal variation of corticotropin-releasing activity in the rat hypothalamus, *Endocrinol. Jap.*, **16**, 465
103. Hume, D. M. (1958). The method of hypothalamic regulation of pituitary and adrenal secretion in response to trauma, *Patho-physiologia Diencephalica*, pp. 217–228, (S. B. Curri and L. Martini, editors) (Wein: Springer-Verlag)
104. Gann, D. S. (1966). Carotid vascular receptors and control of adrenal corticosteroid secretion, *Amer. J. Physiol.*, **211**, 193
105. Urquhart, J. (1965). Adrenal blood flow and the adrenocortical response to corticotropin, *Amer. J. Physiol.*, **209**, 1162
106. L'Age, M., Gonzalez-Luque, A. and Yates, F. E. (1970). Adrenal blood flow dependence of cortisol secretion rate in the unanaesthetized dog. *Amer. J. Physiol.*, **219**, 281
107. Hellman, L., Nakada, F., Curti, J., Weitzman, E. D., Kream, J., Roffwarg, H., Ellman, S., Fukushima, D. K. and Gallagher, T. G. (1970). Cortisol is secreted episodically by normal man, *J. Clin. Endocrinol. Metab.*, **30**, 411
108. Krieger, D. T., Allen, W., Rizzo, F. and Krieger, H. P. (1971). Characterization of the normal temporal pattern of plasma corticosteroid levels, *J. Clin. Endocrinol. Metab.*, **32**, 266
109. Tourniaire, J., Orgiazzi, J., Riviere, J. F., and Rousset, H. (1971). Repeated plasma cortisol determinations in Cushing's syndrome due to adrenocortical adenoma, *J. Clin. Endocrinol. Metab.*, **32**, 666
110. Andrews, R. V. and Folk, G. E. Jr. (1964). Circadian metabolic patterns in cultured hamster adrenal glands, *Comp. Biochem. Physiol.*, **11**, 393
111. Nugent, C. A., Eik-Nes, K., Samuels, L. T. and Tyler, F. H. (1959). Changes in plasma levels of 17-hydroxycorticosteroids during the intravenous administration of adrenocorticotropin (ACTH). IV. Response to prolonged infusions of small amounts of ACTH, *J. Clin. Endocrin. Metab.*, **19**, 334
112. Gibbs, F. P. (1970). Circadian variation of ether-induced corticosterone secretion in the rat, *Amer. J. Physiol.*, **219**, 288
113. Clayton, G. W., Librik, L., Gardner, R. L. and Guillemin, R. (1963). Studies on the circadian rhythm of pituitary adrenocorticotropic release in man. *J. Clin. Endocrinol. Metab.*, **23**, 975
114. Takebe, K., Setaiski, C., Hirama, M., Yamamoto, M. and Horiuchi, Y. (1966). Effects of a bacterial pyrogen on the pituitary–adrenal axis at various times in the 24-hours, *J. Clin. Endocrinol. Metab.*, **26**, 437
115. Motta, M., Fraschini, F. and Martini, L. (1969). 'Short' feedback mechanisms in the

control of anterior pituitary function, *Frontiers in Neuroendocrinology*, pp. 211–253, (W. F. Ganong, and L. Martini, editors) (London: Oxford University Press)

116. Dallman, M. F. and Yates, F. E. (1968). Anatomical and functional mapping of central neural input and feedback pathways of the adrenocortical system, *Mem. Soc. Endocrinol. (London)*, **17**, 39

117. Hodges, J. R. and Vernikos. J. (1959). Circulating corticotropin in normal and adrenalectomized rats after stress, *Acta Endocrinol.*, **30**, 188

118. Kitay, J. I., Holub, D. A., and Jailer, J. W. (1959). Inhibition of pituitary ACTH release: an extraadrenal action of exogenous ACTH, *Endocrinology*, **64**, 475

119. Motta, M., Mangili, G. and Martini, L. (1965). A 'short' feedback loop in the control of ACTH secretion, *Endocrinology*, **77**, 392

120. Motta, M., Sterescu, N., Piva, F. and Martini, L. (1969). The participation of 'short' feedback mechanisms in the control of ACTH and TSH secretion, *Acta Neurol. Belg.*, **69**, 501

121. Plager, J. E. and Cushman, P. Jr. (1962). Suppression of the pituitary–ACTH response in man by administration of ACTH or cortisol, *J. Clin. Endocrinol. Metab.*, **22**, 147

122. Sissman, L., Librik, L. and Clayton, G. W. (1965). Effect of prior ACTH administration on ACTH release in man, *Metabolism*, **14**, 583

123. Vernikos-Danellis, J. and Trigg, L. N. (1967). Feedback mechanisms regulating pituitary ACTH secretion in rats bearing transplantable pituitary tumors. *Endocrinology*, **80**, 345

124. Kastin, A. J., Arimura, A., Schally, A. V. and Miller, M. C. (1971). Mass action-type direct feedback control of pituitary release, *Nature (New Biol.)*, **231**, 29

125. Eik-Nes, K. B. and Brizzee, K. R. (1965). Concentration of tritium in brain tissue of dogs given [2-^{3}H$_2$]cortisol intravenously, *Biochim. Biophys. Acta*, **97**, 320

126. McEwen, B. S., Weiss, J. M. and Schwartz, L. S. (1969). Uptake of corticosterone by rat brain and its concentration by certain limbic structures, *Brain. Res.*, **16**, 227

127. McEwen, B. S., Weiss, J. M. and Schwartz, L. S. (1970). Retention of corticosterone by cell nuclei from brain regions of adrenalectomized rats, *Brain Res.*, **17**, 471

128. McEwen, B. S., Zigmond, R. E., Azmitia, E. C. Jr. and Weiss, J. M. (1970). Steroid hormone interaction with specific brain regions, *Biochemistry of Brain and Behavior*, pp. 123–167, (R. E. Bowman and S. P. Datta, editors) (New York: Plenum Press)

129. Walker, M. D., Henkin, R. I., Harlan, A. B. and Casper, A. G. T. (1971). Distribution of tritiated cortisol in blood, brain, CSF and other tissues of the cat, *Endocrinology*, **88**, 224

130. Stevens. R.. Grosser, B. I. and Reed, D. J. (1971). Corticosteroid-binding molecules in rat brain cytosols: regional distribution, *Brain Res.*, **35**, 602

131. Feldman, S., Todt, J. C. and Porter, R. W. (1961). Effect of adrenocortical hormones on evoked potentials in the brain stem, *Neurology (Minneap.)*, **11**, 109

132. Feldman, S. and Davidson, J. M. (1966). Effect of hydrocortisone on electrical activity, arousal thresholds and evoked potentials in the brain of chronically implanted rabbits, *J. Neurol. Sci.*, **3**, 462

133. Hoagland, H. (1954). Studies of brain metabolism and electrical activity in relation to adrenocortical physiology, *Rec. Prog. Hormone. Res.*, **10**, 29

134. Woodbury, D. M. (1958). Relation between the adrenal cortex and the central nervous system, *Pharmacol. Rev.*, **10**, 275

135. Aus Der Muehlen, K. and Ockenfels, H. (1969). Morphologische Veraenderungen im Diencephalon und Telencephalon nach Stoerungen des Regelkreises Adenohypophyse-Nebennierenrinde. III. Ergebnisse beim Meerschweinchen nach Verabreichung von Cortison und Hydrocortison, *Z. Zellforsch.*, **93**, 126

136. Feldman, S. and Dafny, N. (1966). Effect of hydrocortisone on single cell activity in the anterior hypothalamus, *Israel J. Med. Sci.*, **2**, 621

137. Ruf, K. and Steiner, F. A. (1967). Steroid-sensitive single neurons in rat hypothalamus and midbrain: Identification by microelectrophoresis, *Science*, **156**, 667

138. Slusher, M. A. and Hyde, J. E. (1969). Influence of limbic system and related structures on the pituitary–adrenal axis, *Physiology and Pathology of Adaptation Mechanisms, Modern Trends in Physiological Sciences*, **27**, 146 (E. Bajusz, editor) (Oxford: Pergamon Press)

139. Steiner, F. A., Ruf, K. and Akert, K. (1969). Steroid-sensitive neurons in rat brain: Anatomical localisation and responses to neurohumours and ACTH, *Brain Res.*, **12**, 74

140. Steiner, F. A. (1970). Effects of ACTH and corticosteroids on single neurons in the hypothalamus, *Progress in Brain Res.: Pituitary, Adrenal and the Brain*, **32**, 102

141. Bohus, B. and Endröczi, E. (1964). Effect of intracerebral implantation of hydrocortisone on adrenocortical secretion and adrenal weight after unilateral adrenalectomy, *Acta Physiol. Acad. Sci. Hung.*, **25**, 11

142. Bohus, C., Nyakas, C. and Lissák, K. (1968). Involvement of suprahypothalamic structures in the hormonal feedback action of corticosteroids, *Acta Physiol. Acad. Sci. Hung.*, **34**, 1

143. Bohus, B. and Strashimirov, D. (1970). Localization and specificity of corticosteroid 'feedback receptors' at the hypothalamo-hypophyseal level; comparative effects of various steroids implanted in the median eminence or the anterior pituitary of the rat, *Neuroendocrinol.*, **6**, 197

144. Chowers, I., Feldman, S. and Davidson, J. M. (1963). Effects of intrahypothalamic crystalline steroids on acute ACTH secretion, *Amer. J. Physiol.*, **205**, 671

145. Davidson, J. M. and Feldman, S. (1963). Cerebral involvement in the inhibition of ACTH secretion by hydrocortisone, *Endocrinol.*, **72**, 936

146. Feldman, S., Conforti, N., Chowers, I. and Davidson, J. M. (1969). Differential responses to various ACTH-releasing stimuli in rats with hypothalamic implants of corticosteroids, *Neuroendocrinol.*, **5**, 290

147. Slusher, M. A. (1966). Effects of cortisol implants in the brainstem and ventral hippocampus on diurnal corticosterone levels, *Exp. Brain Res.*, **1**, 184

148. Smelik, P. G. (1969). The effect of a CRF preparation on ACTH release in rats bearing hypothalamic dexamethasone implants: A study on the 'implantation paradox', *Neuroendocrinol.*, **5**, 193

149. Smelik, P. G. (1969). The regulation of ACTH secretion, *Acta Physiol. Pharmacol. Neerl.*, **15**, 123

150. Zimmermann, E., and Critchlow, V. (1969). Effects of intracerebral dexamethasone on pituitary–adrenal functions in female rats, *Amer. J. Physiol.*, **217**, 392

151. Knigge, K. M. (1966). Feedback mechanisms in neural control of adenohypophyseal function: effect of steroids implanted in amygdala and hippocampus (abstract), *2nd Int. Cong. of Hormonal Steroids, Milan, Excerpta Medica Int'l Cong. Series*, **111**, 208

152. McHugh, P. R. and Smith, G. P. (1967). Negative feedback in adrenocortical response to limbic stimulation in *Macaca mulatta*, *Amer. J. Physiol.*, **213**, 1445

153. Takebe, K., Kunita, H., Sakakura, M., Horiuchi, Y. and Mashimo, K. (1971). Suppressive effect of dexamethasone on the rise of CRF activity in the median eminence induced by stress, *Endocrinology*, **89**, 1014

154. Makara, G. B., Stark, E., Palkovits, M., Révész, T. and Mihály, K. (1969). Afferent pathways of stressful stimuli: Corticotrophin release after partial deafferentiation of the medial basal hypothalamus, *J. Endocrinol.*, **44**, 187

155. Makara, G. B., Stark, E. and Palkovits, M. (1970). Afferent pathways of stressful stimuli: corticotrophin release after hypothalamic deafferentation, *J. Endocrinol.*, **47**, 411

156. Diepen, R. (1962). *Handbuch der Mikroskopischen Anatomie des Menschen vol. IV Nervensystem, Teil 7 Der Hypothalamus*, (Berlin: Springer-Verlag)

157. Gann, D. S. and Egdahl, R. H. (1965). Responses of adrenal corticosteroid secretion to hypotension and hypovolemia, *J. Clin. Invest.*, **44**, 1

158. Lorenzen, L. C. and Ganong, W. F. (1967). Effect of drugs related to α-ethyltryptamine on stress-induced ACTH secretion in the dog, *Endocrinology*, **80**, 889

159. Gann, D. S., Ostrander, L. E. and Schoeffler, J. D. (1968). A finite state model for the control of adrenal cortical steroid secretion, *Systems Theory and Biology*, pp. 185–221, (M. D. Mesarović, editor) (New York: Springer- Verlag)

160. Gann, D. S. (1969). Parameters of the stimulus initiating the adrenocortical response to hemorrhage, *Ann. N.Y. Acad. Sci.*, **156**, 740

161. Schally, A. V., Carter, W. H., Hearn, I. C. and Bowers, C. Y. (1965). Determination of CRF activity in rats treated with Monase, dexamethasone, and morphine, *Amer. J. Physiol.*, **209**, 1169

162. Croxatto, H., Zamorano, B., Bazaes, S., Labra, I., san Martin, M. L. and Oritz, S. (1964). Adrenal ascorbic acid depletion produced by polypeptides obtained from the blood serum, *Major Problems in Neuroendocrinology*, pp. 367–378, (E. Bajusz and G. Jasmin, editors) (New York: Karger)

163. Redgate, E. S. (1970). ACTH release evoked by electrical stimulation of brain stem and limbic system sites in the cat: the absence of ACTH release upon infundibular area stimulation, *Endocrinology*, **86**, 806

164. Mandell, A. J., Chapman, L. F., Rand, R. W. and Walter, R. D. (1963). Plasma corticosteroids: changes in concentration after stimulation of hippocampus and amygdala, *Science*, **139**, 1212

165. Mason, J. W. (1959). Plasma 17-hydroxycorticosteroid levels during electrical stimulation of the amygdaloid complex in conscious monkeys, *Amer. J. Physiol.*, **196**, 44

166. Matheson, G. K. (1969). Aspects of forebrain regulation of plasma glucocorticoids, *Dissert. Abstr. (B)*, **30**, 470

167. Salcman, M., Peck, L. and Egdahl, R. H. (1970). Effect of acute and prolonged electrical stimulation of the amygdala of the dog upon peripheral plasma concentrations of corticosteroids, *Neuroendocrinology*, **6**, 361

168. Knigge, K. M. (1961). Adrenocortical response to stress in rats with lesions in hippocampus or amygdala, *Proc. Soc. Exp. Biol. Med.*, **108**, 18

169. Shute, C. C. D. and Lewis, P. R. (1966). Cholinergic and monoaminergic pathways in the hypothalamus, *Brit. Med. Bull.*, **22**, 221

170. Nauta, W. J. H. (1963). Central nervous organization and the endocrine motor system, *Advances in Neuroendocrinology*, pp. 5–28 (A. V. Nalbanov, editor) (Urbana: University of Illinois Press)

171. Nauta, W. J. H. and Kuypers, H. G. J. M. (1958). Some ascending pathways in the brain stem reticular formation, *Reticular Formation of the Brain*, pp. 3–30, (H. H. Jasper, L. D. Proctor, R. S. Knighton, W. C. Noshay and R. T. Costello, editors) (Boston, Mass: Little, Brown and Co)

172. Hedge, G. A. and Smelik, P. G. (1968). Corticotrophin release: inhibition by intrahypothalamic implantation of atropine, *Science*, **159**, 891

173. Dupont, A., Bastarache, E., Endröczi, E. and Fortier, C. (1972). Effect of hippocampal stimulation on the plasma thyrotropin and corticosterone responses to acute cold exposure in the rat, *Can. J. Physiol. Pharm.*, **50**, 364

174. Endröczi, E. and Lissák, K. (1963). Effect of hypothalamic and brain stem structure stimulation on pituitary-adrenocortical function, *Acta Physiol. Acad. Sci. Hung.*, **24**, 67

175. Endröczi, E. and Lissák, K. (1960). The role of the mesencephalon, diencephalon and archicortex in the activation and inhibition of the pituitary–adrenal system, *Acta Physiol. Acad. Sci. Hung.*, **17**, 39

176. Taylor, A. N. and Branch, B. J. (1971). Inhibition of ACTH release by a central inhibitory mechanism in the basal forebrain, *Exp. Neurol.*, **31**, 391

177. Grizzle, W. E., Johnson, R. M., Schramm, L. P. and Gann, D. S. (1973). Localized hypothalamic area related to neural control of ACTH, *Fed. Proc.* (Abstract) (*Fed. Amer. Soc. Exp. Biol.*), **32**, 295 Abs.

178. Van Loon, G. R., Hilger, L., King, A. B., Boryczka, A. T. and Ganong, W. F. (1971). Inhibitory effect of L-dihydroxyphenylalanine on the adrenal venous 17-hydroxycorticosteroid response to surgical stress in dogs, *Endocrinology*, **88**, 1404

179. Van Loon, G. R., Scapagnini, U., Moberg, G. P. and Ganong, W. F. (1971). Evidence for central adrenergic neural inhibition of ACTH secretion in the rat, *Endocrinology*, **89**, 1464

180. Van Loon, G. R., Scapagnini, U., Cohen, R. and Ganong, W. F. (1971). Effect of intraventricular administration of adrenergic drugs on the adrenal venous 17-hydroxycorticosteroid response to surgical stress in the dog, *Neuroendocrinol.*, **8**, 257

181. Ganong, W. F. (1972). Evidence for a central noradrenergic system that inhibits ACTH secretion, *Brain Endocrine Interaction; Median Eminence: Structure and Function*, pp. 254–266 (K. M. Knigge, D. E. Scott and A. Weindl, editors) (Basel: Karger)

182. Nauta, W. J. H. and Haymaker, W. (1969). Hypothalamic nuclei and fiber connections *The Hypothalamus*, pp. 136–209, (W. Haymaker, E. Anderson and W. J. H. Nauta, editors) (Springfield, Ill.: Charles C Thomas)

183. Gurdgian, E. S. (1927). The diencephalon of the albino rat. *J. Comp. Neurol.*, **43**, 1

184. Nauta, W. J. H. (1958). Hippocampal projections and related neural pathways to the midbrain in the cat, *Brain*, **81**, 319

185. Young, M. W. (1936). The nuclear pattern in fiber connections of the non-cortical centers of the telenceophalon of the rabbit, *J. Comp. Neurol.*, **65**, 295

186. Millhouse, O. E. (1967). The Median Forebrain Bundle: A Golgi Analysis, *Ph. D. Thesis*, University of California at Los Angeles
187. Raisman, G. (1970). An evaluation of the basic pattern of connections between the limbic system and the hypothalamus, *Amer. J. Anat.*, **129**, 197
188. Taylor, A. N. (1969). The role of the reticular activating system in the regulation of ACTH secretion, *Brain Res.*, **13**, 234
189. Krieger, H. P. and Krieger, D. T. (1970). Chemical stimulation of the brain: effect on adrenal corticoid release, *Amer. J. Physiol.*, **218**, 1632
190. Smooker, H. H. and Buckley, J. P. (1969). Relationships between brain catecholamine synthesis, pituitary–adrenal function and the production of hypertension during prolonged exposure to environmental stress, *Int. J. Neuropharm.*, **8**, 33
191. Slusher, M. A. (1964). Effects of chronic hypothalamic lesions on diurnal and stress corticosteroid levels, *Amer. J. Physiol.*, **206**, 1161
192. Krieger, D. T., Silverberg, A. I., Rizzo, F., and Krieger, H. P. (1968). Abolition of circadian periodicity of plasma 17-OHCS levels in the cat. *Amer. J. Physiol.*, **215**, 959
193. Liddle, G. W. (1966). Analysis of circadian rhythms in human adrenocortical secretory activity, *Arch. Int. Med.*, **117**, 739
194. Cheifetz, P., Gaffud, N. and Dingman, J. F. (1968). Effects of bilateral adrenalectomy and continuous light on the circadian rhythm of corticotrophin in female rats, *Endocrinol.*, **82**, 1117
195. Scheving, L. E. and Pauly, J. E. (1966). Effect of light on corticosterone levels in plasma of rats, *Amer. J. Physiol.*, **210**, 1112
196. Orth, D. N. and Island, D. P. (1969). Light synchronization of the circadian rhythm in plasma cortisol (17-OHCS) concentration in man, *J. Clin. Endocrinol. Metab.*, **29**, 479
197. Krieger, D. T., Kreuzer, J. and Rizzo, F. A. (1969), Constant light: effect on circadian pattern and phase reversal of steroid and electrolyte levels in man, *J. Clin. Endocrinol. Metab.*, **29**, 1634
198. Krieger, D. T. and Rizzo, F. (1971). Circadian periodicity of plasma 11-hydroxy-corticosteroid levels in subjects with partial and absent light perception, *Neuroendocrinol.*, **8**, 165
199. Dallman, M. F. and Yates, F. E. (1969). Dynamic asymmetries in the corticosteroid feedback path and distribution–metabolism–binding elements of the adrenocortical system, *Ann. N.Y. Acad. Sci.*, **156**, 696
200. Yates, F. E., Leeman, S. E., Glenister, D. W. and Dallman, M. F. (1961). Interaction between plasma corticosterone concentration and adrenocorticotropin-releasing stimuli in the rat: Evidence for the reset of an endocrine feedback controller, *Endocrinol.*, **69**, 67
201. Smelik, P. G. (1963). Relation between blood level of corticoids and their inhibiting effect on the hypophyseal stress response, *Proc. Soc. Exp. Biol. Med.*, **113**, 616
202. Dallman, M. F., Jones, M. T., Vernikos-Danellis, J. and Ganong, W. F. (1972). Corticosteroid feedback control of ACTH sedretion: Rapid effects of bilateral adrenalectomy on plasma ACTH in the rat, *Endocrinology*, **91**, 961
203. Jones, M. T., Brush, F. R. and Neame, R. L. B. (1972). Characteristics of fast feedback control of corticotrophin release by corticosteroids, *J. Physiol. (London)*, **55**, 489
204. Yates, F. E., Brennan, R. D. and Urquhart, J. (1969). Adrenal glucocorticoid control system, *Fed. Proc. (Fed. Amer. Soc. Exp. Biol.)*, **28**, 71
205. Yates, F. E. (1967). Physiological control of adrenal cortical hormone secretion, *The Adrenal Cortex*, pp. 133–183 (A. B. Eisenstein editor) (Boston: Little, Brown and Co.)
206. Motta, M., Schiaffini, O., Piva, F. and Martini, L. (1971). Pineal principles and the control of adrenocorticotropin secretion, *The Pineal Gland; Ciba Foundation Symposium*, pp. 279–291, (G. E. W. Wolstenholme and J. Knight, editors) (Edinburgh: Churchill Livingstone)
207. Urquhart, J. and Li, C. C. (1968). The dynamics of adrenocortical secretion, *Amer. J. Physiol.*, **214**, 73
208. Urquhart, J. and Li, C. C. (1969). Dynamic testing and modeling of adrenocortical secretory function, *Ann. N.Y. Acad. Sci.*, **156**, 756
209. Dallman, M. F. and Jones, M. T. (1973). Corticosteroid feedback control of ACTH secretion: Effect of stress-induced corticosterone secretion on subsequent stress responses in the rat, *Endocrinology*, **92**, 1367

5
Growth Hormone and the Regulation of Metabolism*

E. E. MÜLLER
University of Milan

* The Literature survey for this article was concluded in December, 1972.

5.1 INTRODUCTION

Much new information has accrued in recent years regarding the chemistry, species-specificity and some of the metabolic actions of the growth hormone (GH) molecule. Advances have also been made in the knowledge of factors which influence GH secretion and in the key role played by the central nervous system (CNS) in GH control. In this chapter, far from being exhaustive, we have been rather selective, since we have primarily focused our attention on those aspects of the subject, which, in our view are of special physiological importance. No special emphasis has been placed on the CNS control of GH secretion, a topic which has been extensively covered in Chapter 2 of this volume. Since it is impossible to quote the several hundred references on this subject, the reader is referred to reviews when possible and emphasis is placed on more recent studies and on changes in the overall picture necessitated by the expansion of knowledge in the physiopathology of GH.

A discussion on the chemistry and species-specificity of GH molecules is beyond the scope of this chapter. For these topics the reader is referred to the recently published *Proceedings of the Second International Symposium on Growth Hormone*, Excerpta Medica, Amsterdam, 1972.

5.2 GH SECRETION AND METABOLISM

5.2.1 GH in the pituitary and biological fluids

There is now a vast and rapidly expanding literature on pituitary and plasma levels of GH. The concentration of pituitary GH in laboratory animals and humans is higher than that of other pituitary hormones. Dickerman *et al.*[1] and Burek and Frohman[2] reported values for radioimmunoassayable (RIA)-GH of 40–45 μg mg^{-1} in both adult male and female rats; concentration and content increased significantly with age up to about 80 days in the male and 60 days in the female. Birge *et al.*[3], by contrast, reported that pituitary GH concentration in male rats continued to increase into old age, whereas pituitary concentration in females plateaued at maturity. In the rat, plasma levels of GH are very high at birth, but fall rapidly between 2 and 5 days of age[4]; a constant increase is subsequently observed in both female and male rats from 21 to about 60 days of age, with a significant elevation in the female during oestrus[1]. Calculations of metabolic clearance and secretion rates of GH *in vivo* using injections of ^{131}[I]RGH suggest GH production in adult female rats to be in the range of 60–80 μg day^{-1} [2]. Since it appeared strange that the most rapid phase of body growth in young rats occurs during a time when both pituitary and plasma levels of GH are lowest and the ability to synthesise and release GH is reduced when compared to adult animals[2], it has been proposed that factors other than GH may be more important for body growth during the rapid growth phase of life[5], or that a different end-organ sensitivity may be present during the different stages of the life cycle[6]. In this context, the observation is relevant that *in vitro* the cartilage from rats at weaning shows the highest responsiveness to serum somatomedin[7] (see also Section 5.4). It must, however, be pointed out that results based on content or concentration of a given hormone in plasma or pituitary tissue must be interpreted with caution and that further studies on metabolic clearance and secretion rates of GH at different ages will prove fruitful in this regard.

Precise determinations of GH in anterior pituitary gland from normal or diseased humans have been made possible by RIA techniques. Detectable amounts of human (H) GH were found in the pituitary from human foetuses as early as the 7th–9th gestational week (0.5–13 ng), which progressively increased until the fifth month of gestation (40 μg)[8,9]. In normal anterior pituitary glands from adult individuals of both sexes, the mean GH concentration was 25 μg mg^{-1}[10]; the average gland thus contains 10 mg of HGH, about 10% of its dry weight[11].

Very high levels of plasma HGH are present in the foetus and at parturition (mean 30 ng ml^{-1}). There is subsequent decline, although GH levels in children are higher than in adults[12]. Wide individual variations are present in 2-day-old babies, which subsequently decrease[13]. There is a peak in fasting basal HGH levels in adolescents, especially at the onset of puberty[14], a finding recently corroborated by the more meaningful determination of the integrated concentration of GH over 24 h[15]. Plasma from healthy adult subjects may contain GH at concentrations from 0 to at least 40–50 ng ml^{-1} depending on the sampling conditions (see Section 5.5).

The measurement of GH in urine by the haemaglutination inhibition method and by RIA has already been reported[16,17]. However, further studies showed that many urinary substances, including salt and urea could interfere with the RIA determination of GH in urine and that the removal of these substances by dialysis and gel filtration was necessary[18]. Quite recently, ultrafiltration and lyophilisation of human urine has been employed to demonstrate the presence of intact immunoreactive urinary GH, independent of the presence of salts[19]. In nine normal subjects the calculated excretion rate was between 28 and 53 ng/24 h and was increased in patients with acromegaly or following the administration of HGH to normal and hypopituitary subjects.

The presence of GH has been reported also in thoracic duct lymph[20] and in the cerebrospinal fluid collected from children[21] or acromegalics[22], while there is little placental transport of HGH from mother to foetus and vice versa[23].

The reported molecular size heterogeneity of many polypeptide hormones appears to be also present in circulating and pituitary HGH. Bala et al.[24] were the first to apply gel filtration to the study of plasma GH. They found that over 50% of plasma GH immunoreactivity was less retarded on Sephadex G-75 than pituitary GH. Their endogenous GH was eluted over a very broad range and discrete components were not demonstrated. However, the presence of at least two discrete components of circulating HGH, little and big HGH, which presumably differ in molecular size, has been demonstrated independently by two groups of researchers[25,26]. Little GH migrated almost identically with the major component of radioiodinated human pituitary GH, while big GH was less retarded on the gel and had approximately twice the molecular weight of little GH. In many plasma samples a small and broader peak of immunoreactive GH was eluted between big growth hormone and the void marker. On gel filtration of a preparation of human pituitary GH, two discrete RIA-GH peaks were found which had migration characteristics indistinguishable from those of *little* and *big* RIA-GH in plasma; this suggested that both plasma components may be secreted by the pituitary. Storage of isolated plasma *big* GH resulted in a 50% conversion to a compound indistinguishable from *little* GH, implying that *big* GH consists of *little* GH bound to some dissociable moiety. Induction of insulin hypoglycaemia caused a rise in both plasma *big* GH and *little* GH. Similarly, two distinct peaks of GH immunoreactivity have been reported in freshly prepared extracts of rat, dog and human pituitaries[27].

The chemical nature and physiological significance of *big* GH as well as the biological activities of both molecules are still unknown. The heterogeneity of endogenous plasma and pituitary GH must be taken into account in those physiological and pathological conditions where RIA-GH concentration does not correlate with the expected biological response.

5.2.2 Secretion rate

Because the level of GH is variable throughout the day, depending upon the metabolic state of the individual, isolated measurements cannot give accurate information of total daily secretion. By using the constant infusion technique for metabolic clearance rate (MCR) measurement and a small portable constant withdrawal pump for obtaining continuous blood samples to determine the integrated concentration of GH (ICGH) over 24 h, the secretion rate (SR) has been determined. This provides valuable information concerning anterior pituitary physiology and allows a more precise assessment of pathological states in which HGH production may be altered. In six normal young human males the overall production rate ranged from 211–665 µg day^{-1} (mean 406); the rate of production at night was significantly higher than during daytime activity[28]. Kowarski *et al.* obtained a mean production rate of 660 µg day^{-1} in five normal males and 950 µg day^{-1} in four female subjects and similar values were reported by MacGillivray *et al.* (see Ref. 28). Since the average gland contains about 10 mg of HGH, it can be concluded that the amount of HGH ordinarily secreted over 24 h represents 5 to 10% of the pituitary pool. Clearly elevated production rates (no alteration in MCR) were found in acromegaly (5.6–65 mg day^{-1}) while in hypopituitarism SR were less than normal[28]. The measurement of SR can be profitably applied to the evaluation of the efficacy of a given treatment; in the hands of Burger *et al.*[28], a chronic chlorpromazine treatment was unable to modify GH secretion rates in two acromegalics, despite considerable symptomatic improvement in one of the two.

5.2.2.1 Plasma half-life

Contrary to earlier belief, the turnover of GH in the plasma is rapid. In studies of the disappearance of administered labelled and unlabelled hormone from the plasma (single bolus technique), a half-life of approximately 20 min was observed[29, 30]. In an acromegalic patient following hypophysectomy, however, the half-life of endogenous GH was almost double (49.9 min) that previously reported[30] and was similar to the half-life obtained in the same patient after a constant infusion of exogenous HGH (51.5 min)[31]. These data indicate that the single bolus technique may not be valid for estimating the half-life of polypeptide hormones and that the turnover rate of HGH may be slower than previously suggested'.

5.2.3 Metabolic disposal

Little information is available on the metabolic fate of GH. Studies of the tissue localisation of radioactively labelled HGH gave some indication on the possible sites of action and/or metabolic disposal. Following administration of iodinated or tritiated GH preparations in the rat, significant localisations of radioactivity were demonstrated in the pancreas, adrenal, liver, spleen, thyroid and renal proximal tubular cells[32-34]. Distribution studies of [^{125}I]HGH in the immature hypophysectomised rat by means of whole body autoradiography again revealed a high concentration of radioactive material in the kidney, liver and adrenal cortex and, in addition, high radioactivity, retaining the electrophoretic mobility of GH in the submandibular gland[35]. The latter localisation is particularly intriguing since a potent nerve growth factor and an epithelial growth factor have been extracted from submandibular glands of mice[36] and several mammals, including the rat, have been reported to respond to submandibular adenectomy with a drastically reduced rate of linear growth[37]. Interestingly enough, radioactivity does not accumulate in the epiphyseal cartilage following the injection of tritiated or iodinated GH *in vivo*[34, 38], providing evidence for the physiological role of secondary growth factors mediating the action of GH on cartilage metabolism (see Section 5.4).

   The presence of radioactivity in a given organ does not provide insight into the extent of the clearance of GH by individual organs relative to the overall clearance of the hormone from plasma. Moreover, in none of the studies quoted above, did the data distinguish between radiolabelled GH, radiolabelled GH metabolites and free radioisotope. All or part of these factors were carefully considered in the successive clearance studies. Significant GH clearance by the kidney in dogs was demonstrated by McCormick *et al.*[39], who infused GH at varying rates and determined renal arteriovenous differences. Their conclusion was that the kidney plays a quantitatively major role in GH metabolism. In carefully designed studies, Taylor *et al.*[40], have measured the total and hepatic metabolic clearance of GH in normal individuals and in patients with cirrhosis using [^{131}I]HGH and the constant infusion to equilibrium method. It would appear from their data that the liver is the major site of GH clearance from the plasma in man since hepatic clearance accounted for most (94%) of the total MCR. Animal studies have shown that major localisation occurs in hepatic parenchymal cells rather than in the Kupffer cells[33, 34]. In patients with cirrhosis, despite the reduced hepatic plasma flow, the total MCR and hepatic clearance of GH were normal, implying an increase in the extrahepatic clearance of GH and suggesting that the elevated peripheral levels of GH present in cirrhatic patients[41,42], are not due to altered metabolic disposal. Major roles played by both liver and kidney in the metabolism of HGH in man, have been demonstrated, on the other hand, by the studies of Cameron *et al.*[43], in patients with hepatic or renal failure. The clearance of GH in the isolated perfused pig liver was 24% of that in the intact animal[43].

Investigation of the sites of HGH degradation may provide further information concerning the sites and mechanism(s) of the hormone's manifold actions. In this context, the observation that perfusion of the isolated rat liver with GH results in the production of somatomedin, is of particular interest (see Section 5.4).

5.3 GH AND INTERMEDIARY METABOLISM

GH exerts a multiplicity of metabolic actions which have been extensively reviewed in the past[44-46]. We will consider here mainly observations and advances made in recent years, referring to older articles only to provide essential background information.

5.3.1 Protein metabolism

There is abundant evidence that GH stimulates protein biosynthesis and tissue growth, but the primary action of the hormone has not yet been localised. The overall positive nitrogen balance induced by the administration of the hormone to animals[47] and humans[48] is a reflection of these anabolic effects. As a consequence of GH administration there is a decrease in urinary nitrogen excretion and blood urea nitrogen (BUN) concentration and increased nitrogen retention and serum α-amino nitrogen and amino acid concentrations[12]. The alterations in nitrogen balance are particularly consistent in hypopituitary individuals[49] and the nitrogen-sparing effect of GH has been successfully used as an index of which patients will grow when treated with HGH on a long-term basis[50]. Soon after the administration of GH to a GH-deficient animal, the rate of conversion of amino acids to blood urea is reduced with consequent diminution of serum and urinary urea levels (see above). Attempts to detect a decrease in the activity of liver enzymes responsible for amino acid oxidation (i.e. amino acid oxidase and transaminase) gave inconsistent results[11].

Transfer of amino acids from extracellular to intracellular compartments under the influence of GH was first demonstrated *in vitro* by the use of the non-metabolisable amino acid α-aminoisobutyric acid (α-AIB) and subsequently confirmed with naturally-occurring amino acids[45]. Similarly, studies in human have shown that shortly after a single injection of HGH, especially if given intravenously, serum α-amino nitrogen falls, reflecting a shift of amino acids into the cells[51]. This acute reduction in amino acidaemia, which is not consistent in normal subjects, is very marked in GH-deficient patients and allows a diagnostically useful separation of GH-deficient from non-deficient subjects[52]. There is a dual effect of GH upon amino acid transport both *in vivo* and *in vitro:* the early stimulatory effect is followed by a late inhibitory effect[53, 54].

GH increases amino acid incorporation into newly synthesised protein *in vitro*[55]. Evidence has been presented that these actions of GH upon amino acid transport (early effect) and incorporation are dissociated and that amino acid incorporation into protein is not dependent upon transport[56]. Whereas amino acid transport is a sodium-dependent reaction, amino acid incorporation is not. The effect of GH on amino acid incorporation into protein *in vitro* is abolished by proteolytic enzymes[57], suggesting either an inactivation of specific hormone receptor sites for GH or the enzymatic hydrolysis of some protein which is required for a sequence of events which mediates the action of GH on protein synthesis.

The protein anabolic effect of GH may be related to the stimulated transport of amino acids into liver cells, although not all investigators are in agreement with this[45]. However, in experiments with liver perfusion *in situ*, Jefferson and Korner[58, 59] were able to demonstrate an interesting parallel between the effects of amino acids and those of GH (i.e. greater activity of isolated ribosomes, greater proportion of polysomes, less monomeric ribosomes, etc.), so that more searching comparisons need to be made before identifying the differences in mode of anabolic action of amino acids and GH.

Attempts have been made by many authors to explain GH stimulation of protein synthesis in terms of nucleic acid metabolism. Hypophysectomy induces a fall in hepatic RNA synthesis, while, conversely the administration of GH to hypophysectomised rats increases RNA synthesis in the liver and long-term treatment also increases the RNA content of a number of tissues. Following GH administration the synthesis of all kinds of RNA, including ribosomal and tRNA, appears to be stimulated (for messenger RNA see below) (see Korner[60]). The effect is not shown earlier than 30–60 min after perfusion of the hormone *in vivo*[60], suggesting that the hormone does not act directly on RNA synthesis in this case, but influences other processes which affect the synthesis of RNA in the course of time. It must be pointed out that *in vitro* the stimulating effects of GH on amino acid transport and protein synthesis also do not occur immediately upon contact of the hormone with the cell, but a 15–20 min delay always occurs before an effect of the hormone can be detected[57]. This suggests that the above effects are secondary phenomena triggered by more primary and yet undefined metabolic events taking place during the lag period.

Korner made the important observation that the amino acid incorporating activity of ribosomes isolated from liver, heart or skeletal muscle is less, per unit weight of ribosomal RNA, if they come from hypophysectomised rats rather than from normal ones[60]. Sucrose gradient analyses revealed less polysomes and more monomeric and dimeric ribosomes in ribosome preparations from hypophysectomised rats than from normal rats[60]. All these effects of hypophysectomy could be reversed by treatment of the hypophysectomised rats with GH and the hormone could stimulate the activity of liver ribosomes to greater than normal levels when injected into normal rats. Since mRNA synthesis appears to be required for the stability of the effective ribosomal aggregates, it is tempting to speculate that hypophysectomy might interfere with the synthesis of mRNA and, conversely, that GH might further mRNA synthesis[60]. Unfortunately, no method is available for assaying the m-RNA content of mammalian tissue and from indirect evidence it would appear that GH does not stimulate the synthesis of mRNA as much as that of other types of RNA[60].

Recently, indirect evidence from the assay of total RNA polymerase activity in liver nuclei, has suggested a preferential stimulation of ribosomal RNA synthesis and by implication an action on the nucleolus. In fact, it has been observed by Salaman *et al.*[61] that the first observable effect of GH on liver RNA of normal animals *in vivo* is a stimulation of 45-S ribosomal-precursor RNA synthesis in the nucleolus, followed by a smaller transient stimulation of nucleoplasmic RNA synthesis. The changes in activity of the RNA polymerases of isolated nuclei confirm the early stimulation of nucleolar and nucleoplasmic RNA synthesis. Hypophysectomy induced a gross depletion of all nucleolar RNA species, while administration of GH reversed this and restored the profile to normal. The significance of the hormone-induced stimulation of nucleoplasmic RNA synthesis is still obscure, but the role of this RNA fraction has been the subject of much debate[62, 63]. It is clear that only a very small fraction of this RNA emerges from the nucleus as mRNA, while most of it is degraded within the nucleus[64], and the evidence favours the role of this material in the regulation of gene transcription[62, 63] as well as a precursor of mRNA[63, 64].

It is interesting that the early rises in nucleolar polymerase activity in the liver of hypophysectomised rats following GH treatment are quantitatively very similar to the changes present in regenerating liver following partial hepatectomy[65], although the time course is different. However, the strong similarity suggests that in both these examples of anabolic stimulation of RNA and protein synthesis a common intracellular mechanism may be involved.

It has been assumed for steroid hormones that the nuclear receptor–hormone complex interacts with the genetic repressor resulting in derepression, increased RNA polymerase and mRNA synthesis which leads to protein synthesis in the cytoplasm at the ribosomes[66]. As described above, nuclear RNA polymerase activity goes up after treatment with GH; thus, the possibility cannot be excluded of a primary action of GH at the level of the genes by a classic derepression mechanism.

5.3.1.1   Insulin and the action of GH on protein synthesis

A protein anabolic effect of insulin in the whole animal is difficult to demonstrate because its well-known hypoglycaemic action induces considerable metabolic and hormonal changes which obscure its action in stimulating protein synthesis. However, insulin appears to share many of the actions of GH, in this respect (see Wool *et al.*[67]). *In vitro* insulin promotes the incorporation of a variety of amino acids into the protein of isolated rat diaphragm and perfused rat heart by mechanisms which are independent of the known effects of insulin in stimulating glucose uptake by muscle. The stimulating action of insulin is present also in diaphragms from hypophysectomised or hypophysectomised-diabetic rats. Ribosomes isolated from muscle of diabetic rats are less efficient at incorporting amino acids into protein *in vitro* than normal ones; injection of insulin into the diabetic rats restores this impairment, an effect which is reminiscent of that of GH in the hypophysectomised rat. Some years ago Young and his pupils proposed that GH acted indirectly to produce an anabolic state by virtue of its capacity to stimulate insulin release from the pancreas (see Manchester and Young[68]). In support of this concept were the observations that the anabolic action of GH are poorly demonstrable in pancreatectomised animals and that hypophysectomy decreases and GH increases the insulin-like activity in plasma (see Knobil and Hotchiss[45]). However, results of further investigations favoured a direct action of GH on processes leading to the stimulation of protein synthesis. Thus, the GH-induced amino acid incorporation into protein of diaphragm from hypophysectomised rats was not abolished by the addition of anti-insulin serum to the system[45] and the effect of GH in promoting a-AIB acid transport in diaphragms was present both in hypophysectomised control and in alloxan-diabetic animals[45]. Moreover, Jefferson and Korner[58] showed that perfusion of isolated liver with GH stimulated protein and RNA synthesis in a system devoid of pancreatic insulin. Despite these latter observations on a direct role for GH in the anabolic processes, Young's original concept that GH acts through the agency of insulin appears now to be, even if in modified form, vigorously revived. Somatomedin, the GH-dependent plasma sulphation factor responsible for many of the metabolic effects of GH, is in fact, a potent insulin-like substance (see Section 5.4).

5.3.2 Lipid metabolism

In contrast to the role of GH in sustaining the process of growth in the immature animal, is the developing concept of its participation in maintaining metabolic homeostasis in the adult organism. This is reflected by the profound effects exerted on lipid and carbohydrate metabolism.

Available evidence indicates that non-esterified fatty acids (NEFA) are the active form in which lipids are transported from fat depots to the sites of utilisation. Among the many hormonal factors which influence the balance of uptake and liberation of NEFA in adipose tissue, GH plays an important role (see Weil[69]). HGH has a twofold action in NEFA metabolism: (1) an immediate increase in NEFA uptake by muscle and (2) a significant but delayed increase of NEFA output from adipose tissue[80]. These findings appear to provide a plausible explanation for the early fall and delayed rise in plasma NEFA that follow systemic administration of HGH. In summarising the investigations of the effect of GH on NEFA levels in plasma, it appears that a single dose of hormone produces in man at first a consistent fall of NEFA levels lasting from 15 to 45 min, which is usually accompanied by a similar slight decrease in blood glucose concentration, then a slow increase culminating in a maximum rise to many fold after 4–8 h, and finally a slow decrease to normal after 24 or more hours depending on the dose of GH used[69]. In the animal the initial depression of fatty acids in the blood is usually not seen, but a lag of several hours in fatty acid mobilisation is demonstrable[71]. Diffusion studies have indicated that this lag in metabolic effects after acute administration of GH is not due to delay in diffusion into the extravascular space[20]. The property of GH to mobilise NEFA is extremely sensitive to the blood glucose level being completely suppressed by administration of glucose or food and conversely enhanced by fasting[72, 73]. HGH raises the fasting values of plasma NEFA not only in normal but also in hypopituitary subjects; in these latter the effect is clearly enhanced and of longer duration[72]. In normal fasting individuals, the hormone is capable of increasing the fatty acid concentration far beyond the elevated levels of fasting alone[74], suggesting that GH controls the rate of adipokinesis in the post-absorptive period and accelerates fat mobilisation beyond the rate induced by fasting in the absence of the pituitary[72]. Despite its prominent lipid-mobilising activity, the presence of GH does not appear to be critical for the occurrence of this process. Hypophysectomy, in fact, does not abolish the increase in NEFA mobilisation usually seen during fasting, even if the magnitude of the response is reduced following the operation[45]. An identical increase in plasma NEFA levels was present in normal and hypopituitary subjects during fasting[75]. It would appear, therefore, that an increased secretion of GH does not account for the fatty acid mobilisation taking place upon the institution of fasting. The same conclusion can be applied to the early changes in blood glucose and NEFA levels that occur in response to hypoglycaemia[76]. Also in this instance the slow action of GH does not appear quick enough to accomplish this task and most probably GH serves only to prolong these effects in the later phase acting in concert with other factors.

GH mobilises fat not only *in vivo* but also *in vitro*; however, the concentration of the hormone which is necessary to produce this effect is, in most cases, far beyond the physiological levels, so that a physiologically significant effect on fat mobilisation *in vitro* is not yet firmly established (see Goodman[77]). In studies on human adipocytes *in vitro*, the addition of HGH in concentrations a thousand-fold greater than those in normal fasting serum and/or shown to be optimal for lipolysis stimulation in rat fat cells did not show any acute stimulatory effect[78, 79].

The large amounts of GH necessary to elicit direct lipolytic effects *in vitro* on rat epididymal fat (up to 1000 µg ml^{-1}) may be contrasted with the small amounts required for potentiation of lipolysis in response to theophylline[77]. In fact, GH is effective in this regard when as little as 10 ng ml^{-1} are present in the incubation medium, although a 3 h incubation period is required. Since after exposure to the same low dose, no changes in the basal lipolytic activity of the tissues are apparent, it has been proposed that 'GH conditions the lipolytic machinery of adipose cells, but may not signal the initiation of the lipolytic process'[77]. Such an indirect role for GH in the process of lipolysis is also suggested by the observation that its fat-mobilising activity *in vivo* depends on the dietary regimen of the animals, the hormone being extremely active in either fasting animals or those fed *ad lib.*, practically ineffective in animals fed once daily[73]. Here again, it would appear that, rather than acting as a direct lipolytic agent, GH simply potentiates endogenous signals for fat mobilisation.

Even though little can be said of how GH affects the lipolytic process, the permissive action on theophylline-induced lipolysis suggests its implication in some way in the production, activity or destruction of cyclic-AMP in adipose tissue. Thus, it is possible that GH may affect lipolysis through alteration of a cyclic AMP-sensitive lipase. The ubiquity of cyclic AMP and the recognition of its role as an intermediate in hormonal action[80], in conjunction with the widespread effects of GH led Goodman[77] to suggest that GH may possibly affect the metabolism of cyclic AMP in tissues other than adipose tissue. The hypothesis has been proposed that some other metabolic effects of GH might be related to this phenomenon.

The metabolic disposal of long-chain fatty acids released into the blood stream and captured mainly by the liver takes place along two major pathways: esterification to neutral fat and oxidative breakdown to acetyl-CoA. A single injection of GH induces after 2–6 h a new formation of triglycerides from fatty acids in the liver. The resultant fatty infiltration of the liver cells subsides after a few days (see Weil[69]). However, in animals treated with GH, the fatty acid concentration in liver is very high and this lowers the ratio glucose/fatty acids—the limiting factor in the new formation of lipids—to a point where hepatic lipogenesis from fatty acids is limited. Thus, the majority of fatty acids taken up by the liver is disposed of through the second channel: β oxidation to acetyl-CoA, a process which is not restricted by the supply of glucose[69]. In both man and animals the respiratory quotient (R.Q.) falls following HGH adminstration, suggesting an increase in the oxidation of fatty acids. Investigators, however, failed to demonstrate any stimulation in the oxidation of infused labelled fatty acids after administration of GH into fed or fasted rats or into man[44]. Brown and Bennet[81] by studying the oxidation of infused palmitate 1-^{14}C in human forearm muscle made the observation that despite the lowering by GH of the R.Q. of the tissue *in situ*, the specific activity of the produced CO_2 fell, an indication that the plasma NEFA was not the major source of the additional fatty acids oxidised by forearm tissue after GH administration. The results obtained, in the author's opinion, were amenable to the interpretation that *intracellular* lipolysis was the major source of the fatty acids oxidised. Rabinowitz *et al.*[70], on the other hand, in studies of human forearm metabolism following intra-arterial injection of HGH, interpreted their results as evidence of an increase in fatty acid oxidation by muscle in response to the infusion (see Knobil and Hotchkiss[45]).

5.3.3 Carbohydrate metabolism

The initial effect of GH administration on carbohydrate metabolism is intimately intertwined with the alterations induced in lipid metabolism. The GH-induced triglyceride catabolism in adipose tissue enhances NEFA formation in the cytoplasm[82], a process which, in turn, stimulates their re-esterification to glycerides[83]. Glucose is needed for the lipid synthesis; thus, the sudden demand for carbohydrate induced by the lipid catabolic effect of GH, results in an initial reduction in the intracellular glucose content and in the lowering of its blood level[84]. The degree of the hypoglycaemic response to GH appears to be dependent upon the dose of the hormone and the animal species. Marked hypoglycaemia leading to convulsions and shock up to death has been reported in the hypophysectomised dog and monkey[69]. On the other hand, in the studies of Rabinowitz *et al.*[70], on human forearm metabolism, in which lower doses (500 µg) of the hormone were used, the early insulin-like action of GH on glucose uptake by both muscle and subcutaneous tissue was lacking. Blockade of the utilisation of glucose and consequently depression of its uptake by muscle and other tissues mainly characterise the second stage of GH action. The large quantity of 2C-units coming from fat depots inhibits the inflow of acetyl-CoA derived from carbohydrate into the common pool[85]; accumulated pyruvate inhibits the glycolytic pathway, so that glucose entering the pathway cannot be adequately broken down for oxidation, but takes the alternate route to glycogen, the glycostatic effect of GH[86]. This effect has more recently been, instead, attributed to the increase availability of circulating insulin following GH[87]. Glucose-6-phosphate accumulates and hinders the phosphorylation of intracellular glucose with consequent piling up of free glucose within the cell, and in the blood, depression of glucose uptake and impairment of glucose tolerance Reduced sensitivity to the hypoglycaemic effect of injected insulin and impaired glucose tolerance are two concomitant metabolic features of the GH-induced depression of glucose uptake which have been amply documented in normal human subjects[69].

More recently, the possibility of determining plasma immunoreactive insulin precisely has provided an additional dimension to the understanding of the GH effects on carbohydrate metabolism[87]. In the normal dog, administration of bovine GH for several days, besides a mild hyperglycaemic effect, markedly elevated endogenous glucose production and overall glucose uptake (designated as turnover) and induced a striking increase in the plasma insulin concentration. Calculations of the glucose uptake during a similar hyperglycaemia, produced in this instance, by infusion of glucose, showed, however, that despite the observed rise in uptake, the actual effect of the GH regimen was to induce a relative inhibition of glucose uptake. The rather limited increase in glucose uptake in the presence of high concentrations of insulin was further proof of the action of GH to decrease the effectiveness of insulin on glucose uptake. Additional clarification of the effects of GH was derived by the study of its action in the fasting state[87]. In the fasted dog the injection of GH for a few days, had little effect on the plasma glucose concentration or on glucose production and uptake, and this in marked contrast to the effects in the dog fed daily. Although lacking significant effect on glucose turnover, GH administration, nevertheless, significantly reduced the effectiveness of injected insulin to increase glucose uptake and produced a significant rise in plasma insulin levels. This latter effect of GH in the starved dog, in the absence of changes in plasma glucose concentration and glucose turnover is an indication of a direct stimulation of insulin secretion.

Direct evaluation of insulin in plasma has also permitted a better insight into the biochemical events leading to GH diabetes[87]. In dogs, the early effects of a GH regimen at high doses (3 mg day^{-1}), as those observed with the smaller dose, consist in moderate hyperglycaemia, increase in glucose production and uptake and high levels of plasma insulin concentration. As GH administration is continued, there is a further rise in the plasma glucose concentration, unaccompanied by a further rise in glucose production, which suggests an exacerbation of the inhibitory effect of GH on glucose uptake. This metabolic situation does not result from an exhaustion of insulin secretion, since plasma insulin concentration is high and can be increased further in.

response to a glucose load, and appears to be reversible, since all parameters described above return to normal a few days after GH injection is terminated (idiohypophyseal diabetes)[69].

More sustained administration of GH prompts the third stage of the response of carbohydrate metabolism; higher fasting blood sugar levels, glycosuria, ketonaemia and ketonuria are the major metabolic features[88]. If the cells lose their power of recovery, the idiohypophyseal diabetes is changed to a true diabetic condition (metahypophyseal diabetes), whose production, however, cannot be achieved in all classes of animals by GH alone[69]. Animals behave under these conditions exactly like depancreatised ones, and like diabetic patients.

In the human, a condition similar to the idiohypophyseal diabetes of the laboratory animal has been induced by the administration of GH (20 mg for 2–3 days) to hypophysectomised non-diabetic patients[89]. The diabetogenic effect is also very evident in the hypophysectomised-diabetic[90]. Non-diabetic hypopituitary patients and normal subjects may show modest increases in urinary ketones and acetone following GH administration but this acetonuria is not sustained even though the hormone is continued[91]. Most likely, insulin secreted in response to GH may counteract the excess production of ketone bodies[92].

It must be pointed out, however, that the concept of the true diabetogenicity of HGH in the human has been reappraised in recent years, especially in the light of a better knowledge of the prediabetic condition (see Luft and Cerasi[93]). HGH certainly decreases the peripheral utilisation of glucose, but in the presence of a pancreas capable of responding to its insulin-stimulating effect is not diabetogenic. It is so, only in prediabetic subjects, where compensatory hyperinsulinism cannot occur[93]. It is apparent, therefore, that HGH may be regarded as an additional factor for the development of diabetes, the major determinant being a pre-existing prediabetic state.

5.4 SOMATOMEDIN

GH is undoubtedly a prime determinant of postnatal growth in man. Pituitary dwarfism at one end of the secretory spectrum and gigantism and acromegaly at the other are well-known clinical disorders of abnormal GH secretion. In the last 15 years, investigations into the mechanisms of action of GH on skeletal tissue have provided evidence that the control is not direct but involves the participation of a secondary hormonal mediator. In 1956–1957, the possibility of such an indirect control of cartilage metabolism by GH was firmly established by Daughaday and Salmon[94] after a series of negative attempts to stimulate sulphate uptake directly with GH in cartilage segments from hypophysectomised rats—the active incorporation of sulphate into chondroitin sulphate providing a simple index of anabolic activity. They made the basic observation that when GH is administered to hypophysecto-mised rats, their plasma after a few hours becomes capable of stimulating sulphate uptake *in vitro*. GH itself or plasma from untreated hypophysecto-mised rats could not reproduce this effect. In the light of these findings, they suggested that the GH-dependent stimulator of sulphate uptake, to which the operation term sulphation factor was given[94], was responsible for the action of GH on skeletal tissue. Subsequent work has established the presence of a sulphation factor in normal human serum, and semi-quantitative bio-assays have been developed for its measurement[95].

The metabolic effects of the sulphation factor are not confined to the sulphation of chondroitin sulphate. A general stimulation of the protein synthetic machinery can be demonstrated by measuring the incorporation of uridine into RNA and amino acids into chondromucoprotein[96]. The sulpha-tion factor was shown to be a potent stimulus for chondrocyte replication, as demonstrated by the incorporation of thymidine into DNA in rat cartilage segments[97]. The recognition that the biological actions of the sulphation or thymidine factor are not limited to cartilage but also include non-skeletal tissues (see below), prompted recently the substitution of these operational terms with the more general designation of somatomedin[98], which connotes both its hormonal relationship to somatotrophin and also to the soma.

Somatomedin is present not only in plasma, since fractions prepared from a number of tissues (kidney, pancreas, heart, pituitary and skeletal muscle) have significant activity[99, 100]. Following hypophysectomy in the rat, somato-medin disappears from the plasma within 24 h, with a half-life of approxi-mately 3–4 h[101]. There is evidence that somatomedin generation may occur in both liver and kidney[102, 103, 104]: isolated perfused rat livers or rat liver slices, perfused rat kidney and kidney slices after addition of bovine GH gave rise to somatomedin activity in the effluent or the medium. Adult rat livers were less responsive to bovine GH than livers from normal or hypo-physectomised 3-week-old rats; this is in keeping both with the greater ^{35}S-uptake in cartilage from young rats[7] and the reported higher effectiveness of GH *in vitro* on tissue from young animals[6].

Blood levels of somatomedin were reduced, following partial hepatectomy in 4–6 h and returned to normal as the liver regenerated[105]. So far, the identity of liver somatomedin with plasma somatomedin, has not been proved. Unlike GH, somatomedin does not appear to be so species-specific[106]. When plasmas of various animal species were tested for their somatomedin activity, plasma from man, monkey, pig, cow, dog and rat proved to be effective in the rat, monkey and pig. However, pigeon plasma was inhibitory and fish plasma had no effect, suggesting that the induction of plasma soma-tomedin is involved in the mechanism by which the GH species-specificity comes about.

Although somatomedin activity reflects GH secretion in most normal situ-ations, dissociation of this relationship has been reported. Substances other than GH, give rise to somatomedin. Infestation of rodents with spargana of the tape worm, *Spirometra mansonoides* induced in mice and hamsters a massive obesity, but true skeletal growth in rats with hypothyroidism and hypopituitarism[95]. The stimulation of growth by spargana in hypophysecto-mised rats corresponded closely to that induced by GH, with the exception that it was sustained only for a few weeks after infestation[107, 109].

When serum from actively growing infested rats was tested in the standard somatomedin assay, it was found to contain only about six-tenths of the somatomedin activity of normal rat serum[108], in spite of the fact that it was far more potent than normal rat serum in stimulating growth when injected into non-infested hypophysectomised rats[107]. This finding was hard to reconcile with the possibility of spargana producing a somatomedin-like material, but suggested that, instead, they released a material different from GH, i.e. a worm factor, immunologically unrelated to GH, which in turn stimulated somatomedin generation and skeletal growth. In the infested-hypophysectomised rats, growth ceased when antibodies developed able to neutralise the primary worm product (see Daughaday[95]). In addition to stimulating growth *in vivo*, the worm factor, when present in normal rats inhibited GH storage and release, either directly or through somatomedin generation[109] (see Section 5.6).

Isolation of somatomedin from plasma has been a difficult task because of the time consuming and expensive bioassays. The original assay has also been modified by a dual labelling technique to permit simultaneous measurements of sulphate and thymidine uptake[109-111].

Chromatography on Sephadex G-100 of either native human plasma or human plasma partially purified on diethylaminoethanol cellulose suggested a molecular size of 50 000 daltons or larger for somatomedin. Efforts were made to separate somatomedin from other plasma proteins and to recover activity in a smaller peptide fraction[111]. After extraction of the whole plasma with acid ethanol, a procedure which had been previously employed successfully to extract from plasma a small molecular weight component of the non-suppressible insulin-like activity (NSILA)[112], the recovery of somatomedin activity from native plasma was 30%–40%, whereas over 99% of the original proteins were removed. The dose–response curves obtained were parallel with those of the native plasma both for plasma sulphation factor (PSF) and plasma thymidine factor (PTF), suggesting the similarity of the substances extracted. Subsequent chromatography of the acid ethanol extracts on Sephadex G-50 revealed the molecular weight to be >6000 and $<11\,000$. These data suggested that in native plasma the peptide(s) containing PSF and PTF activities were either aggregated or bound to a larger carrier protein. The combined procedure of acid ethanol extraction, cation exchange chromatography and gel chromatography allowed the purification of PSF and PRF 6200 X and 15 000 X respectively, over their activities in native plasma. Assuming, for the active material a molecular weight of 8000, it proved to be active *in vitro* at 1×10^{-8} M, an activity which compares favourably with that of other hormones. Further purification has been achieved by ion exchange chromatography, partition chromatography on Sephadex L-20 and a variety of electrophoretic separations. Using a combination of these techniques, Hall *et al.* obtained a small amount of somatomedin purified 1 million-fold (see Van Wyk *et al.*[113]).

Although some differences are evident, somatomedin and insulin are strikingly similar in their qualitative effects. This has become increasingly clear with the recognition of the extra skeletal effects of the peptide. Purified preparations of somatomedin exhibit insulin-like effects in at least four different bioassay systems. Salmon and Du Vall[114] showed that both insulin and somatomedin stimulate incorporation of [³H]leucine into TCA-insoluble protein by diaphragm and costal cartilage of hypophysectomised rats. In intact epididymal fat pads, somatomedin, like insulin, increased the conversion of [¹⁴C]glucose into labelled CO_2[115], an effect which was also duplicated in isolated fat cells[113]. In addition, somatomedin has also been shown to stimulate HeLa cell replication[116]; all these are insulin-like effects. Quite recently, Underwood et al.[117], reported a further insulin-like effect of somatomedin, i.e. inhibition of *in vitro* glycerol release in epinephrine-stimulated rat epididymal fat pad segments, and Hintz et al.[118] were able to show that somatomedin, at physiological concentrations, competes with [^{125}I]insulin for receptor sites on isolated fat cells, liver membranes and isolated chondrocytes, an action which was previously shown only for insulin, proinsulin and substituted insulins[119]. The competitive binding of somatomedin and insulin is suggestive of a structural as well as functional homology between the two molecules. In this context, it must be remembered that Hall and Uthne[115] were unable to dissociate somatomedin activity from non-suppressible insulin-like activity during purification from human plasma; at each purification step there was about 100–300 μU of NSILA per somatomedin unit activity.

Although NSILA has not been previously considered to be GH-dependent, plasma ILA levels decrease to undetectable levels after hypophysectomy and pancreatectomy and increase a few hours after i.v. injection of HGH[120]. These observations imply a pituitary control mechanism since it has been demonstrated that NSILA does not originate in pancreatic islets[121]. A tentative hypothesis is that somatomedin are resident in the same molecule[113, 115].

Although the biological significance of the insulin-like effect of somatomedin is not entirely apparent, at present, it could account for much of the anabolic effects of GH on skeletal and extra-skeletal tissue and also provide an explanation for the great difficulty in demonstrating direct *in vitro* effects of GH commensurate with the magnitude of GH effects *in vivo*. Differently from GH, somatomedin, in fact, acts directly not only on cartilage receptors but also on fat and liver receptors at levels which are well below the concentration normally found in plasma.

The above and cognate observations emphasise the need for re-investigating some of the metabolic effects ascribed to GH in order to dissociate the direct effect of the hormone on target tissue from those attributable to the induction of somatomedin.

5.5 STIMULI FOR GH SECRETION

With the development of the radioimmunoassays of plasma GH, extensive investigations performed in both laboratory animals and man have indicated the existence of a variety of factors for the release of GH (see also Root[12]). Based on these studies, it has been postulated that three major separate mechanisms of control exist and these are summarised in Figure 5.1. One appears to be concerned with maintaining circulating energy substrate levels when there is an actual or threatened decrease in the substrate for energy production in the cells (glucoprivation, fasting, lowering of the NEFA levels, etc.), the second is associated with changes in plasma amino acids, and the third operates under a variety of stresses of various types (emotional, surgical, febrile, etc.). All of these stimuli require the integrity of the hypothalamic–pituitary axis and the majority of them appear to act by activating the brain

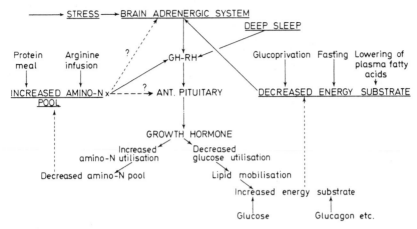

Figure 5.1 Control mechanisms postulated for the control of growth hormone secretion. (Redrawn from Baylis *et al.*[128] by courtesy of Excerpta Medica, Amsterdam)

adrenergic system (see also Müller[122]). Besides these, the stimulant effect on GH secretion induced by deep sleep must be considered in addition, a mechanism in which the noradrenergic pathways do not appear to be operative.

5.5.1   Energy-feed-back control

5.5.1.1   Glucoprivation

In 1963, Roth *et al.*[123, 124], made the crucial observation that insulin-induced hypoglycaemia was associated with a rapid rise of plasma HGH values, whereas administration of glucose resulted in their fall to undetectable levels. The secretion of HGH in response to hypoglycaemia follows a circadian rhythm being greater in the morning than at night, being possibly related to the basal level of plasma HGH when insulin is administered[125], The observations of Roth and associates have been repeatedly confirmed and in addition to hypoglycaemia, similar results were obtained when intracellular glucose metabolism was blocked with 2-deoxy-D-glucose (2-DG) administration in the human[124, 126] or the monkey[127]. In normal individuals, fructose, which can substitute for glucose in the receptors, suppressed insulin-induced GH secretion and even prevented the stimulant action of insulin hypoglycaemia on GH secretion[128]. Falling blood glucose, even in the absence of hypoglycaemia is a stimulus for GH secretion[124], however, the infusion of glucose has to be maintained for 10 or more minutes prior to termination in order for a subsequent fall in blood glucose to be an effective stimulus[129]. This control mechanism operates on the negative feed-back principle, HGH secretion bearing a reciprocal relationship not to the level of circulating energy substrate, but to its intracellular availability. The secretion of GH in response to glucoprivation, would thus, appear particularly suited to maintain homeostasis by its ability to increase lipid mobilisation and decrease peripheral glucose utilisation, protecting the brain from glucose deficiency. The possibility that in the human the secretion of GH under such circumstances may be merely the result of a non-specific response to the stress of glucoprivation[130, 131], seems to be contradicted by the findings of Luft et al.[132]. They reported that falls in blood glucose of only 10 mg (100 ml)$^{-1}$ which were asymptomatic, were associated with significant elevations of plasma GH, a finding supported also by the experiments of Greenwood et al.[133], but not confirmed in later studies[134, 135]. In a study in which frequency and magnitude of plasma GH increases and their relationship to symptomatic hypoglycaemic stress was investigated during insulin reactions and insulin infusion test, Molnar et al.[136], concluded that symptomatic hypoglycaemic stress was the phenomenon most consistently related to GH release.

The specificity of the shortage of carbohydrate substrate as a stimulus for GH secretion is, however, supported by the demonstration of glucoreceptor neurones which control the secretion of GH. Available evidence indicates, in fact, that specific glucosensitive elements in the hypothalamus are involved and that the response is mediated by a growth hormone-releasing factor or hormone (GRF or GH-RH) liberated into the hypothalamic-pituitary portal vascular tract. Thus, in the monkey, electrolytic lesions of anterior and central median eminence and pituitary stalk[137], or microinjections of glucose into the hypothalamus[138] prevented the normal GH response to hypoglycaemia. Conversely, unilateral microinjections of minute amounts of 2-DG into the lateral hypothalamic area alongside the midpart of the ventromedial nucleus were followed by a rise of plasma GH comparable in magnitude and duration to that provoked by hypoglycaemia[139]. In the human, pituitary stalk section prevented the GH response to hypoglycaemia[140, 141] and similar results were obtained in patients with pituitary or hypothalamic dysfunction[128]. In the rat, depletion of both pituitary bioassayable (BA) and hypothalamic GRF and appearance of a circulating GRF in the plasma of hypophysectomised rats have been reported following the induction of hypoglycaemia, a finding not confirmed by other authors for pituitary and plasma RIA-GH (see Ref. 122 and also Chapter 2).

Granted that in the hypothalamus, possibly in the ventrolateral area, chemoreceptors exist sensitive to a lack of metabolisable glucose, which initiate secretion of GH during hypoglycaemia, it would appear that their activation requires the integrity of the brain adrenergic system. In the rat, among many CNS-active drugs, reserpine and chlorpromazine, known for their anti-adrenergic effects, were the most effective in blocking insulin-induced depletion of pituitary BA-GH[131]. In addition to reserpine, other brain norepinephrine depletors suppressed insulin-induced GH release[122]. In the baboon, α-adrenergic blockade with phentolamine significantly depressed and β-adrenergic blockade with propranolol induced a prompt rise in GH secretion[142]. Studies done in the human showed that phentolamine significantly reduced the increase in plasma GH that follows insulin-induced hypoglycaemia[143], while conversely propranolol augmented the levels of GH in hypoglycaemic[143] and normal subjects[144]. The bulk of these and many other studies not reported here are compatible with the view that an α-adrenergic tone within the hypothalamus modulates the activity of the glucosensitive receptors for GH secretion, while β-adrenergic tone exerts an opposite effect. Suppression of the adrenergic tone results in a blunted GH response to glucoprivation. In contrast to adrenergic blockade, suppression of cholinergic tone with atropine did not influence the GH response to insulin-induced hypoglycaemia in healthy adult males[145].

5.5.1.2 Fasting

A slow plasma GH rise has been reported in the human during prolonged fasting[124, 146, 147]. However, the great variability in GH levels observed in a careful metabolic and hormonal evaluation of prolonged starvation in the human[148] casts some doubt on its importance as a metabolic regulator during fasting. Similarly, in the monkey no evidence was obtained by Knobil and Meyer[149] which would support the view that prolonged fasting is a stimulus to GH secretion. In the latter study the characteristic alterations of NEFA and glucose associated with fasting were divorced from changes in plasma GH concentration, a finding not particularly unexpected in view of the earlier finding that hypophysectomy in the monkey and the rat does not abolish the increase in plasma NEFA concentration during fasting[45]. Also in subprimate species it would appear that fasting does not alter either plasma GH levels or pituitary GH content[150-152], although increased levels of plasma GH during fasting have been reported by Machlin et al.[153], in the pig and by Garcia and Geschwind[154] in the mouse and the rabbit.

The above evidence tends to exclude the role of GH as the primary metabolic regulator during fasting; however, an ancillary action in this metabolic condition cannot be denied. The normal metabolic adaptation seen in the adult organism to prolonged starvation consists in accelerated lipolysis reflected in an elevated plasma NEFA level. The data available are compatible with the hypothesis that the glucose–insulin feed-back mechanism may be the primary control process regulating the release of peripheral fuel to provide energy for metabolism during fasting[148]. The decrease in plasma insulin present during starvation is inversely correlated with the NEFA levels; however, when insulin decreases in the plasma of the hypophysecto-mised rat, the rise in plasma NEFA is much slower and significantly smaller than that present in the normal animal[155]. Thus, the presence of GH seems to influence the level of lipolytic activity seen at any given insulin concentration.

5.1.2.1 Protein-calorie malnutrition

The consistent increase of GH concentration in plasma of protein-calorie malnourished children with low serum protein levels (Kwashiorkor) (see Pimstone et al.[156],), stands in contrast to the erratic rises of plasma GH levels present during fasting. The elevated levels of GH are not suppressed by in-duced hyperglycaemia, do not correlate with fasting blood glucose or drop with carbohydrate refeeding without protein. Although there is a significant inverse correlation between serum albumin and fasting HGH, artificial elevation of the serum albumin levels does not suppress GH release. Instead, the return of fasting HGH and glucose-induced suppressibility to normal is evident within 3 days of initiation of oral protein feeding, before any change in albumin concentration is recorded. An inverse correlation is also present between the fasting HGH levels and certain plasma amino acids; infusion of amino acids, however, fails in most cases to lower the concentration of GH. Interestingly enough, no increase in basal levels of GH is present in healthy young men kept for 25 days on a protein-deficient but calorically adequate diet[157] or in patients with only short-term protein depletion[158].

The increased GH levels in protein-calorie malnutrition might be simply explained by an impairment of the degradative enzymes for HGH, or by an intracellular glucose deficit[156]. However, it seems more likely that it is factors related to the relative protein deficit rather than starvation itself which stimulate secretion of GH.

Determination of somatomedin levels in blood of simply starved or protein-calorie-deficient children might provide useful information on the long-term stimulus to the secretion of GH (see Section 5.6).

5.5.1.3 Lowering of plasma fatty-acid levels

If GH plays a major role in energy metabolism by providing NEFA as a fuel during hypoglycaemic states and thus protecting amino acids from being burned, one would expect the existence of some kind of feed-back mechanism between plasma NEFA concentration and HGH secretion. The finding that GH elevations following nicotinic acid administration might be due to lowering of NEFA concentrations suggested that NEFA depression might be responsible in part for GH elevations after insulin administration[159]. However, in experiments in which attempts were made to maintain plasma NEFA levels (by administering heparin or through the ingestion of cream) without influencing the hypoglycaemic response to an insulin tolerance test, the expected inverse relationship between NEFA and GH levels was not apparent[128]. On the other hand, Quabbe et al.[160], by decreasing plasma NEFA levels with nicotinic acid, observed a delayed rise in HGH, even during persistent hyperglycaemia. However, the delay of 2 h between NEFA decrease and HGH increase made it unlikely that NEFA concentration was a direct signal for HGH secretion, but suggested that secondary changes were triggered off which then influenced HGH release. A more direct inter-relationship was suggested by the results of Buber et al.[161], who observed a sharp rise in plasma HGH after a 2 h infusion of β-pyridylcarbinol, a drug which lowers plasma NEFA levels. More recent experiments have provided substantial evidence that plasma NEFA concentrations and HGH release are inter-related[162]. Apparent differences were also shown between the ability of NEFA to suppress HGH secretion stimulated by arginine infusion as compared with that stimulated by hypoglycaemia. Elevated NEFA concentrations induced by administration of corn oil and heparin abolished release after arginine and merely inhibited release resulting from hypoglycaemia. NEFA suppression of amino acid-initiated HGH release appeared to be independent of glucose concentrations.

If spontaneously falling concentrations of NEFA do stimulate HGH release the available evidence indicates, however, that these increases are quantitatively small. In fact, when NEFA concentrations were acutely increased in the human to a mean concentration of more than 2 mM l^{-1} and then fell to 40% of this peak level, only small and statistically insignificant increases in mean HGH concentrations were observed[162].

In monkey, infusion of a soybean oil emulsion or of sodium octanoate which markedly increased NEFA concentration inhibited insulin-induced GH elevations[163]; however, infusion of a ketone, a substrate metabolised by the brain during starvation[148], did not block the effect of insulin hypoglycaemia.

5.5.2 Amino-acid proteins

Since GH release results in a phase during which protein anabolism exceeds the rate of its catabolism, a control of GH secretion by some aspects of protein metabolism might be foreseen. The observation that infusion of l-arginine provoked a striking rise in plasma insulin concentration with modest changes in blood glucose[164] suggested the simultaneous release of a contra hormone, possibly HGH. Studies from two laboratories showed, in fact, that intravenous administration of certain amino acids (arginine, histidine, lysine, phenylalanine, leucine, valine, methionine and threonine) resulted in elevated plasma HGH levels[165, 166], a finding which has been amply confirmed in the following years (see also Root, 1972)[12]. The GH response following amino acids would maintain amino-N homeostasis by increasing amino acid incorporation into protein and thus restoring the elevated plasma amino-N levels to normal. GH and insulin simultaneously released might have 'the dual effect of buffering changes in blood glucose concentration, while encouraging incorporation of amino acid into protein'[167]. Arginine, the direct precursor or urea in the Krebs–Henseleit cycle has been the amino acid most extensively investigated. Plasma HGH levels rising to values in excess of 20 ng ml^{-1} between 30 and 60 min after the start of arginine HCl infusion (1/6 and 1/4 g per pound of body weight) were almost constantly observed in normal females[165-167] while the response in the normal post pubertal male was quite poor and unpredictable[167]. Pretreatment of the non-responding males with oestrogen (diethylstilboestrol) induced a female pattern of response[167]. In contrast to that induced by glucoprivation, the release of GH evoked by arginine remains, although not invariably, competent in the face of hyperglycaemia produced from both an endogenous or exogenous source[167, 168] and is not depressed by cortisone pretreatment[167]. The reported differences between hypoglycaemia-induced and arginine-induced GH release appeared to suggest different pathways used by the two stimuli in eliciting GH discharge. Experiments performed in the rat showed, however, that at least the final pathway is the same for both stimuli, since amino acids also depleted hypothalamic stores of GRF[169]. Activation of the sympatheticoadrenal system also appears to take place during the arginine-induced GH release as implied by the blunting effect exerted by phentolamine[170].

Recently, studies of arginine and normal saline as stimuli to GH release have suggested that GH rise following arginine infusion are not specific, but may be related to features of the investigation, since comparable levels were found in control subjects[171, 172]. Variability in the GH response to arginine infusion has been reported in the same individual[173]. According to other investigators, however, the arginine stimulus is usually effective[173, 174] and particularly suitable for evaluating GH production in children[175, 176]. The controversy is still open and the problem of the specificity of arginine as a stimulus for GH secretion may be resolved by integrated plasma HGH sampling. Certainly, spontaneous fluctuations and occasional elevation of plasma GH associated with saline infusions emphasises that any study of HGH levels must be performed under controlled conditions which minimise the influence of other metabolic or physical factors.

In agreement with the action of amino acids, administration to female subjects of a high protein meal (beef tenderloin) resulted in an increment in plasma insulin and in plasma HGH 1 1/2 to 4 h postprandially, whereas a mixed substrate meal comprising protein and glucose induced an exaggerated rise in plasma insulin, but the HGH response was markedly blunted[177]. Administration of glucose, as expected, induced an early rise in plasma insulin and a delayed rise in plasma HGH.

From these and other observations a concept has been formulated of the interaction between GH and insulin during the time of food intake and during the post-absorptive period. The three-phase cycle comprises: Phase I—immediate postprandial period—when insulin, secreted in response to exogenous carbohydrate increases the rate of glucose uptake and encourages storage of carbohydrate and fat; Phase II—delayed post prandial phase—during which GH, secreted in response to the falling blood glucose, acts synergistically with insulin mainly to direct production of protein digestion towards protein synthesis while its lipid mobilising activity is cancelled by the secreted insulin; Phase III—the remote post-absorptive period in which HGH acts exclusively as a fat-mobilising agent, since the low circulating levels of insulin do not allow either an inhibition of NEFA or a stimulation of the anabolic action of GH.

As a consequence of the sequential release of insulin and GH, carbohydrate, fat and protein storage is promoted during the postprandial period and lipid mobilisation and oxidation with preservation of carbohydrate takes place during the post-absorptive period. The cycle would start anew with the next intake of food. In accord with this hypothesis, marked postprandial increases in plasma GH were found after the administration of protein meals to male subjects[178, 179], and in some but not all males 3–4 h after meals[180].

The hormonal and metabolite-modulated mechanism proposed by Rabinowitz et al.[177] undoubtedly provides a plausible picture of the day-to-day role of HGH and insulin in the economy of the normal adult organism. However, the role of GH appears to be questionable from the variable results on plasma GH produced by meal ingestion. Contrary to the above finding, Bayliss et al.[128] were unable to show a GH response to protein ingestion. Quite recently, Baker et al.[181] in a careful study on the effects of a 3-day regimen in six healthy adults, two females and four males, who continued their usual sedentary activities, found that the peaks of GH concentration had no consistent temporal relationship to meals. The mean plasma GH concentration between meals was unrelated to the meal content except that it was lowest after the high carbohydrate meal in the females. Moreover, the patterns in the females were not reproducible when identical high protein meals were given again after an interval of 6 months.

In the three-phase cycle proposed above, the increased secretion of GH in the remote post-absorptive period by stimulating an increased breakdown of fat would steer the organism away from further utilisation of carbohydrate and from substitution of protein for carbohydrate, with the result that carbohydrate and protein are conserved. Such an action of GH would be exacerbated during fasting, a situation in which protein conservation appears to be the main bodily requirement[182].

However, the role of GH both as a substrate regulator following feeding and as a primary hormonal mediator of the metabolic response to fasting appears to be denied by the reported experimental evidence. Its physiological role in the mobilisation of NEFA is doubtful (see Section 5.3.2). The fasting-induced NEFA rise has been found to be normal in dwarfs with isolated GH deficiency[215], hypophysectomised monkeys[73] and treated hypopituitary humans[75]. In addition, the dissociation of the NEFA rise from GH secretion during exercise[184] (see following subsection), the lack of a direct action of GH on lipolysis *in vitro*[77], and on the contrary, the demonstrated antilipolytic effect of somatomedin[107] make it unlikely that GH plays an important role in NEFA mobilisation and substrate regulation.

5.5.3 Stressful procedures

GH levels can increase in response to a number of psychologically or physically stressful situations. In the human, studies of the effects of stress on GH secretion initially dealt with the effects of walking[140, 185], but have since been extended to include other types of stress[186]. GH rises have been described on the occasion of a visit to the dentist or after repeated venipuncture, or by the thought that insulin had been given, whereas the injection was of saline[128]. Significant increases in plasma GH levels were present in adult subjects shortly after naturally-occurring or induced physical trauma; the levels usually fell after therapy[186-188]. Surgery has been reported to elicit the secretion of GH in children also, but the response is less reproducible[12]. Electroconvulsive therapy causes a small but significant rise in plasma GH[186, 189], a finding, however, not confirmed by subsequent studies[190]. Cold exposure, a stimulus effective in releasing GH in non-primate species[131, 153], had no effect on normal adult humans[191], ether-anaesthetised infants[192], or pentobarbital-anaesthetised monkeys[193]. In the restrained monkey, painful stimuli, haemorrhage, injection of epinephrine, histamine or chlorpromaline, minimal environmental disturbances, and arousal from pentobarbital anaesthesia, all induced significant increases in plasma GH[130]. The GH response to capture and ether anaesthesia in the squirrel monkey was blocked by small lesions in either anterior or posterior median eminence[194].

Administration of vasopressin stimulated GH release both in restrained monkeys[195] and in the human[128], a finding subsequently confirmed by many investigations (see Root[12]). Catecholamines were also shown to be implicated in the vasopressin-induced release since phentolamine was effective in

suppressing the increased GH secretion which follows vasopressin administration to the human[122]. From the available data, the GH response to vasopressin does not appear to be a suitable test for pateints with suspected
hypopituitarism[196].

The administration of bacterial endotoxin pyrogens stimulated the secretion of GH[128, 197, 198]. In the human, following the intravenous injection of
Pseudomonas endotoxin (Pyromen) or *pyrogen E*, both plasma HGH and
cortisol levels rise and there is a pyrexial response after an initial delay of
about 60 min. The mechanism by which pyrogen administration stimulates
GH secretion remains to be elucidated. The rise in GH is not produced by the
fever itself, because the GH rise usually precedes the rise in temperature,
and is not prevented by antipyretic drugs[128]. Moreover, the delay of the
pyrexial response suggests that the hormonal responses are not directly due
to pyrogen but probably relate to some metabolic consequences of its administration, i.e. release of epinephrine[197]. The GH response to pyrogen appears to
be a more reliable indication of pituitary and/or hypothalamic damage than
is plasma cortisol[197, 198].

GH concentration tends to increase during and after strenuous exercise.
The studies of Roth *et al.*[140], revealed that 30 min of walking at 1–4 m.p.h.
by normal subjects was followed by an elevation of plasma HGH; feeding
of glucose to subjects who had been fasting for 12–15 h prior to exercise,
resulted in a blunted GH response. Analogous results were reported by
Hunter *et al.*[185]. A marked rise in plasma GH was observed in young adults
engaged in playing either basketball or lacrosse; similarly climbing stairs
induced a rise in plasma GH[186].

The increase in base-line plasma GH concentration, present in the various
forms of physical stress, occurred coincidentally with elevations in glucose
and NEFA concentrations, which have been shown to be associated with
stressful stimuli[199]. However, HGH does not appear to play a major role in
fat mobilisation during exercise, which seems secondary to activation of the
sympathetic nervous system[200]. A different time pattern in the rise of HGH
and NEFA levels was present in fasting adult males[185]; both GH and NEFA
increased during the first hour of walking. The NEFA levels, however,
remained high for several hours, while in the second hour GH levels fell.
Similarly, bicycle riding induced fat mobilisation within 5–10 min, while
plasma GH levels rose only after 20 min[184].

Although GH secretion does not account for early exercise-induced fat
mobilisation, a feed-back action of increased NEFA levels on GH release
during exercise cannot be disregarded. Following administration of nicotine,
which abolished NEFA changes, but left unimpaired the initial GH response,
a continuous rise rather than a fall of GH levels was found during the
second hour of exercise[184], implying that the decline of GH levels observed
under control conditions may be related to increased fatty-acid concentrations.

The stimulus to GH secretion during exercise stress is clearly unrelated to a
direct effect of blood glucose levels. One may speculate on the existence of
humoral agents released from muscle, on a reflex stimulation of the CNS, and
on possible metabolites released as the result of exercise which stimulate the
sensitive centre[187]. None of these speculations, however, are based on any

firm evidence. Whatever the mechanism involved, it requires the participation of the adrenergic system. In both normal and diabetic subjects,
phentolamine suppressed exercise-induced GH release, while propranolol
magnified it[201].

5.5.4 Adrenergic drugs

The evidence that suppression of central adrenergic tone was responsible for
a reduction of the stimulated release of GH and the recognition that most of
the stimuli for GH secretion involved an adrenergic mechanism, implied as an
irrefutable corollary the GH-stimulant action of adrenergic compounds (see
also Chapter 2 and Müller[122]). In contrast to the positive effects of the direct
infusion of catecholamines (CA) into the lateral ventricle of the rat or the
monkey[122], systemic infusions of epinephrine in the human gave either no
results or inconsistent results on GH release[123, 167]. The poor penetrability
of the blood–brain barrier by CA[202], was circumvented by administering high
doses of the immediate precursor of dopamine, L-DOPA a drug which crosses
the blood–brain barrier easily and increases brain levels of both dopamine
and norepinephrine[203]. Administration of L-DOPA to normal or Parkin-
sonian patients, who required gram amounts of the substance, induced a
significant increase in plasma GH levels. The stimulatory effect on GH-secre-
tion of L-DOPA was not blocked by either oral or intravenous glucose, but
considerably reduced by concomitant infusion of phentolamine, stressing the
involvement of a-adrenergic receptors in the regulation of GH secretion.
Recently, the use of L-DOPA has been proposed as a provocative test for the
diagnosis of hyposomatotropism, even if the unpredictable time of the
response (between 30 and 120 min) after drug administration may limit its
use as a diagnostic test in the evaluation of growth deficiency (see Ref. 122).
In contrast to a-adrenergic receptors, the β-receptor system appears to be
inhibitory to GH release[144], and this could account, besides the impenetra-
bility of the blood–brain barrier, for the inconsistency of epinephrine, a drug
endowed with both a- and β-stimulant effects[200] resulted, in fact, in increased
GH levels in the human[204]. In this instance the stimulatory effect of epinephrine as a GH releaser. Concomitant administration of propranolol, the
β-blocking agent and epinephrine on plasma HGH in the presence of propranolol was probably the result of unopposed a-receptor activity, since
β-stimulation would be expected to inhibit GH secretion. Quite recently, an
increased GH secretion not suppressed by glucose has been observed in
two patients with excessive serotonin secretion from a carcinoid[205]. Decreasing
the serotonin secretion by chemotherapy or blocking its action by methy-
sergide restored GH secretion to normal.

Much more information is needed, however, before the role of serotonin,
another brain neurotransmitter, in the GH-releasing mechanism can be
definitively established.

5.5.5 Deep sleep

In 1966, Quabbe et al.[206], were the first to report in the adult human the
occurrence of a pattern of intermittent bursts of GH secretion during the

time of deeper sleep; this observation was confirmed in children and adolescents[14]. Since then, much more information is available on the sleep-induced GH peaks[122]. The elevation of plasma GH at night during sleep might be considered to represent a late post-absorptive phase rise and it is suggested that the brain in some way monitors the nutritional state of the body[207, 239] However, these rises have been found to correlate with the time of onset and the depth of sleep[208, 240] and appear to be unrelated to the time lapse after the last meal.

Takahashi et al.[208] and Sassin et al.[209], correlated the changes in plasma GH with the electroencephalographic-determined stages of sleep. From these studies a great uniformity in the pattern of GH secretion during sleep than had previously been recognised was evident. There was a greater clearly defined peak plasma GH which reached its highest values about 70 min after onset of sleep. Delay of sleep allowed a delayed peak of GH to be shown, which appeared, even though of lower magnitude, when sleep was re-initiated. The correlation of onset of GH peaks with the level of sleep favoured an association of GH peaks with the deeper encephalographic stages of sleep (3 and 4). At first, no correlation could be demonstrated between the GH peaks and period of rapid eye movement sleep (REM sleep)[208]. However, Sassin et al.[210] were able to show that REM sleep deprivation increased GH secretion, while REM sleep appeared to inhibit GH levels. In the last few years the various patterns of GH secretion during sleep have been described at different ages or in subjects with endocrinopathies (see Müller[122]). No correlation between plasma HGH levels and sleep–wake cycles during a 3 h period were found in 2-, 4- and 8-day-old infants[13]; such a correlation was present after the third month of life[211].

The sleep-related GH peaks were absent in aged normal subjects and in acromegaly[212]. The persistence of normal GH responses to insulin-induced hypoglycaemia in elderly persons[213] suggests that the age-related loss of GH-sleep peaks cannot be attributable to a generalised hyporesponsiveness to all GH provocative stimuli. From the evidence cited in the preceding subsections, the final activation of the adrenergic mechanism following most of the GH-releasing stimuli was apparent. It would appear, however, that brain CA do not play a major role in the sleep-induced peak of GH secretion. Neither phentolamine nor propranolol, in fact, significantly after the GH secretory pattern typical of deep sleep[214]. Only with imipramine, a tricyclic antidepressant which inhibits the uptake of both norepinephrine and serotonin into the storage granules in the nerve terminal, was an inhibition noted[208]. This would imply that the activity of a neurotransmitter with inhibitory effects on GRF was enhanced. Because of the lack of correlation between the nocturnal secretion of GH and plasma concentration of glucose, insulin and NEFA[206, 208], it has been assumed that the sleep peak of GH is controlled by CNS rhythms which are independent of the availability of metabolic substrate. However, obese individuals secrete little HGH at night[206, 207] and even in normal individuals treated with heparin to increase plasma NEFA levels, HGH output after onset of sleep was considerably reduced[215]. In addition, a suppressive action on the sleep-induced GH peaks has been reported after acute administration of high doses of glucose[214]. This suggests that the nocturnal secretion of HGH may not be totally independent of metabolic regulation. In the light of these last observations one cannot completely disregard the concept that the CNS in some way monitors the nutritional state of the body. Additional information is needed to clarify this point.

5.6 SHORT FEED-BACK MECHANISM IN THE CONTROL OF GH SECRETION

The lack of the usual feed-back mechanism for the control of GH secretion operated by the secretion product of a peripheral target gland made the postulate of the existence of a *short* or *auto* feed-back mechanism likely, in which the controlling signal which acts on hypothalamic and/or pituitary receptors is represented by the pituitary trophic hormone itself. Evidence that GH may inhibit its own secretion has been accumulated rapidly especially on the basis of animal studies. Transplantation of GH secreting tumours, the implantation of bovine or HGH into the hypothalamus of rats, or pretreatment of rats with GH were associated with the lowering of pituitary GH content and weight or blockade of the insulin-induced GH release. Intravenous infusions of GH in monkeys for 2 h inhibited GH responsiveness to insulin-induced hypoglycaemia or pitressin administration[122]. Recent reports in normal man are essentially in accordance with the findings of the animal studies. Merimee et al.[216], reported a failure of GH to rise in response to arginine administration in normal females after a 20 min walk which had raised GH levels at the beginning of the infusion, Abrams et al.[217] prevented hypoglycaemic-induced elevations in GH by the exogenous administration of GH for 6 days in healthy man. Rises in GH levels induced, either by a provocative stimulus or by infusing HGH at a constant rate, dampened or prevented the expected hypothalamo–pituitary response to the known provocative stimuli of exercise, arginine administration or insulin-induced hypoglycaemia[218].

From these studies it is assumed that elevated titres of circulating GH exert such an *auto* feed-back at the level of the hypothalamic GRF centre and/or at pituitary level[122]. The basic nature of the GH *auto* feed-back mechanism, however, remains obscure and the above studies do not answer the question of whether the observed effects were due to GH itself or to some metabolic consequence of the hormone. The possibility that the feed-back operates on the basis of somatomedin plasma levels, with high levels of the peptide inhibiting, and, conversely, low levels increasing, GH secretion, although unproved, is nevertheless, highly appealing. Though Abrams et al., did not actually imply somatomedin in the feed-back mechanism, the time relations in their study would fit very well with this explanation. The ability of their subjects to secrete GH in response to insulin hypoglycaemia began to return about 12 h after the exogenous HGH was stopped and was back to normal in about 48 h. Similarly, in the study of Hagen et al.[218], arginine or insulin testings were performed after a time lapse sufficient to allow a GH-dependent increase of somatomedin in plasma[101].

The existence of a somatomedin feed-back system is also supported by other observations; high concentrations of plasma HGH are present in children who are unable to produce somatomedin[219, 251] and, conversely, decreased pituitary GH concentrations are found in rats infested with spargana of *Spirometra mansonoides*[109] (see Section 5.4). The elevated HGH levels of the somatomedin-deficient children are reminiscent of similar elevated levels of trophic hormones seen in thyroidectomised and adrenalectomised patients and raise the possibility of a long-loop feed-back of GH acting through somatomedin to inhibit GH secretion.

Thus, although in a modified way due to the peculiarity of the hormonal target, a long-loop feed-back system might be operative also for GH secretion. The somatomedin feed-back system might alter the sensitivity of the hypothalamic GRF centre and thus serve to modulate its response to a variety of a short-term metabolic and neurogenic stimuli. As to its actual role in the process of growth, we are still very much in the dark.

5.7 CONCLUDING REMARKS

It would be difficult and perhaps unnecessary to summarise the contents of this article, perhaps more appropriate would be to place emphasis on certain aspects which deserve special attention in the future.

The fundamental site of action of GH is still unknown. By and large it exerts a multiplicity of metabolic actions, but some of them, once considered of primary importance for the bodily requirements, have recently been re-evaluated. Thus, the experimental evidence tends to exclude the role of GH both as a substrate regulator following feeding and as a primary hormonal mediator during fasting, and suggests, at the most, its intervention in the state of severe protein deprivation.

GH is undoubtedly the prime determinant of postnatal growth in man. Several lines of evidence support the hypothesis that it does not act directly on cartilage, but through the mediation of a secondary hormonal agent, i.e. somatomedin. Although there are few published studies concerning concentrations of somatomedin in normal children in relation to age, the correlation present between somatomedin levels in plasma and growth rate in GH-treated hypopituitary dwarfs is evidence that somatomedin and not GH is the true growth-promoting factor. The somatomedin mechanism appears to account for GH function in the long-range strategic objective of orderly skeletal growth more logically than the intermittent daily bursts of GH which occur in response to a variety of metabolic and neurogenic stimuli. Perhaps, the net effect of the isolated GH bursts may be integrated by the somatomedin mechanism to provide a modulated system suitable for skeletal growth regulation. If there is a long-term homeostatic mechanism linking GH in growth, it is likely to link the plasma level of somatomedin with the GH-releasing factor of the hypothalamus.

Evidence has now been accumulated that somatomedin has marked insulin-like actions in non-skeletal as well as in skeletal tissue. These facts, while posing again the ancient problem of the GH-insulin inter-relationship, call for the re-investigation of the metabolic effects of GH in order to dissociate the direct effects of GH on target tissues from those attributable to the induction of somatomedin. Further insight into the metabolic role of GH might be derived by the determination of plasma levels of somatomedin under different metabolic conditions as well as by the assessment of somatomedin–insulin competition at receptor sites.

Despite recent advances in knowledge, much requires to be learned about the physiological factors which influence GH secretion. A negative feed-back mechanism exists between the availability of intracellular glucose and GH secretion which operates under physiological conditions. This mechanism involves the participation of specific glucosensitive elements in the hypo-thalamus and the mediation of a GRF. Nonetheless, the physiological signifi-cance of the hormone secreted is open to question, since in GH-deficient individuals no obvious consequences can be observed, other than those of lack of body growth. A number of other stimuli have been described which include stresses of several kinds, infusion of amino acids or protein ingestion, falling free fatty acid levels, etc., but their function and significance in the control of GH release is still unknown. On the basis of the acquired know-ledge, to the list of these stimuli we might add a decrease of blood somato-medin. Most of the GH-releasing stimuli demand the presence of a central a-adrenergic tone and the GH response are blunted following a-adrenergic blockade. CNS participation in the regulation of GH secretion is also supported by the large peak of GH secretion associated with deep sleep. Undoubtedly, the studies mentioned here have posed more questions than definite answers to the many problems connected with the physiology of GH. However, there is every reason to suppose that within the next few years many problems at present unanswered will be solved.

References

1. Dickerman, E., Dickerman, S. and Meites, J. (1972). *Growth and Growth Hormone, Influence of age, sex and estrous cycle on pituitary and plasma GH levels in rats*, ICS **244**, 252 (A. Pecile and E. E. Müller, editors) (Amsterdam: Excerpta Medica)
2. Burek, C. L. and Frohman, L. A. (1970). Growth hormone synthesis by rat pituitary *in vitro*: effect of age and sex. *Endocrinology*, **86**, 1361
3. Birge, C. A., Peake, G. T., Mariz, I. K. and Daughaday, W. H. (1967). Radio-immunoassayable growth hormone in the rat pituitary gland: effects of age, sex and hormonal state. *Endocrinology*, **81**, 195
4. Wilson, J. T. and Frohman, L. A. (1972). Concomitant association between liver drug metabolism and plasma levels of growth hormone (GH) in the young rat (1972). (Abstracts) *Vth Int. Congr. Pharmacol.*, San Francisco, 254
5. Jost, A. (1947). Experiences de decapitation de l'embryon du lapin. *C.R. Soc. Biol.* (*Paris*), **225**, 322
6. Daughaday, W. H. and Kipnis, D. M. (1966). The growth promoting and anti-insulin actions of somatotropin. *Rec. Prog. Horm. Res.*, **22**, 49
7. Heins, J. N., Garland, J. T. and Daughaday, W. H. (1970). Incorporation of ^{35}S-sulphate into rat cartilage explants '*in vitro*': Effects of aging on responsiveness to stimulation by sulfation factor. *Endocrinology*, **87**, 688
8. Gitlin, D. and Biasucci, A. (1969). Ontogenesis of immunoreactive growth-hormone, follicle stimulating hormone, thyroid stimulating hormone, luteinizing hormone, chorionic prolactin and chorionic gonadotropin in the human conceptus. *J. Clin. Endocrinol.*, **29**, 926
9. Matsuzaki, F., Irie, M. and Shizume, K. (1971). Growth hormone in human fetal pituitary gland and cord blood. *J. Clin. Endocrinol.*, **33**, 908
10. Lloyd, H. M., Donald, K. I., Catt, K. J. and Burger, H. G. (1969). Growth hormone concentration in human pituitary tumours. *J. Endocrinol.*, **45**, 133

11. Daughaday, W. H. (1968). *Textbook of Endocrinology*, 27 (R. H. Williams, editor) (Philadelphia: Saunders Company)
12. Root, A. W. (1972). *Human Pituitary Growth Hormone* (I. N. Kugelmass, editor) (Springfield: Charles Thomas)
13. Shaywitz, B. A., Finkelstein, J., Hellman, L. and Weitzman, E. D. (1971). Growth hormone in newborn infants during sleep-wake periods. *Pediatrics*, **48**, 103
14. Hunter, W. M. and Rigal, W. M. (1966). The diurnal pattern of plasma growth hormone concentration in children and adolescents. *J. Endocrinol.*, **34**, 147
15. Thompson, R. G., Rodriguez, A., Kowarski, A., Migeon, C. J. and Blizzard, R. M. (1972). Integrated concentrations of growth hormone correlated with plasma testosterone and bone age in preadolescent and adolescent males. *J. Clin. Endocrinol.*, **35**, 334
16. Geller, J. and Loh, A. (1963). Identification and measurement of growth hormone in extracts of human urine. *J. Clin. Endocrinol.*, **23**, 1107
17. Sakuma, M., Irie, M., Shizume, K., Tsushima, T. and Nakao, K. (1968). Measurement of urinary human growth hormone by radioimmunoassay. *J. Clin. Endocrinol.*, **28**, 103
18. Girard, G. and Greenwood, F. C. (1968). The absence of intact growth hormone in urine as judged by radioimmunoassay. *J. Endocrinol.*, **40**, 493
19. Hanssen, K. F. (1972). Immunoreactive growth hormone in human urine. *Acta Endocrinol.*, (Kbh) **71**, 665
20. Santis, M. R., Lowrie, E. G., Hampers, C. L. and Soeldner J. S. (1969). *Diffusion of growth hormone into thoracic duct lymph in man*. 51*st Meet. Endocrinol. Soc.*, 108
21. Root, A. W. and Russ, J. (1972). unpublished data
22. Linfoot, J. A., Garcia, J. F., Wei, W., Fink, R., Sarisi, R., Born, J. L. and Lawrence, J. W. (1970). Human growth hormone levels in cerebrospinal fluid. *J. Clin. Endocrinol.*, **31**, 230
23. Gitlin, D., Kumate, J. and Morales, C. (1965). Metabolism and maternofetal transfer of human growth hormone in the pregnant woman at term. *J. Clin. Endocrinol.*, **25**, 1599
24. Bala, R. M., Ferguson, K. A. and Beck, J. C. (1970). Plasma biological and immunoreactive human growth hormone-like activity. *Endocrinology*, **87**, 506
25. Goodman, A. D., Tanebaum, R. and Rabinowitz, D. (1972). Existence of two forms of immunoreactive growth hormone in human plasma. *J. Clin. Endocrinol.*, **35**, 868
26. Gorden, P., Hendricks, C. M. and Roth, J. (1972). Evidence for 'big' and 'little' components of human plasma and pituitary growth hormone. *J. Clin. Endocrinol.*, **36**, 178
27. Frohman, L. A., Burek, L. and Stachura, M. (1972). Characterization of growth hormone of different molecular weights in rat, dog and human pituitaries. *Endocrinology* **91**, 262
28. Burger, H. G., Alford, F. P. and Cameron, D. P. (1973). *Proc. IVth. Int. Congr. Endocrinol., The secretion rate and metabolism of human growth hormone*, (Amsterdam: Excerpta Medica) (in press)
29. Parker, M. L., Utiger, R. D. and Daughaday, W. H. (1962). Studies on human growth hormone. II. The physiological disposition and metabolic fate of human growth hormone in man. *J. Clin. Invest.*, **41**, 262
30. Glick, S. M., Roth, J. and Lonergan, E. T. (1964). Survival of endogenous human growth hormone in plasma. *J. Clin. Endocrinol.*, **24**, 501
31. Refetoff, S. and Sonksen, P. H. (1970). Disappearance rate of endogenous and exogenous human growth hormone in man. *J. Clin. Endocrinol.*, **30**, 386
32. Sonenberg, M., Money, W. L., Dorans, J. F., Lucas, V. and Bourque, L. (1954). The distribution of radioactivity in the tissues of the rat after the administration of radioactive growth hormone preparation. *Endocrinology*, **55**, 709
33. Collip, R. J., Patrick, J. R., Goodheart, C. and Kaplan, S. A. (1966). Distribution of tritium labelled human growth hormone in rats and guinea pigs. *Proc. Soc. Exp. Biol. Med.*, **121**, 173
34. De Kretser, D. M., Catt, K. J., Burger, H. G. and Smith, G. C. (1969). Radioautographic studies on the localization of ^{125}I labelled human luteinizing and growth hormone in immature male rats. *J. Endocrinol.*, **43**, 105
35. Mayberry, H. E., Van Den Brande, J. L., Van Wyk, J. J. and Waddel, W. J. (1971). Early localization of ^{125}I labelled human growth hormone in adrenal and other organs

of immature hypophysectomized rats. *Endocrinology*, **88**, 1309

36. Levi-Montalcini, R. and Cohen, S. (1960). Effect of the extract of the mouse sub-maxillary salivary glands on the sympathetic systems of mammals. *Ann. N.Y. Acad. Sci.*, **85**, 324

37. Narasimhan, M. J. Jr. and Gonla, V. G. (1968). The regulatory influence of the sub-mandibular salivary gland on growth. *Ann Endocrinol. (Paris)*, **29**, 513

38. Sonenberg, M. and Money, W. L. (1955). The fate and metabolism of anterior pituitary hormones. *Rec. Prog. Horm. Res.*, **11**, 43

39. McCormick, J. R., Sonksen, P. H., Soeldner, J. S. and Egdahl, R. H. (1969). Renal handling of insulin and growth hormone in hemorrhagic shock. *Surgery*, **66**, 175

40. Taylor, A. L., Lipman, R. L., Salam, A. and Mintz, D. H. (1972). Hepatic clearance of human growth hormone. *J. Clin. Endocrinol.*, **34**, 395

41. Becker, M. D., Cook, G. C. and Wright, A. D. (1969). Paradoxical elevation of growth hormone in active chronic hepatitis, *Lancet*, **11**, 1035

42. Samaan, N. A., Stone, D. B. and Eckhardt, R. D. (1969). Serum glucose, insulin and growth hormone in chronic hepatic cirrhosis. *Arch. Int. Med.*, **24**, 149

43. Cameron, D. P., Burger, H. G., Catt, K. J., Gordon, E. and Mck Watts, J. (1972). Metabolic clearance of human growth hormone in patients with hepatic and renal failure, and in the isolated perfused pig liver. *Metabolism*, **21**, 895

44. Daughaday, W. M. and Parker, M. L. (1965). Human pituitary growth hormone. *Ann. Rev. Med.*, **16**, 47

45. Knobil, E. and Hotchkiss, J. (1964). Growth hormone. *Ann. Rev. Physiol.*, **26**, 47

46. Matsuzaki, F. and Raben, M. S. (1965). Growth hormone. *Ann. Rev. Pharmacol.*, **5**, 37

47. Knobil, E., Wolf, R. C., Greep, R. O. and Wilhelmi, A. E. (1957). Effect of a primate pituitary growth hormone preparation on nitrogen metabolism in the hypophysecto-mized Rhesus monkey. *Endocrinology*, **60**, 166

48. Beck, J. C., McGarry, B. E., Dyrenfurth, I. K. and Venning, E. H. (1958). The meta-bolic effects of human and monkey growth hormone in man. *Ann. Int. Med.*, **49**, 1090

49. McGarry, E. and Beck, J. C. (1972). *Human Growth Hormone, Metabolic effects of Human Growth Hormone.* 25 (A. Stuart Mason, editor) (London: W. Heinemann Medical Books Ltd.)

50. Prader, A., Zachmann, M., Poley, J. R. and Illig, R. (1968). The metabolic effect of a small uniform dose of human growth hormone in hypopituitary dwarfs and in control children. I. Nitrogen, α-amino-N, inorganic phosphorus and alkaline phosphatase. II. Blood glucose response to insulin-induced hypoglycaemia. *Acta Endocrinol.*, (Kbh) **57**, 115

51. Rabinowitz, D., Merimee, T. J., Rimoin, D. L., Hall, J. G. and McKusick, V. A. (1968). Peripheral subresponsiveness to human growth hormone in a proportionate dwarf. *J. Clin. Invest.*, **47**, 82a

52. Zachmann, M., Prader, A. Ferrandez, A. and Illig, R. (1972). *Growth and growth hormone, Evaluation of growth deficiency by metabolic tests*, ICS **244**, 421 (A. Pecile and E. E. Müller, editors) (Amsterdam: Excerpta Medica)

53. Ahren, K. and Hjalmarson, A. (1968). *Growth Hormone, Early and late effects of growth hormone on transport of amino acids and monosaccharides in the isolated rat diaphragm*, ICS **158**, 143 (A. Pecile and E. E. Müller, editors) (Amsterdam: Excerpta Medica)

54. Dawson, K. G. and Beck, J. C. (1968). Early and late effects of growth hormone on the rat diaphragm. *Proc. Soc. Exp. Biol. Med.*, **127**, 617

55. Kostyo, J. L. and Knobil, E. (1959). The effects of growth hormone on the '*in vitro*' incorporation of leucine 2-^{14}C into the protein of rat diaphragm. *Endocrinology*, **65**

56. Kostyo, J. L. (1964). Separation of effects of growth hormone on muscle amino acid transport and protein synthesis. *Endocrinology*, **75**, 113

57. Rillema, J. A. and Kostyo, J. L. (1970). Studies on the delayed action of growth hormone on the metabolism of the rat diaphragm. *Endocrinology*, **88**, 240

58. Jefferson, L. S. and Korner, A. (1967). A direct effect of growth hormone on the incorporation of precursors into proteins and nucleic acids of perfused rat liver. *Biochem. J.*, **104**, 826

59. Jefferson, L. S. and Korner, A. (1969). Influence of amino acid supply on ribosomes and protein synthesis of perfused rat liver. *Biochem. J.*, **111**, 703

60. Korner, A. (1970). *Control Processes in Multicellular Organisms, Insulin and Growth*

Hormone Control of Protein Biosynthesis, 86 (G. E. W. Wolstenholme and J. Knight, editors) (London: Churchill)

61. Salaman, D. F., Betteridge, A. and the late Korner, A. (1972). Early effects of growth hormone on nuclear and nucleoplasmic RNA synthesis and RNA polymerase activity in normal rat liver. *Biochem. Biophys. Acta*, **272**, 382

62. Britten, R. J. and Davidson, E. H. (1969). Gene regulation for higher cells: a theory. *Science*, **165**, 349

65. Scherrer, K., Spohr, G., Granboulan, N., Morel, C., Grosclaude, J. and Chezzi, C. (1970). *Cold Spring Harbor Symp. Quant. Biol.*, **35**, 539

64. Darnell, J. E., Pagoulatos, G. N., Lindberg, V. and Balint, R. (1970). *Cold Spring Harbor Symp. Quant. Biol.*, **35**, 555

65. Kenney, F. T. (1965). *J. Cell Physiol.*, **66**, Suppl 1, 69

66. Karlson, P. (1970). *Schering Workshop on Steroid Hormone Receptor, Mechanism of Hormone Action* (G. Raspé, editor) (Wieweg: Pergamon Press)

67. Wool, I. G., Stirewalt, W. S., Kurihara, K., Low, R. B., Bailey, P. and Oyer, D. (1968). Mode of action of insulin in the regulation of protein biosynthesis in muscle. *Rec. Prog. Horm. Res.*, **24**, 139

68. Manchester, K. L. and Young, F. G. (1961). Insulin and protein metabolism. *Vit. Horm.*, **19**, 95

69. Weil, R. (1965). Pituitary growth hormone and intermediary metabolism. *Acta Endocrinol.*, (Kbh). Suppl. 98, **49**, 5

70. Rabinowitz, D., Klassen, G. A. and Zierler, K. L. (1965). Effect of human growth hormone on muscle and adipose tissue metabolism in the forearm of man. *J. Clin. Invest.*, **44**, 51

71. Swislocki, N. I. and Szego, C. M. (1965). Acute reduction of plasma nonesterified fatty acid by growth hormone in hypophysectomized and Houssay rats. *Endocrinology*, **76**, 665

72. Raben, M. S. and Hollenberg, C. H. (1959). Effect of growth hormone on plasma fatty acids. *J. Clin. Invest.*, **38**, 484

73. Goodman, H. M. and Knobil, E. (1959). The effect of fasting and of growth hormone administration on plasma fatty acid concentration in normal and hypophysectomized Rhesus monkey. *Endocrinology*, **65**, 451

74. Van der Laan, W. P. and Simpson, D. P. (1960). Restoration by growth hormone of normal responses to fasting in pituitary dwarfs. *J. Clin. Invest.*, **39**, 1037

75. Sawin, C. T. and Willard, D. A. (1970). Normal rise in plasma free fatty acids during fasting in patients with hypopituitarism. *J. Clin. Endocrinol.*, **31**, 233

76. Williams, R. H. (1968). *Textbook of Endocrinology*, 803 (R. H. Williams, editor) (Philadelphia: Saunders Company)

77. Goodman, H. M. (1960). Effects of growth hormone on the lipolytic response of adipose tissue to theophylline. *Endocrinology*, **82**, 1027

78. Galton, D. J. and Bray, G. A. (1967). Studies on lipolysis in human adipose cells (1967). *J. Clin. Invest.*, **46**, 621

79. Bjorntorp, P., Karlsson and Hovden, A. (1969). Quantitative aspects of lipolysis and reesterification in human adipose tissue *in vitro*. *Acta Med. Scand.*, **185**, 89

80. Sutherland, E. W., Øye, I. and Butcher, R. W. (1965). The action of epinephrine and the role of the adenyl cyclase system in hormone action. *Rec. Prog. Horm. Res.*, **21**, 623

81. Brown, J. and Bennet, L. R. (1964). Effect of growth hormone on fatty acid utilization in human subjects. *Clin. Res.*, **12**, 263 (Abstract)

82. Buckle, R. M. (1962). The stimulating effects of adrenaline and anterior pituitary hormones on the release of free fatty acids from adipose tissue. *J. Endocrinol.*, **25**, 189

83. Ashmore, J., Cahill, G. F. Jr and Hastings, A. B. (1960). Effect of hormones on alternate pathways of glucose utilization in isolated tissues. *Rec. Prog. Horm., Res.* **16**, 547

84. Dominguez, J. M., Greenberg, E., Pazianos, A. O., Ray, B. S. and Pearson, O. H. (1960). Diabetogenic and hypoglycemic effects of human growth hormone. *Acta Endocrinol.*, (Kbh). Suppl. **51**, 241

85. Garland, P. B. and Randle, P. J. (1964). Control of pyruvate dehydrogenase in the perfused rat heart by the intracellular concentration of acetyl-Coenzyme A. *Biochem. J.*, **91**, 6

86. Randle, P. J. and Morgan, H. E. (1962). Regulation of glucose uptake by muscle. *Vit. Horm.*, **20**, 199

87. Altszuler, N., Steele, R., Rathgeb, I. and De Bodo, R. C. (1968). *Growth Hormone, Influence of growth hormone on glucose metabolism and plasma insulin levels in the dog*, ICS **158** (A. Pecile and E. E. Müller, editors) (Amsterdam: Excerpta Medica)

88. Campbell, J., Chaikoff, L., Wrenshall, G. A. and Zemel, R. (1959). Effects of growth hormone on metabolic and endocrine factors in hypophysectomized dogs. *Can. J. Biochem.*, **37**, 1313

89. Ikkos, S. and Luft, R. (1960). 'Idiohypophyseal' diabetes mellitus in two hyposectomized women. *Lancet, II*, 897

90. Luft, R., Ikkos, D., Gemzell, C. A. and Olivecrona, H. (1959). The effect of human growth hormone in hypophysectomized diabetic subjects. *Acta Endocrinol.*, **32**, 330

91. Henneman, D. H. and Henneman, P. H. (1960). Effects of human growth hormone on levels of blood and urinary carbohydrates and fat metabolites in man. *J. Clin. Invest.*, **39**, 1239

92. Schwarz, F., der Kinderen, J., van Riet, H. G., Thissen, J. H. H. and van Wayjen, R. G. A. (1972). Influence of exogenous human growth hormone on the metabolism of fasting obese patients. *Metabolism*, **21**, 297

93. Luft, R. and Cerasi, E. (1968). *Growth Hormone, Human growth hormone in blood glucose homeostasis*, ICS **158**, 373 (A. Pecile and E. E. Müller, editors) (Amsterdam: Excerpta Medica)

94. Salmon, W. D. Jr and Daughaday, W. H. (1957). A hormonally controlled serum factor which stimulates incorporation by cartilage *in vitro. J. Lab. Clin. Med.*, **49**, 825

95. Daughaday, W. H. (1971). Sulphation factor regulation of skeletal growth. A stable mechanism dependent on intermitent growth hormone secretion. *Amer. J. Med.*, **50**, 277

96. Salmon, W. D. Jr and Du Vall, M. R. (1970). A serum fraction with 'sulfation factor activity' stimulates *in vitro* incorporation of leucine and sulfate into protein polysaccharide complexes, uridine into RNA and thymidine into DNA of costal cartilage from hypophysectomized rats. *Endocrinology*, **86**, 721

97. Daughaday, W. M. and Reeder, C. (1966). Synchronous activation of DNA synthesis in hypophysectomized rat cartilage by growth hormone. *J. Lab. Clin. Med.*, **68**, 357

98. Daughaday, W. H., Hall, K., Raben, M. S., Salmon, W. D. Jr, Van den Brande, J. L. and Van Wyk, J. J. (1972). Somatomedin: proposed designation for sulphation factor *Nature (London)*, **235**, 107

99. Salmon, W. D. Jr (1972). *Growth and Growth Hormone, Investigation with a partially purified preparation of serum sulphation factor: lack of specificity for cartilage sulphation* ICS **244**, 180 (A Pecile, E. E. Müller, editors) (Amsterdam: Excerpta Medica)

100. Hall, K., Holmgren, A. and Lindahl, U. (1970). Purification of a sulphation factor from skeletal muscle of rat. *Biochem. Biophys. Acta*, **201**, 398

101. Daughaday, W. H., Heins, J. N., Srivastava, L. and Hammer, C. (1968). Sulphation factor: studies of its removal from plasma and metabolic fate in cartilage. *J. Lab. Clin. Med.*, **72**, 803

102. McConaghey, P. and Sledge, C. B. (1970). Production of 'sulphation factor' by the perfused liver, *Nature (London)*, **225**, 1249

103. McConaghey, P. (1972). The production of 'sulphation factor' by rat liver. *J. Endocrinol.*, **52**, 1

104. McConaghey, P. and Muller, J. (1971). *Abstr. 2nd Int. Symp. Growth Hormone, Sulphation factor: its production by the rat liver and kidney*, ICS **236**, 26 (Amsterdam: Excerpta Medica)

105. Uthne, K. and Uthne, T. (1972). Influence of liver resection and regeneration on somatomedin (sulphation factor) activity in sera from normal and hypophysectomized rats. *Acta Endocrinol.*, **71**, 255

106. Van den Brande, J. L., Koote, F., Tielenburg, R., Van Der Wilk, M. and Koot, T. (1971). *Abstr. 2nd Int. Symp. Growth Hormone, Plasma sulphation factor (PSF) in different animal species*, ICS **236**, 26 (Amsterdam: Excerpta Medica)

107. Steelman, S. L., Morgan, E. R., Cuccaro, A. J. and Glitzer, M. S. (1970). Growth hormone-like activity in hypophysectomized rats implanted with *Spirometra mansonoides* sparnga. *Proc. Soc. Exp. Biol. Med.*, **133**, 269

108. Garland, J. T., Reugamer, W. R. and Daughaday, W. H. (1971). Induction of sulphation factor activity by injection of hypophysectomized rats with *Spirometra Mansonoides. Endocrinology*, **88**, 924

109. Daughaday, W. H. and Garland, J. T. (1972). *Growth and Growth Hormone, The Sulphation Factor Hypothesis: recent observations*, ICS **244**, 168 (A. Pecile and E. E. Müller, editors) (Amsterdam: Excerpta Medica)
110. Van den Brande, J. L., Van Wyk, J. J., Weaver, R. R. and Mayberry, H. E. (1971). Partial characterization of sulphation and thymidine factors in acromegalic plasma. *Acta Endocrinol.*, (Kbh.) **66**, 65
111. Van Wyk, J. J., Hall, K., Vand den Brande, J. L., Weaver, R. P., Uthne, K., Hintz, R. L., Harrison, J. H. and Mathewson, P. (1972). *Growth and Growth Hormone, Partial purification from human plasma of small peptide with sulfation factor activities*, ICS, **244**, 148 (A. Pecile and E. E. Müller, editors) (Amsterdam: Excerpta Medica)
112. Jacob, A., Hauri, C. H. and Froesch, E. R. (1968). Non suppressible insulin-like activity in human serum. III Differentiation of two distinct molecules with non-suppressible ILA. *J. Clin. Invest.*, **47**, 2678
113. Van Vyk, J. J., Hintz, R. L., Clemmons, D. R., Hall, K. and Uthne, K. (1973). *Proc. IVth Int. Congr. Endocrinol.*, *Human somatomedin, the growth hormone dependent sulfation and thymidine factor*, (in press) (Amsterdam: Excerpta Medica)
114. Salmon, W. D., Jr and Du Vall, M. R. (1970). '*In vitro*' stimulation of leucine incorporation into muscle and cartilage by a serum fraction with sulphation factor activity. Differentiation of effects from those of growth hormone and insulin. *Endocrinology*, **87**, 1168
115. Hall, K. and Uthne, K. (1972). *Growth and Growth Hormone, Human growth hormone and sulphation factor*, ICS **244**, 192 (A. Pecile and E. E. Müller, editors) (Amsterdam: Excerpta Medica)
116. Salmon, W. D., Jr and Hosse, B. R. (1971). Stimulation of HeLa cell growth by a serum factor with sulfation factor activity. *Proc. Soc. Exp. Biol. Med.*, **136**, 805
117. Underwood, L. E., Hintz, R. L., Voina, S. J. and Van Wyk J. J. (1972). Human somatomedin, the growth hormone dependent sulphation factor, is anti-lipolytic. *J. Clin. Endocrinol.*, **35**, 194
118. Hintz, R. L., Clemmons, D. R., Underwood, L. E. and Van Wyk, J. J. (1972). Competitive binding of somatomedin to the insulin receptor of adipocytes, chondrocytes and liver membranes. *Proc. Nat. Acad. Sci. USA*, **69**, 2351
119. Cuatrecasas, P. (1971). Insulin-receptor interactions in adipose tissue cells: direct measurements and properties. *Proc. Nat. Acad. Sci. USA*, **68**, 1264
120. Randle, P. J. and Young, F. G. (1956). The influence of pituitary growth hormone on plasma insulin activity. *J. Endocrinol.*, **13**, 335
121. Poffenbarger, P. L., Espinosa De Los Monteros Mena, A. and Steinke, J. (1970). Nonsuppressible insulin-like activity: immunochemical and physicochemical evidence against its pancreatic origin. *Metabolism*, **19**, 509
122. Muller, E. E. (1973). Nervous control of growth hormone secretion. *Neuroendocrinology*, **11**, 338
123. Roth, J., Glick, S. M., Yalow, R. S. and Berson, S. A. (1963). Hypoglycaemia: a potent stimulus to secretion of growth hormone. *Science*, **140**, 987
124. Roth, J., Glick, S. M., Yalow, R. S. and Berson, S. A. (1963). Secretion of human growth hormone: physiologic and experimental modification. *Metabolism*, **12**, 577
125. Takebe, K., Kunita, H., Sawano, S., Horiuchi, Y. and Mashimo, K. (1969). Circadian rhythms of plasma growth hormone and cortisol after insulin. *J. Clin. Endocrinol.*, **29**, 1630
126. Wegienka, L. C., Grodsky, G. M., Karam, J. H., Grasso, S. G. and Forsham, P. H. (1967). Comparison of insulin and 2-deoxy-D-glucose-induced glucopenia as stimulators of growth hormone secretion. *Metabolism*, **16**, 245
127. Smith, G. P. and Root, A. W. (1969). Effects of feeding on hormonal responses to 2-deoxy-D-glucose in conscious monkeys. *Endocrinology*, **85**, 963
128. Baylis, E. M., Greenwood, F., James V., Jenkins, J., Landon, J., Marks, V. and Samols, E. (1968). *Growth Hormone, An examination of the control mechanisms postulated to control growth hormone secretion in man*, ICS **158**, 89 (A. Pecile and E. E. Müller, editors (Amsterdam: Excerpta Medica)
129. Irie, M. M., Sakuma, T., Tsushima, F., Matsuzaki, K., Shizume, K. and Nakao, K. (1967). Effect of acute glucose infusion on plasma concentration of human growth hormone. *Proc. Soc. Exp. Biol. Med.*, **125**, 1314

130. Meyer, V. and Knobil, E. (1967). Growth hormone secretion in the unanesthetized Rhesus monkey in response to noxious stimuli. *Endocrinology*, **80**, 163
131. Müller, E. E., Saito, A., Arimura, A. and Schally, A. V. (1967). Hypoglycemia, stress and growth hormone release: blockade of growth hormone release by drugs acting on the central nervous system. *Endocrinology*, **80**, 109
132. Luft, R., Cerasi, E., Madison, L. L., von Euler, U. S., Della Casa, L. and Roovete, A. (1966). Effect of a small decrease in blood-glucose on plasma growth hormone and urinary excretion of catecholamines in man. *Lancet*, **II**, 254
133. Greenwood, F. C., Landon, J. and Stamp, T. C. B. (1966). The plasma sugar, free fatty acid, cortisol, and growth hormone response to insulin. I. In control subjects. *J. Clin. Invest.*, **45**, 429
134. Koh, C. S., Kohn, J., Catt, K. J. and Burger, H. G. (1968). Lack of relation between plasma growth hormone levels and small decrements in blood sugar. *Lancet*, **II**, 13
135. Fatourechi, V., Molnar, G. D., Service, F. J., Ackerman, E., Rosevear, J. E., Moxness, K. E. and Taylor, W. F. (1969). Growth hormone and glucose interrelationships in diabetes: Studies with insulin infusion during continuous blood glucose analysis. *J. Clin. Endocrinol.*, **29**, 319
136. Molnar, G. D., Fatourechi, V., Service, F. J., Ackerman, E., Rosevear, J. E. and Taylor, W. F. (1971). *Abstr. 2nd Int. Symp. on Growth Hormone, Stress and growth hormone release during continuously monitored hypoglycaemia*, ICS **236**, 50 (Excerpta Medica: Amsterdam)
137. Abrams, R. L., Parker, M. L., Blanco, S., Reichlin, S. and Daughaday, W. H. (1966). Hypothalamic regulation of growth hormone secretion. *Endocrinology*, **78**, 605
138. Blanco, S. D., Schalch, S. and Reichlin, S. (1966). Control of growth hormone secretion by glycoreceptors in the hypothalamic-pituitary unit. *Fed. Proc.*, **25**, 191 (Abstract)
139. Himsworth, R. L., Carmel, P. W. and Frantz, A. G. (1972). The location of the chemoreceptor controlling growth hormone secretion during hypoglycaemia in primates. *Endocrinology*, **91**, 217
140. Roth, J., Glick, S. M., Yalow, R. S. and Berson, S. A. (1964). The influence of blood glucose on the plasma concentration of growth hormone. *Diabetes*, **13**, 355
141. Antony, G. J., Van Wyk, J. J., French, F. S., Weaver, R., Dugger, G. S., Timmons, R. L. and Newsome, J. F. (1969). Influence of pituitary stalk section on growth hormone and TSH secretion in women with metastatic breast cancer. *J. Clin. Endocrinol.*, **29**, 1238
142. Werbach, J. H., Gale, C. C., Goodner, C. J. and Conway, M. J. (1970). Effects of autonomic blocking agents on growth hormone, insulin, free fatty acids and glucose in baboons, *Endocrinology*, **86**, 77
143. Blackard, W. G. and Heidingsfelder, S. A. (1968). Adrenergic receptor control mechanisms for growth hormone secretion. *J. Clin. Invest.*, **47**, 1400
144. Imura, K., Kato, Y. Ikeda, M., Morimoto, M., Yawata, M. and Fukase, M. (1968). Increased plasma levels of growth hormone during infusion of propranolol. *J. Clin. Endocrinol.*, **28**, 1079
145. Blackard, W. G. and Waddel, C. C. (1969). Cholinergic blockade and growth hormone responsiveness to insulin hypoglycemia. *Proc. Soc. Exp. Biol. Med.*, **131**, 192
146. Hunter, W. M. and Greenwood, F. C. (1964). Studies on the secretion of human-pituitary growth hormone. *Brit. Med. J.*, **1**, 804
147. Hunter, W. M., Rigal, W. M. and Sukkar, M. Y. (1968). *Growth Hormone, Plasma growth hormone during fasting*, ICS **158**, 408 (A. Pecile and E. E. Müller, editors) (Amsterdam: Excerpta Medica)
148. Cahill, J. F. Jr, Herrera, M. G., Morgan, A. P., Soeldner, J. S., Steinke, J., Levy, P. L., Reichard, G. A. Jr, and Kipnis, D. M. (1966). Hormone fuel interrelationships during fasting. *J. Clin. Invest.*, **45**, 1751
149. Knobil, E. and Meyer, V. (1968). Observations on the secretion of growth hormone, and its blockade in the Rhesus monkey. *Ann. N.Y. Acad. Sci. USA*, **148**, 459
150. Trenkle, A. (1970). Effect of starvation on pituitary and plasma growth hormone in rats. *Proc. Soc. Exp. Biol. Med.*, **135**, 77
151. Müller, E. E., Miedico, D., Giustina, G. and Cocchi, D. (1971). Ineffectiveness of hypoglycaemia, cold exposure and fasting in stimulating GH secretion in the mouse. *Endocrinology*, **88**, 345

152. Kokka, N., Garcia, J. F., Morgan, M. and George, R. (1971). Immunoassay of plasma growth hormone in cats following fasting and administration of insulin, arginine, 2-deoxyglucose and hypothalamic extract. *Endocrinology*, **88**, 359

153. Machlin, L. J., Takahashi, Y., Horino, M., Hertelendy, F., Gordon, R. S. and Kipnis, D. (1968). *Growth Hormone, Regulation of growth hormone secretion in non-primate species*, ICS **158**, 292 (A. Pecile, E. E. Müller, editors) (Amsterdam: Excerpta Medica)

154. Garcia, J. F. and Geschwind, I. I. (1968). *Growth Hormone, Investigation of growth hormone secretion in selected mammalian species*, ICS **158**, 267 (A. Pecile, E. E. Müller, editors) (Amsterdam: Excerpta Medica)

155. Tarrant, M. E., Mahler, R. and Ashmore, R. (1964). Studies in experimental diabetes IV. Free fatty acid mobilization. *J. Biol. Chem.*, **239**, 1714

156. Pimstone, B. L., Becker, D. J. and Hansen, J. D. L. (1972). *Growth and Growth Hormone, Human growth hormone in protein-calorie malnutrition*, ICS **244**, 389 (A. Pecile, E. E. Müller, editors) (Amsterdam: Excerpta Medica)

157. Merimee, T. J. and Fineberg, S. E. (1972). Inadequate protein intake and hormonal secretion. *J. Clin. Endocrinol.*, **34**, 441

158. Adibi, S. S. and Drash, A. L. (1970). Hormone and amino acid levels in altered nutritional states. *J. Lab. Clin. Med.*, **76**, 722

159. Irie, M., Sakuma, M., Tsushima, T., Shizume, K. and Nakao, K. (1967). Effect of nicotinic acid administration on plasma growth hormone concentrations. *Proc. Soc. Exp. Biol. Med.*, **126**, 708

160. Quabbe, H. J., Elban, K., Siegers, V. and Bratzke, H. J. (1971). *Abstract 2nd Int. Symp. Growth Hormone, Studies on a possible feedback mechanism between plasma free fatty acid concentration and human growth hormone*, ICS **236**, 49 (Amsterdam: Excerpta Medica)

161. Büber, V., Felber, P. J. and Vannotti, A. (1971). *Abstr. 2nd Int. Symp. Growth Hormone, Stimulation of GH by decrease of FFA*, ICS **236**, 49 (Amsterdam: Excerpta Medica)

162. Fineberg, S. S., Horland, A. A. and Merimee, T. J. (1972). Free fatty acid concentration and growth hormone secretion in man. *Metabolism*, **21**, 491

163. Blackard, W. G., Boylen, C. T., Hinson, T. C. and Nelson, N. C. (1969). Effect of lipid and ketone infusions on-insulin induced growth hormone elevations in rhesus monkeys. *Endocrinology*, **85**, 1180

164. Floyd, J. C., Fajans, S. S., Conn, J. W., Knopf, R. F. and Rull, J. A. (1966). Stimulation of insulin secretion by amino acids. *J. Clin. Invest.*, **45**, 1487

165. Knopf, R. F., Conn, J. W., Fajans, S. S., Floyd, J. C., Guntsche, E. M. and Rull, J. A. (1965). Plasma growth hormone response to intravenous administration of amino acids. *J. Clin. Endocrinol.*, **25**, 1140

166. Merimee, T. J., Lillicrap, D. A. and Rabinowitz, D. (1965). Effect of arginine on serum levels of growth hormone. *Lancet*, *II*, 668

167. Rabinowitz, D., Merimee, T. J., Nelson, I. K., Schultz, R. B. and Burgess, J. A (1968). *Growth and Growth Hormone, The influence of proteins and amino acids on growth hormone release in man*, ICS **158**, 105 (A. Pecile, E. E. Müller, editors) (Amsterdam: Excerpta Medica)

168. Tyson, J. and Fiedler, A. (1969). Hyperglycemia and arginine-initiated growth hormone release during pregnancy. *Obstet. Gynec.*, **34**, 319

169. Pecile, A., Müller, E. E., Felici, M. and Masarone, M. (1971). Partecipazione del sistema nervoso nella liberazione di ormone somatotropo dall'ipofisi indotta da aminoacidi. *Riv. Farm. Terap.*, **I**, 471

170. Buckler, J. H. M., Bold, A. M., Taberner, M. and London, D. R. (1969). Modification of hormonal responses to arginine by α adrenergic blockade. *Brit. Med. J.*, **3**, 153

171. Best, J. B., Catt, K. J. and Burger, H. G. (1968). Non-specificity of arginine infusion as a test for growth hormone secretion, *Lancet*, *II*, 124

172. Baker, H. W. G., Best, J. B. and Burger, H. G. (1970). Arginine infusion test for growth hormone secretion. *Lancet*, *II*, 1193

173. Penny, R., Blizzard, R. M. and Davis, W. T. (1970). Sequential study of arginine monochloride and normal saline as stimuli to growth hormone release. *Metabolism*, **19**, 165

174. Nakagawa, K., Horiuchi, Y., Mashimo, K. (1969). Specific and non-specific factors in arginine test. *Lancet*, *I*, 1320

175. Parker, M. L., Hammond, J. M. and Daughaday, W. H. (1967). The arginine provocative test: an aid in the diagnosis of hyposomatotropism. *J. Clin. Endocrinol.*, **27**, 1129
176. Carnelutti, M., del Guercio M. J. and Chiumello, G. (1970). Influence of growth hormone on the pathogenesis of obesity in childhood. *J. Pediat.*, **77**, 285
177. Rabinowitz, D., Merimee, T. J., Maffezzolo, R. and Burgess, J. A. (1966). Patterns of hormonal release after glucose, protein and glucose plus protein. *Lancet, II*, 454
178. Pallotta, J. A. and Kennedy, P. J. (1968). Response of plasma insulin and growth hormone to carbohydrate and protein feeding. *Metabolism*, **17**, 901
179. Sukkar, M. Y., Hunter, W. M. and Passmore, R. (1968). The effect of a protein meal with and without subsequent exercise on plasma insulin and growth hormone. *Quart. J. Exp. Physiol.*, **53**, 206
180. Hunter, W. M., Friend, J. A. R. and Strong, J. A. (1966). The diurnal pattern of growth hormone concentration in adults. *J. Endocrinol.*, **34**, 139
181. Baker, H. W. G., Best, J. B., Burger, H. G. and Cameron, D. P. (1973). Plasma human growth hormone levels in response to meals: a reappraisal. *Austr. J. Exp. Biol.*, (in press)
182. Russell, J. A. (1957). Effects of growth hormone on protein and carbohydrate metabolism. *Amer. J. Clin. Nutr.*, **5**, 404
183. Merimee, T. J., Felig, P., Marliss, E., Fineberg, S. E. and Cahill, G. G. (1971). Glucose and lipid homeostasis in the absence of human growth hormone. *J. Clin. Invest.*, **50**, 574
184. Hartog, M., Havel, R. J., Copinschi, G., Earll, J. M. and Ritchie, B. C. (1967). The relationship between changes in serum levels of growth hormone and mobilization of fat during exercise in man. *Quart. J. Exp. Physiol.*, **52**, 86
185. Hunter, W. M., Fonseka, C. C. and Passmore, R. (1965). The role of growth hormone in the mobilization of fuel for muscular exercise. *Quart. J. Exp. Physiol.*, **50**, 406
186. Schalch, D. S. and Reichlin, S. (1968). *Growth and Growth Hormone, Stress and growth hormone release*, ICS **158**, 211 (A. Pecile and E. E. Müller, editors) (Amsterdam: Excerpta Medica)
187. Glick, S. M., Roth, J., Yalow, R. S. and Berson, S. A. (1965). The regulation of growth hormone secretion. *Rec. Prog. Horm. Res.*, **21**, 241
188. Charters, A. C., Odell, W. D. and Thompson, J. C. (1969). Anterior pituitary function during surgical stress and convalescence. Radioimmunoassay of blood TSH, LH, FSH and growth hormone. *J. Clin. Endocrinol. Metab.*, **29**, 63
189. Takahashi, K. S., Takahashi, Y., Honda, K., Shizume, M., Irie, M., Sakuma, M. and Tsushima, T. (1967). Secretion of human growth hormone during insulin coma and electroshock therapies. *Folia Psychiatr. Neurol. Jap.*, **21**, 87
190. Ryan, R. J., Swanson, D. W., Faiman, C., Mayberry, W. E. and Spadoni, A. J. (1970). Effects of convulsive electroshock on serum concentration of follicle stimulating hormone, luteinizing hormone, thyroid stimulating hormone and growth hormone in man. *J. Clin. Endocrinol.*, **30**, 51
191. Berg, G. R., Utiger, R. D., Schalch, D. S. and Reichlin, S. (1966). Effect of central cooling in man on pituitary-thyroid function and growth hormone secretion. *J. Appl. Physiol.*, **21**, 1791
192. Baum, D. C., Gale, C. and Dillard, D. M. (1967). *Abstr. 1st. Int. Symp. Growth Hormone, Hyperglycemia with deep hypothermia: the roles of growth hormone and insulin*, ICS **142**, 49 (Amsterdam: Excerpta Medica)
193. Glick, S. M. (1968). Normal and abnormal secretion of growth hormone. *Ann. N.Y. Acad. Sci.*, **148**, 471
194. Brown, G. M., Schalch, D. S. and Reichlin, S. (1971). Hypothalamic mediation of growth hormone and adrenal stress response in the squirrel monkey. *Endocrinology*, **89**, 694
195. Meyer, V. and Knobil, E. (1966). Stimulation of growth hormone secretion by vasopressin in the rhesus monkey. *Endocrinology*, **79**, 1016
196. Quabbe, H-J. (1969). Plasma growth hormone response to vasopressin in normal subjects and in patients with intra and supra sellar tumours. *Acta Endocrinol.*, *Suppl.* **138**, 142
197. Frohman, L. A., Horton, E. S. and Lebowitz, H. E. (1967). Growth hormone releasing action of a pseudomonas endotoxin (Piromen). *Metabolism*, **16**, 57
198. Kohler, P. O., O'Malley, B. W., Rayford, P. L., Lipsett, M. B. and Odell, W. D.

(1967). Effect of pyrogen on blood levels of pituitary trophic hormones. Observations on the usefullness of the growth hormone response in the detection of pituitary disease. *J. Clin. Endocrinol.*, **27**, 219

199. Bogdonoff, M. D., Estes, R. H., Harlan, W. R., Trout, D. L. and Kirshner, N. (1960). Metabolic and cardiovascular changes during a state of acute central nervous system arousal. *J. Clin. Endocrinol.*, **20**, 1333

200. Himms-Hagen, J. (1967). Sympathetic regulation of metabolism. *Pharmac. Rev.*, **19**, 367

201. Hansen, A. P. (1971). *Abstr. 2nd Int. Symp. Growth Hormone, The effect of α and β blocking agents on the exercise induced growth hormone release in normal subjects and juvenile diabetics*, ICS **236**, 53 (A. Pecile and E. E. Müller, editors) (Amsterdam: Excerpta Medica)

202. Axelrod, J. (1965). The metabolism, storage and release of catecholamines. *Rec. Prog. Horm. Res.*, **21**, 597

203. Anden, N. E., Corrodi, H., Dahlstrom, A., Fuxe, K. and Hökfelt, T. (1966). Effect of tyrosine hydroxylase inhibition on the amine levels of central monoamine neurons. *Life Sci.*, **5**, 561

204. Massara, F. and Strumia, E. (1970). Increase in plasma growth hormone concentration in man after infusion of adrenaline-propranolol. *J. Endocrinol.*, **47**, 95

205. Feldman, J. M. and Lebowitz, H. E. (1972). *Abstr. IVth Int. Congr. Endocrinol., Control of insulin and growth hormone secretion by serotonin and dopamine*, ICS, **256**, 35 (Amsterdam: Excerpta Medica)

206. Quabbe, H-J., Schilling, E. and Helge, H. (1966). Pattern of growth hormone secretion during a 24-hour fast in normal adult. *J. Clin. Endocrinol.*, **26**, 1173

207. Vanderlaan, W. P., Parker, D. C., Rossman, L. G. and Vanderlaan, E. F. (1970). Implications of growth hormone release in sleep. *Metabolism*, **19**, 891

208. Takahashi, Y., Kipnis, D. M. and Daughaday, W. H. (1968). Growth hormone secretion during sleep. *J. Clin. Invest.*, **47**, 2079

209. Sassin, J. F., Parker, D. C., Mace, J. W., Gotlin, W. R., Johnson, L. C. and Rossman, L. G. (1969). Human growth hormone release: relation to slow-wave sleep and sleep-waking cycles. *Science*, **165**, 513

210. Sassin, J. F., Parker, D. C., Johnson, L. C., Rossman, L. G., Mace, J. W. and Gotlin, R. W. (1969). Effect of slow wave sleep deprivation on human growth hormone release in sleep: preliminary study. *Life Sci.*, **8**, 1299

211. Vigneri, R. and D'Agata, R. (1971). Growth hormone release during the first year of life in relation to sleep-wake periods. *J. Clin. Endocrinol.*, **33**, 561

212. Carlson, H. E., Gillin, J. C., Gorden, P. and Snyder, F. (1971). Absence of sleep related growth hormone peaks in aged normal subjects and in acromegaly. *J. Clin. Endocrinol.*, **34**, 1102

213. Sachar, E. J., Finkelstein, J. and Hellman, L. (1971). Growth hormone response in depressive illness. *Arch. Gen. Psychiat.*, **25**, 253

214. Lucke, C. and Glick, S. M. (1971). Experimental modification of the sleep induced peak of growth hormone secretion. *J. Clin. Endocrinol.*, **32**, 729

215. Lucke, C., Adelman, N. and Glick, S. M. (1972). The effect of elevated free fatty acids (FFA) on the sleep induced human growth hormone (HGH) peak. *J. Clin. Endocrinol.*, **35**, 407

216. Merimee, T. J., Rabinowitz, D. and Fineberg, S. E. (1969). Arginine-initiated release of human growth hormone. *New Engl. J. Med.*, **280**, 1434

217. Abrams, R. L., Grumbach, M. M. and Kaplan, S. L. (1971). The effect of administration of human growth hormone on the plasma growth hormone, cortisol, glucose and free fatty acid response to insulin: evidence for growth hormone autoregulation in man. *J. Clin. Invest.* **50**, 940

218. Hagen, T. C., Lawrence, A. M. and Kirsteins, L. (1972). Autoregulation of growth hormone secretion in normal subjects. *Metabolism*, **21**, 603

219. Laron, Z., Pertzelan, A. and Mannheimer, S. (1966). Genetic pituitary dwarfism with high serum concentrations of human growth hormone: a new inborn error in metabolism. *Israel J. Med. Sci.*, **2/1**, 152

6
The Pancreas as a Regulator of Metabolism*

R. H. UNGER

Veterans Administration Hospital, University of Texas Southwestern Medical School, Dallas

* Supported by NIH Grant AM 02700–13; Hoechst Pharmaceutical Company, Somerville, N.J.; The Upjohn Company, Kalamazoo, Michigan; Pfizer Laboratories, New York, N.Y.; Bristol Myers Company, New York; Mead Johnson Research Center, Evansville, Indiana; Lilly Research Laboratories, Indianapolis, Indiana; Wm. S. Merrell and Company, Cincinnati, Ohio; and Dallas Diabetes Association, Dallas, Texas.

6.1 MOLECULAR STRUCTURE

The pancreas of all vertebrates studied contains glucagon, a 29 amino acid polypeptide with the amino acid sequence shown in Figure 6.1[1]. Although this is the sequence for beef and pork glucagon, it is believed that rat, rabbit and human glucagon are very similar, if not identical[2-4]. The biosynthesis of glucagon, like that of insulin and several other polypeptide hormones, probably involves the formation of a precursor, 'large glucagon immunoreactivity' (LGI)[5] or 'pro-glucagon'[6], which has a molecular weight at least twice that of glucagon (Figure 6.2). LGI, which has no demonstrable hyperglycaemic or glycogenolytic activity *in vivo* or *in vitro* (Figure 6.3), constitutes $< 5\%$ of the total immunoreactivity extractable from the pancreas. It has also been found in the circulation in approximately the same proportion as in the pancreas (Figure 6.4). The pro-glucagon molecule is believed to contain the entire amino acid sequence of glucagon[5] but its precise biochemical and/or physiological significance is not understood.

In considering the physiology of pancreatic glucagon, it is important to make the distinction between 'pancreatoglucagon' and 'enteroglucagon' ('glucagon-like immunoreactivity', 'GLI'). The latter terms refer to a group of at least two polypeptides, which originate from the A-cells in the gastro-intestinal tract, described by Orci *et al.*[7]. Because of their morphological similarity to pancreatic a-cells, these workers have suggested that they are the probable source of gut GLI, a suspicion recently verified by means of immunofluorescent staining techniques by Polak *et al.*[8], who renamed them 'EG cells'. The physiological role or roles of GLI have not been established, and, on the basis of immunological and biological differences from pancreatic glucagon, GLI is believed to differ structurally from pancreatoglucagon, and certainly responds differently to physiological stimuli. For these reasons it would seem prudent to exclude further discussion of this substance from a review of pancreatic glucagon.

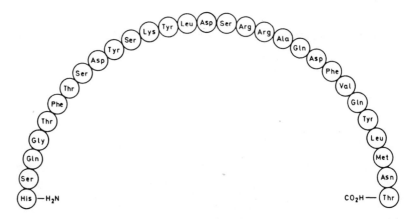

Figure 6.1   The molecular structure

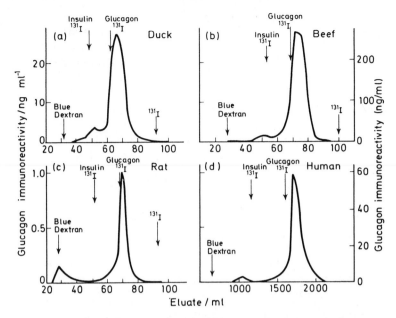

Figure 6.2 Elution patterns of extractable pancreatic glucagon immunoreactivity (Bio-Gel-P-10) in four species showing 'large glucagon immunoreactivity' ('LGI)'. (From Rigopoulou et al.[5] by courtesy of *Journal of Biological Chemistry*.)

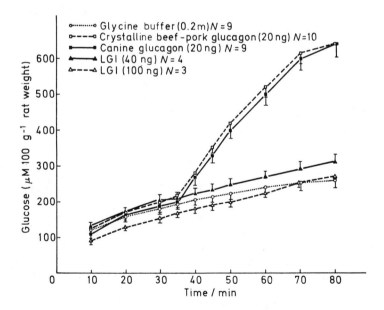

Figure 6.3 The glycogenolytic activity of large glucagon immunoreactivity in the perfused rat liver system, (From Rigopoulou et al.[5] by courtesy of *Journal of Biological Chemistry*.)

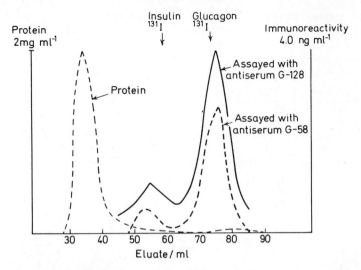

Figure 6.4 Elution pattern of extractable pancreatic glucagon immuno-reactivity (assayed with pancreatoglucagon-specific antiserum G-58) and total immunoreactivity (assayed with the less specific antiserum G-128) of plasma obtained from a dog during a-cell stimulation by amino acid infusion. (From Valverde *et al.* by courtesy of *Diabetes*.)

The similarity and perhaps identity of the primary structure of glucagon in many species suggests that the structure shown in Figure 6.1 may be essential to its biological actions. Indeed it appears that almost the entire glucagon molecule is required for the full biological properties of this hor-mone[9]. According to Rodbell[10], the intensely hydrophobic C-terminal region of the glucagon molecule may interact with a phospholipid receptor in the cell membrane having a regulatory function in a two component adenylate cyclase system. This specific interaction, coupled with an allosteric type of action by nucleotides, ultimately results in activation of the catalytic components of the adenylate cyclase system, and thence to the genera-tion of cyclic AMP, which is believed to mediate all of the intrahepatic actions of glucagon and, in all probability, its action in fat cells as well.

6.2 ACTIONS OF GLUCAGON ON THE LIVER: GLYCOGENOLYSIS

Glucagon secreted by the pancreatic a-cells reaches the liver by the portal blood and binds to specific receptors on the surface of hepatic cells having both a high affinity and specificity for this hormone. As a result of this interaction, the enzyme adenylate cyclase is activated to catalyse the conversion of ATP to c-AMP. It now appears that all of the metabolic processes activated by glucagon are mediated by the increase in cyclic AMP which it generates, in accordance with the suggestions of Sutherland *et al.*[11]. The increase in hepatic glucose output caused by glucagon follows or coincides with the increase in cyclic AMP production, is enhanced by theophylline, a phosphodiesterase inhibitor, and can be duplicated by exogenous cyclic AMP or its analogues[12]. At the present time, therefore, it seems reasonable to attribute the hepatic actions of glucagon to the increase in cyclic AMP, which in turn activates glycogenolysis, inhibits glycogen synthesis, and stimulates gluconeogenesis to degrees which vary greatly with the physiological circumstances. The activation of glycogenolysis by glucagon occurs within seconds after its contact with the liver and results in a dramatic increase in hepatic glucose production to provide an immediate defence against hypoglycaemia. This response probably involves the activation of a group of enzymes called protein kinases, which activate the phosphorylase–kinase which activates phosphorylase, the rate-limiting enzyme in the conversion of glycogen to glucose[12]. At the same time, cyclic AMP leads to inactivation of glycogen synthetase so as to prevent a futile cycle of simultaneous synthetic and degradative reactions between glucose 6-phosphate and glycogen[13].

It should be noted that the enzymatic steps which result in the activation of glycogenolysis and inactivation of glycogenesis represent a 'cascade', which provides a remarkable amplification of the glucagon signal, i.e. an enormous change in catalytic power. An estimate of the number of glucagon molecules carried to the liver and the increase in glucose molecules leaving the liver suggests that one glucagon molecule stimulates the production of 3×10^6 molecules of glucose. About half of this enormous amplification occurs at the glucagon receptor–adenylate cyclase activation stage[12].

6.3 ACTIONS OF GLUCAGON ON THE LIVER: GLUCONEOGENESIS

The increase in hepatic cyclic AMP is believed to mediate the stimulatory effect of glucagon upon gluconeogenesis[14], although the mechanism is unknown. The rise in nucleotide concentration precedes glucagon-stimulated gluconeogenesis, which can also be stimulated by exogenous cyclic AMP. In the isolated perfused liver preparation, the sensitivity to glucagon is about the same as that of glycogenolysis and is well within the concentration range of glucagon reported to exist in human plasma.

In addition to its action on the gluconeogenic pathway, possibly between lactate and phosphoenolpyruvate, Mallette et al. report that glucagon and cyclic AMP activate the transport of certain gluconeogenic amino acids across the plasma membrane of the liver[15]. It should be kept in mind that virtually all of the evidence for the gluconeogenic action of glucagon has been obtained in in vitro systems and that clear-cut evidence that glucagon is a gluconeogenic hormone in vivo has yet to be presented[16].

The summations of the actions of glucagon and insulin on the liver may be the major force governing moment-to-moment hepatic glucose production, perhaps through their diametrically opposing actions on the tissue levels of cyclic AMP. Insulin lowers hepatic cyclic AMP thus reducing glycogenolysis and gluconeogenesis[17]. The concept that the rate of hepatic glucose production is governed by the relative concentrations of insulin and glucagon is extremely attractive from the teleologic standpoint and is in accord with a host of in vitro and in vivo experimental observations.

Exton *et al.*[18] have demonstrated that in the absence of cortisol, glucagon has little effect on gluconeogenesis, despite the fact that it stimulates a normal increase in cyclic AMP. The gluconeogenic action of glucagon and of cyclic AMP can be restored by treatment with glucocorticoids.

6.4 ACTIONS OF GLUCAGON ON ADIPOSE TISSUE

Glucagon is a powerful lipolytic hormone capable of enhancing the release of glycerol and free fatty acids from adipose tissue in concentrations as low as 100 pg ml^{-1}, which are well within the range of plasma glucagon[19, 20]. However, there appears to be a wide species variation with respect to the sensitivity of adipose tissue to the lipolytic action of glucagon. It has been proposed that glucagon binds to a specific protein receptor situated on the outer surface of the plasma membrane of the adipocyte. This union, in turn, results in the activation of the enzyme adenylate cyclase, and thus increases intracellular cyclic AMP, which activates the hormone-sensitive lipase, the rate-limiting enzyme of lipolysis[21]. The validity of this proposed mechanism is supported by the fact that lipolysis induced by glucagon follows an increase in intracellular cyclic AMP, and correlates positively with the intracellular levels of the nucleotide[22]; moreover, the lipolytic action of glucagon is enhanced by the phosphodiesterase inhibitor theophylline as shown by Rodbell and Jones[23] and LeFebvre and Luckyx[24]. Insulin, which lowers cyclic AMP in fat cells, opposes the lipolytic action of glucagon. Although the precise physiological importance of glucagon as a lipolytic hormone is a controversial question, it appears possible that in fat cells, as in liver cells, the relative concentrations of insulin and glucagon may determine the direction and magnitude of substrate balance.

6.5 THE INSULIN : GLUCAGON MOLAR RATIO

The actions of glucagon are in diametric opposition to those of insulin in target tissues common to both hormones[25, 26]. According to this view, a high glucagon concentration relative to that of insulin would increase the release into the extracellular space of fuels such as glucose and free fatty acids. Conversely, when the concentration of insulin is high relative to that of glucagon, as is normally the case after a meal, the synthesis of the ingested nutrients into macromolecules, i.e. glycogen, fat and protein, will be enhanced. In keeping with the notion that these two hormones have the biological properties required to govern on a moment-to-moment basis the disposition of endogenous and exogenous fuels in accordance with the requirements of the organism, it has been proposed that the α- and β-cells be viewed as a single bicellular bihormonal functional unit, a highly-efficient 'push–pull' regulatory system; the molar ratio of insulin to glucagon has been proposed as the most valid index of the state of functional activity of this organ[27]. The recent studies of Orci *et al.*[28] reveal the existence of intercellular channels, known as 'gap junctions' which connect α- and β-cells to one another in what may actually be a 'functional synctitium' of Langerhans. This provides a morphological basis for the physiological concept of an α–β cell couple.

6.6 a-CELL FUNCTION: GLUCOSE NEED

Under normal circumstances glucose is an obligatory substrate for the tissues of the central nervous system, and normal cerebral function depends on the adequacy of glucose delivery. This fact may explain the seemingly obligatory responsiveness of a- and β-cells to all circumstances which threaten the glucose supply to the brain. Whenever the availability of glucose is reduced or

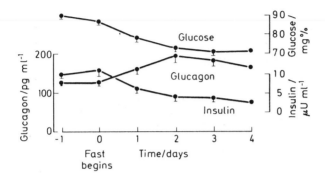

Figure 6.5 The effect of starvation on plasma levels of pancreatic glucagon, insulin and glucose in normal human volunteers. (From Aguilar-Parada *et al.*[30], by courtesy of *Diabetes*.)

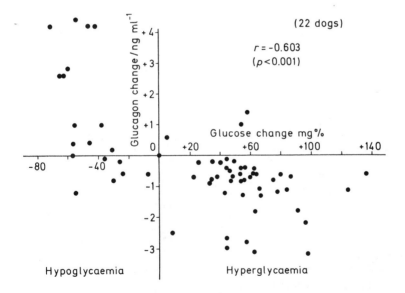

Figure 6.6 The relationship between change in plasma glucose levels and change in pancreaticoduodenal vein glucagon levels in normal dogs made hypoglycaemic by infusion of glucagon-free insulin and hyperglycaemic by glucose infusion. (From Ohneda *et al.*[34], by courtesy of *Diabetes*.)

threatened, as during restriction of dietary carbohydrate, in total starvation, during violent exercise and during artificially-induced hypoglycaemia, glucagon secretion rises above its usual basal level. In normal human subjects, after an overnight fast, plasma glucagon averages 75 pg ml^{-1} [29], but if the fast

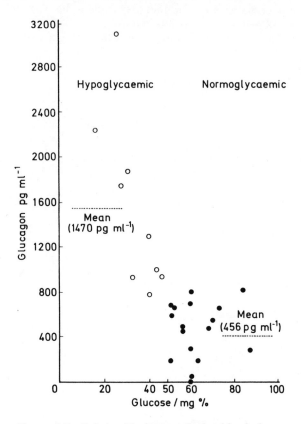

Figure 6.7 Relationship between fasting blood glucose and the pancreaticoduodenal vein plasma glucagon levels of hypoglycaemic (open circles) and normoglycaemic dogs treated with phloridzin. A statistically-significant negative relationship was observed. (From Lefebvre and Unger (eds.)[55], by courtesy of *Journal of Clinical Investigation* and Pergamon Press.)

continues for an additional 48 h, glucagon rises *ca*. 50 pg ml^{-1} higher, while insulin declines reciprocally (Figure 6.5)[30]. The insulin: glucagon ratio, which averages *ca*. 3 after an overnight fast, declines to 0.4 after 48 h of starvation[27]. It is believed that these bihormonal changes contribute to a major degree to the maintenance of plasma glucose concentration at a level compatible with full cerebral function, pending the readjustment of the brain to the use of ketones as a fuel, an adaptation which may require 5–7 days[31]. It is proposed that during this period of readjustment to starvation, glucagon plays an important role in maintaining the production of endogenous glucose, initially by means of increased glycogenolysis and subsequently by means of increased gluconeogenesis. The importance of the contribution of glucagon is supported by the experiments of Gray et al.[32] and more recently by those of Rocha et al.[33], in which rats fasted for 48 h developed hypoglycaemia when treated with antiglucagon serum.

Acute hypoglycaemia caused by the administration of insulin[34] or of a sulphonylurea[35] is followed by an increase in glucagon secretion, which varies with the magnitude of the decline in glucose concentration and becomes

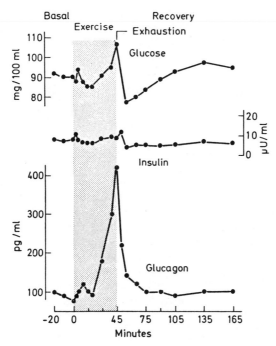

Figure 6.8 Mean plasma glucose, insulin, and glucagon levels in a group of 7 dogs before and after treadmill running to collapse. Open circles represent significant changes ($p < 0.02$) by paired analysis from the baseline. (From Boettger et al.[37], by courtesy of the Journal of Endocrinology and Metabolism.)

obligatory whenever plasma glucose declines below 60 mg $(100 \text{ ml})^{-1}$. This inverse relationship between glucose and glucagon concentrations is depicted in Figures 6.6 and 6.7, in which the glucose–glucagon relationship during chronic phloridzin-induced hypoglycaemia is represented[36].

It is clear that as glucose concentration falls to levels which threaten the adequacy of glucose delivery to the brain, the α–β cell couple responds in a manner which increases hepatic glucose production to whatever level is necessary to maintain adequate cerebral glucose delivery; at the same time, the reduction in insulin restricts entry of glucose into insulin-dependent tissues for which it is not an obligatory substrate.

When acute glucose need is induced by strenuous exercise, as in dogs exercised on a treadmill to collapse (Figure 6.8), the bihormonal response consists of a striking fourfold increase in glucagon without any change in insulin[37]. Interestingly, the insulin: glucagon ratio declines to 0.4, approximately the same level observed in starvation. The exercise-induced fall in insulin: glucagon ratio, which must satisfy an urgent need for increased glucose production, is not the result of arterial hypoglycaemia which did not occur. Rather it would seem to be the consequence of the increased levels of epinephrine and norepinephrine which occur in exhaustive exercise[38, 39]. Iversen and others have demonstrated that glucagon secretion is stimulated by catecholamines[40], and the studies of Luckyx and LeFebvre[41] and Harvey *et al.*[42] have shown in rats that exercise-induced hyperglucagonaemia can be abolished by adrenergic blockade.

6.7 *a*-CELL FUNCTION: GLUCOSE ABUNDANCE

Hyperglycaemia elicits a reciprocal bihormonal response of the islet cell hormones, which is opposite in direction to that of glucose need, the insulin: glucagon ratio rising dramatically. A rising blood glucose concentration induced by the intravenous infusion of glucose is accompanied by a proportional decline in plasma glucagon level (Figure 6.9)[34, 43] and, of course, a proportional increase in insulin (Figure 6.9). The result is a change in insulin: glucagon ratio from the normal basal level of *ca.* 3 to as high as 20 within 30 min of the start of a glucose infusion[27]. Ingested carbohydrate exerts an even more powerful effect, presumably through augmentation by an enteric signal to the islets of Langerhans released during the absorption of glucose. As a result of this 'entero-insular' signal, the rise in insulin and the decline in glucagon are considerably greater than can be attributed to the hyperglycaemia[44] (Figure 6.11), and as a result the insulin: glucagon ratio rises as high

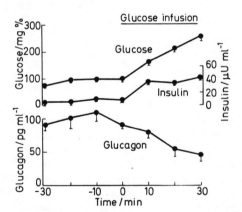

Figure 6.9 The effect of intravenously induced hyperglycaemia on the plasma levels of pancreatic glucagon and insulin in normal males. (From Lefebvre and Unger (eds.)[55], by courtesy of the *Journal of Clinical Investigation* and Pergamon Press.)

as 70[27]. Moreover, the hormonal changes actually appear to anticipate the influx of glucose, commencing at the very start of glucose absorption. This may explain the fact that peak arterial glycaemia is not proportional to the amount of glucose absorbed, a 300 g oral glucose load causing only a slightly greater peak level than a 30 g load[45]. The immediate release of an anticipatory signal from the gut proportional to the amount of glucose absorbed may provide an early warning of the magnitude of the incoming load, permitting the β-cells to secrete the appropriate quantity of insulin. The entero-insular signal has not been specifically identified, but it is believed to be humoral.

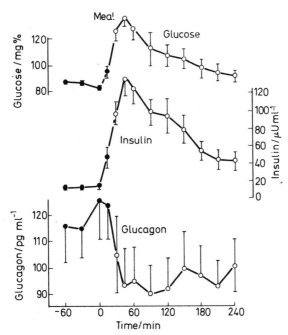

Figure 6.10 The effect of a large carbohydrate meal upon the plasma concentration of pancreatic glucagon, insulin and glucose in 11 normal human volunteers. (From Lefebvre and Unger (eds.)[55], by courtesy of *New England Journal of Medicine* and Pergamon Press.)

Secretin, which is reportedly released during the absorption of glucose[47], has the biological properties to serve as such a signal; not only does it cause the release of insulin within minutes after its injection[46], but, at least in dogs, is capable of suppressing glucagon secretion[49] (Figure 6.11).

The mechanism by which glucose suppresses glucagon secretion is unknown at the present time. It would seem that, in contrast to the low level of insulin secretion which prevails in the basal state, the a-cell under basal conditions maintains a relatively high secretory rate, which is further increased by a dearth of glucose, a highly appropriate behaviour for a cell which maintains the output of endogenous fuels. Whenever the a-cell is deprived of glucose, whether through hypoglycaemia or because of a block in intracellular entry or metabolism of glucose, glucagon secretion rises, irrespective of the extracellular glucose concentration. Mannoheptulose and 2-deoxyglucose, which block intracellular glucose metabolism, increase glucagon secretion despite a rising plasma glucose level[50] (Figure 6.12). In addition, a similar paradoxical rise in glucagon secretion during hyperglycaemia occurs in experimental insulin

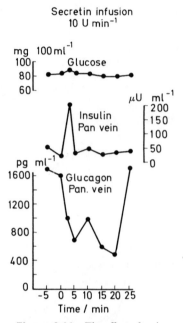

Figure 6.11   The effect of an infusion of purified secretin upon the pancreaticoduodenal vein plasma levels of glucagon and insulin in a conscious dog. (From Lefebvre and Unger (eds.)[55], by courtesy of Pergamon Press.)

deficiency[50] whether produced either with anti-insulin serum (Figure 6.13) or by alloxan (Figure 6.14) or streptozotocin treatment[51], presumably because of deficient entry of glucose into the α-cell in the absence of insulin[50]. This paradoxical hyperglucagonaemia is promptly suppressed by insulin repletion (Figure 6.14). Edwards and Taylor[52] have recently postulated that the suppressive effect of glucose upon the release of glucagon from isolated islets is correlated with ATP formation, and that metabolic poisons which block the generation of ATP, such as cyanide, dinitrophenol, iodoacetate and malonate, completely block the suppressive action of glucose on glucagon secretion. It would thus appear that the release of glucagon from the α-cell is an obligatorily continuing process which is interrupted only during an intracellular abundance of energy-yielding fuels, the same abundance which stimulated

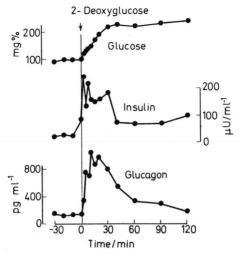

Figure 6.12 The effect of a 2-deoxyglucose injection upon the peripheral venous plasma levels of glucagon, insulin and glucose in a conscious dog. (From Lefebvre and Unger (eds.)[55], by courtesy of the *Journal of Clinical Investigation* and Pergamon Press.)

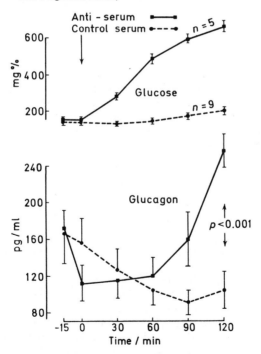

Figure 6.13 The effect of guinea pig anti-insulin serum and non-immune control serum on the plasma glucagon and glucose levels of rats. (From Lefebvre and Unger (eds.)[55], by courtesy of The *Journal of Clinical Investigation* and Pergamon Press.)

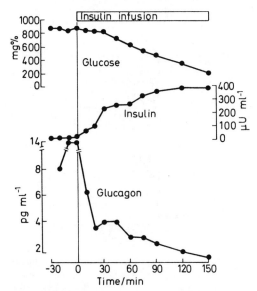

Figure 6.14   Extreme elevation of plasma glucagon and its response to insulin infusion in a dog with severe alloxan diabetes. (From Muller and Unger[50], by courtesy of *Journal of Clinical Investigation*.)

insulin secretion. It is possible that the continuous secretion of glucagon, which is capable of effecting the distribution of *ca.* 700 g of glucose per day in a starving human, requires remarkably little energy expenditure. It seems likely that in order to reduce its secretion in a manner appropriate to the prevailing glucose needs of the organism, the a-cell requires the unimpeded entry and metabolism of glucose, and this, in turn, requires the presence of insulin. Otherwise the a-cell is 'blind' to extracellular glucose and functions autonomously, releasing glucagon at a relatively high rate, even when extracellular glucose is abundant. As will be pointed out later, autonomous a-cell hyperfunction now seems to be a potential contributing factor to the 'protein catabolic state' observed in diabetes mellitus, severe infection, burns, trauma, and perhaps other diseases of man.

6.8 a-CELL FUNCTION: RESPONSE TO FREE FATTY ACIDS

The lipolytic action of glucagon has prompted a search for evidence of negative feed-back control of glucagon by products of lipolysis. Seyfert and Madison[53] have demonstrated that an increase in plasma-free fatty acids caused by the simultaneous administration of a triglyceride emulsion and heparin is associated with a slight decline in peripheral plasma glucagon levels, experiments confirmed by Luckyx and LeFebvre[54]. In addition, the latter group reported that hypolipacidaemia produced with nicotinic acid is associated with an increase in pancreaticoduodenal venous plasma glucagon[55].

In vitro studies by Edwards and Taylor also indicate a powerful inhibitory effect of octanoate and palmitate, as well as β-hydroxybutyrate, upon the glucagon release from isolated guinea-pig islets of Langerhans[52]. Despite the abundance of *in vitro* evidence indicating the suppressive effects of free fatty acids and ketone bodies, the physiological importance of this suppression in the intact organism seems doubtful. Not only is the demonstrated suppressive effect of hyperlipacidaemia very slight *in vivo*, but in clinical circumstances in which free fatty acids and ketone bodies are elevated, hyperglucagonaemia is usually present, e.g. starvation, exercise and diabetic ketoacidosis. It appears that control by glucose overpowers any competing influences on alpha cell function by other substrates.

6.9 α-CELL FUNCTION: EFFECTS OF AMINO ACIDS

Most amino acids stimulate the secretion of glucagon; Assan in 1967 first demonstrated the effect of arginine[56]. As shown in Figure 6.15, normal human subjects uniformly exhibit within 5 min an increase in glucagon to values approximately twice the basal concentrations; at its peak 40 min after the start of the infusion glucagon averages approximately three times the basal concentration. Failure of plasma glucagon to rise at least 75 pg ml^{-1} during the 40 min arginine infusion is regarded as evidence of α-cell insufficiency and

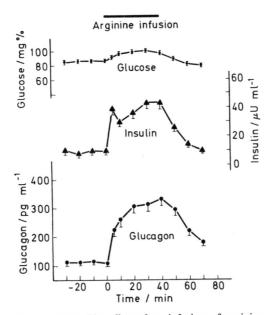

Figure 6.15 The effect of an infusion of arginine at a rate of 11.7 mg kg^{-1} min^{-1} on the peripheral venous plasma levels of pancreatic glucagon, insulin and glucose in normal subjects. (From Lefebvre and Unger (eds.)[55], by courtesy of the *Journal of Clinical Investigation* and Pergamon Press.)

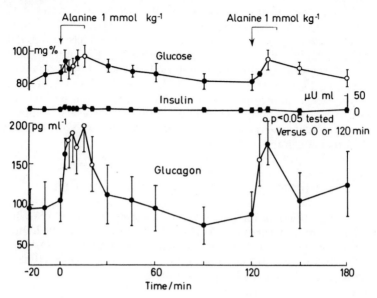

Figure 6.16 The response of glucagon, insulin and glucose in the peripheral venous plasma of four normal dogs during the infusion of alanine. (From Lefebvre and Unger (eds.)[55], by courtesy of the *Journal of Clinical Investigation* and Pergamon Press.)

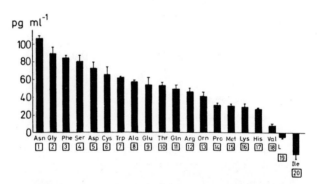

Figure 6.17 Glucagon-stimulating activity (GSA) of l mmol kg^{-1} of 20 L-amino acids in the dog in decreasing order of activity. Numbers refer to rank of GSA. (From Rocha *et al.*[59], by courtesy of *Journal of Clinical Investigation*.)

has been encountered clinically only in patients with extensive chronic pancreatitis[43] and in the patient of Levy et al.[57] believed to have an isolated glucagon deficiency. Alanine, which is far more important than arginine as a glucose precursor, also is a powerful stimulus of glucagon secretion (Figure 6.16)[58]. Most of the 20 amino acids tested in dogs so far appear to stimulate

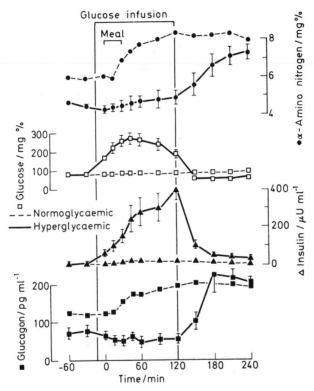

Figure 6.18 Prevention of the glucagon response to a protein meal by glucose infusion in non-diabetic human volunteers. (From Müller et al.[44], by courtesy of *New England Journal of Medicine* and Pergamon Press.)

glucagon to a varying degree[59]. Figure 6.17 shows the relative glucagon stimulating activity of these amino acids. It should be noted, that the three branched chain amino acids, valine, leucine and isoleucine, are virtually devoid of glucagon-stimulating activity, and it would appear that isoleucine actually suppresses glucagon secretion. All other amino acids tested share to a varying degree the ability to stimulate glucagon. The mechanism is, of course, not known, but the enormous structural difference in the R-chain of the active amino acids speaks against an obvious structure–activity relationship.

At the teleologic level aminogenic glucagon secretion is believed to prevent hypoglycaemia as a consequence of aminogenic insulin secretion[60]. Amino acids stimulate the release of insulin[61], which is regarded as essential for their incorporation into protein, and glucose concomitantly enters cells under the influence of the increased insulin levels. The absence of hypoglycaemia under these circumstances can be attributed to parallel glucagon secretion which increases hepatic output sufficiently to replace the glucose leaving the extracellular space; i.e. although glucose concentration has not changed, glucose turnover has increased. The parallelism of the insulin and glucagon responses to protein loads is of obvious importance in carnivores, and

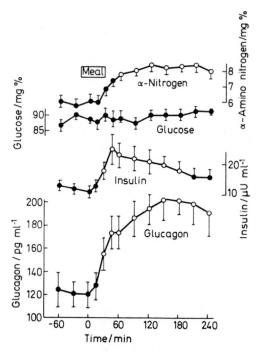

Figure 6.19 The effect of a large protein meal on the peripheral venous levels of pancreatic glucagon, insulin, glucose, and amino nitrogen in 14 normal human volunteers. (From Müller *et al.*[44], by courtesy of the *New England Journal of Medicine* and Pergamon Press.)

probably in human subjects as well. The patient of Levy *et al.*[57], who was reported to have a deficiency of glucagon, experienced hypoglycaemia episodes in response to arginine infusion and to protein ingestion. Aminogenic glucagon secretion is abolished whenever entry of exogenous glucose accompanies the influx of amino acids, as when carbohydrate is ingested or infused with a protein meal, as in Figure 6.18. In other words, when endogenous glucose is not needed to prevent hypoglycaemia, aminogenic glucagon secretion does not occur.

The ingestion of a large protein meal is normally associated with a brisk rise in glucagon averaging 80 pg ml^{-1} above the fasting level at its peak 150 min after the start of the meal; insulin increases by *ca.* 15 μU ml^{-1} [44] (Figure

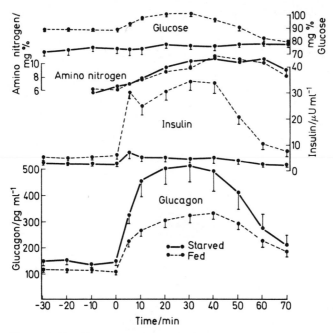

Figure 6.20 The mean response of glucagon, insulin, glucose, and a-amino nitrogen to arginine infusion after 3 or 4 days' total starvation compared with that of normal subjects. (From Aguilar-Parada et al.[30], by courtesy of *Diabetes*.)

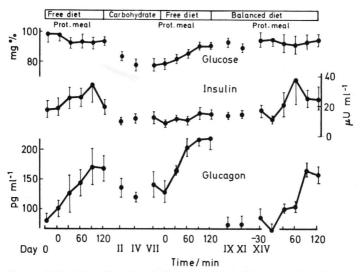

Figure 6.21 The effect of carbohydrate content of the antecedent diet on the glucagon, insulin and glucose response to a beef meal (1 g kg[-1]) in five normal subjects. (From Lefebvre and Unger[55], by courtesy of *The New England Journal of Medicine* and Pergamon Press.)

6.19). The net bihormonal change induced by protein under normal circumstances consists of a rise of the insulin:glucagon ratio to approximately
twice the usual basal value[61], an 'anabolic' change which should favour the
utilisation of a substantial fraction of the ingested amino acids for synthesis
of new protein. However, the bihormonal response is altered profoundly by a
change in nutrient needs. For example, an arginine infusion, which normally
increases the insulin:glucagon ratio by a factor of 2, as a consequence of a
fourfold increase in insulin coupled with a twofold increase in glucagon, will
after 3 days of starvation[30] actually reduce the insulin:glucagon ratio to
approximately 20% of its basal level (Figure 6.20)[31]. Thus, during the first few

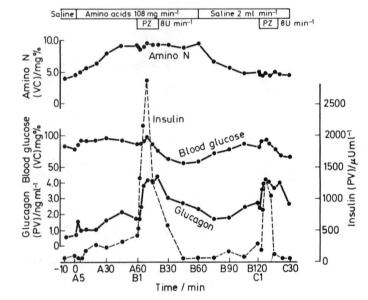

Figure 6.22 The effect of pancreozymin upon the pancreaticoduodenal
venous plasma levels of glucagon and insulin in conscious dogs during
intravenously induced hyperaminoacidaemia and during normoamino-
acidaemia. (From Lefebvre and Unger (eds.)[55], by courtesy of *The Journal of
Clinical Investigation* and Pergamon Press.)

days of total starvation, the islets of Langerhans respond to an influx of exogenous amino acids, not with the normal 'anabolic' bihormonal response, but
rather with a 'catabolic' response which would favour the utilisation of amino
acids for new glucose production. A low carbohydrate diet for 7 days also
abolishes the normal anabolic rise in insulin:glucagon ratio in response to a
protein meal[62]. The catabolic response under these circumstances is presumed
to favour the use of the absorbed amino acids for new glucose production
which may explain the 15 mg (100 ml)$^{-1}$ rise in glucose concentration observed. (Figure 6.21). Thus, the direction of the bi-hormonal response of the
islets of Langerhans to the same amino acid load will, in the same individual,

vary sharply according to the prior availability of nutrients. Influx of protein in a period of carbohydrate abundance will result in an anabolic response and pre-empt a larger share of amino acids for protein synthesis, while in a period of carbohydrate deprivation it will elicit a catabolic response and a greater share of the amino acids will be employed for gluconeogenesis at the expense of protein synthesis.

As shown in Figure 6.18, an abundance of exogenous glucose produced by glucose infusion exaggerates the protein-induced rise in insulin:glucagon ratio by a factor of 8 and rises as high as 170 are observed. This is the result of marked augmentation of the insulin response to protein coupled with almost complete suppression of aminogenic glucagon secretion. This intensely-anabolic bihormonal response to protein must completely shut off gluconeo-genesis and conserve the amino acids for protein synthesis. This may be the explanation for the well known protein-sparing effect of glucose and for the efficacy of the intravenous hyperalimentation regimen of Dudrick[63] in individuals unable to take food by mouth.

As in the case of carbohydrate ingestion, there is evidence that protein ingestion causes a greater rise of insulin and glucagon than can be accounted for by the rise in plasma amino nitrogen. In addition, as in the case of carbohydrate loads, the response of the islet cell hormones appears to anticipate the rise in a-amino nitrogen levels (Figure 6.19). On this basis, one can again implicate an entero-insular signal. The hormone pancreozymin, known to be released during the absorption of amino acids, certainly qualifies for such a role, since it appears to be a powerful and almost instantaneous stimulus of insulin and glucagon release[46] (Figure 6.22).

6.10 THE EFFECT OF A FAT MEAL ON ISLET CELL HORMONES

The intraduodenal administration of emulsified long-chain triglycerides elicits within 10 min a marked increase in plasma glucagon which lasts for 90 min[64] (Figure 6.23). A very small and short-lived increase in insulin is observed during the first 15 min but is not statistically significant. Since the infusion of chyle has no effect on glucagon secretion (Figure 6.24), the response to a fat meal must be attributed entirely to an enteric signal from the intestine to the islets of Langerhans. Indeed, in dogs with thoracic duct fistulae, in whom the absorbed lipids are excluded completely from the circulation, the absorption of fat is accompanied by the same rise in glucagon as in intact dogs[64]. Again, the entero-insular signal has not been identified. However, pancreozymin is known to be released during the absorption of fat[65] and is known to stimulate glucagon secretion[46]. Moreover, the absorption of medium chain triglycerides which, according to Go and Summerskill[66] do not stimulate the release of pancreozymin, fails to stimulate glucagon secretion[65]. Yet, if pancreozymin is the enteric signal released during fat absorption, it is difficult to explain the relatively trivial insulin response. Equally difficult to explain is the lack of a hyperglycaemic response to the hyperglucagonaemia when unaccompanied by an appropriate degree of hyperinsulinaemia.

The physiological implications of fat-induced hyperglucagonaemia remain to be established. It has been known, however, that glucagon is a powerful

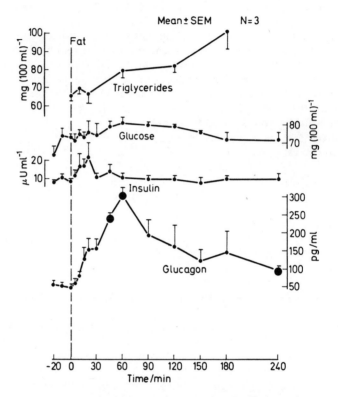

Figure 6.23 The effect of 3 g kg^{-1} of intraduodenally administered peanut oil emulsified with egg yolk upon glucagon and insulin in a group of three conscious dogs. The large circles represent points which differ statistically ($p < 0.02$) from the mean of the three baseline values. (From Boettger[66], by courtesy of the *Journal of Clinical Investigation*.)

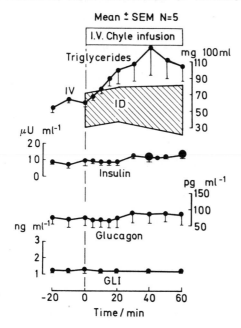

Figure 6.24 The effect of canine chyle infused intravenously at a rate of 1.1–2.1 ml min⁻¹ for 60 min upon glucagon, insulin and GLI in a group of five conscious dogs. The large circles represent points which differ statistically ($p < 0.02$) from the mean of the three baseline values. (From Boettger[66], by courtesy of the *Journal of Clinical Investigation.*)

hypolipaemic hormone[67, 68] and recent work suggests that this action involves cyclic AMP-mediated inhibition of VLDL release from the liver[10], perhaps through inhibition of apoprotein synthesis. One can therefore speculate that the function of the hyperglucagonaemia which occurs during absorption of exogenous fat particles may be to inhibit the formation of endogenous particles by the liver. Because glucose can inhibit hyperglucagonaemia induced by fat absorption, just as it inhibits protein-induced hyperglucagonaemia, one can speculate that induction of hyperlipoproteinaemia by carbohydrate is the result of its suppression of the hyperglucagonaemia which occurs during the absorption of protein and fat.

6.11 SUMMARY

The metabolic functions of the pancreatic islets thus embrace a broad area of metabolic control, playing a major role in the disposition of nutrients and the regulation of fuel balance across tissues. Their normal function seems to be a critical factor in the remarkable ability of organisms to maintain the fuel needs of vital tissues such as the brain in time of famine as in time of plenty, and to prevent wasteful excretion or disposal of valuable substrates after a feast. It has become increasingly clear that human diseases characterised by an inability to conserve ingested nutrients, such as diabetes mellitus, and other catabolic states such as severe infection[29], trauma[70] and burns[70] are also characterised by 'abnormal' islet cell function. Hyperglucagonaemia is generally present together with diminished or absent ability to raise appropriately the lowered insulin: glucagon ratio, either by reducing glucagon or raising the insulin. Such patients are in a hormonal and metabolic sense, 'frozen' in a state of continuous starvation—even when exogenous fuels are abundant. Consequently, the abundance is not exploited adequately and glucose and/or the most valuable metabolic currency, nitrogen, is wasted. This can be partially or completely reversed if the insulin: glucagon ratio can somehow be raised. It seems increasingly clear that glucagon, in addition to its metabolic adversary insulin, appears to occupy an important if not essential role in moment-to-moment metabolic regulation.

References

1. Bromer, W. W., Sinn, L. and Behrens, O. K. (1957). Hydrolysis of glucagon by trypsin. *J. Amer. Chem. Soc.*, **79**, 2801
2. Sundby, F. and Markussen, J. (1971). Isolation, crystallization and amino acid composition of rat glucagon. *Horm. Metab. Res.*, **3**, 184
3. Sundby, F. and Markussen, J. (1972). Rabbit glucagon: isolation, crystallization and amino acid composition. *Horm. Metab. Res.*, **4**, 56
4. Thomsen, J., Kristiansen, K. and Brunfeldt, K. (1972). The amino acid sequence of human glucagon. *FEBS Lett.*, **21**, 315
5. Rigopoulou, D., Valverde, I., Marco, J., Faloona, G. R. and Unger, R. H. (1970). Large glucagon immunoreactivity. *J. Biol. Chem.*, **245**, 496
6. Noe, B. D. and Bauer, G. E. (1971). Evidence for precipitation of precursors in glucagon biosynthesis. *Diabetes*, **20**, 238
7. Orci, L., Pictet, R., Forssmann, W. G., Renold, A. E. and Rouiller, C. (1968). Structural evidence for glucagon producing cells in the intestinal mucosa of rat. *Diabetologia*, **4**, 56
8. Polak, J. M., Bloom, S., Coulling, I. and Pearse, A. G. E. (1971). Immunofluorescent localization of enteroglucagon cells in the gastrointestinal tract of a dog. *Gut*, **12**, 311
9. Spiegel, A. M. and Bitensky, M. W. (1969). Effects of chemical and enzymatic modifications of glucagon on its motivation of hepatic adenyl cyclase. *Endocrinology*, **85**, 638
10. Rodbell, M. (1972). *Glucagon: Molecular Physiology*. Regulation of glucagon action at its receptors. Chap. 5, pp. 61. (P. Lefebvre and R. H. Unger, editors) (Oxford: Pergamon Press)
11. Sutherland, E. W., Robison, G. A. and Butcher, R. W. (1968). Some aspects of the biological role of Adenosine 3′,5′-monophosphte (cyclic AMP). *Circulation*, **37**, 279
12. Parke, C. R. and Exton, J. H. (1972). *Glucagon: Molecular Physiology*, Glucagon and the metabolism of glucose, Chap. 6, pp. 77. (P. Lefebvre and R. H. Unger, editors) (Oxford: Pergamon Press)
13. Larner, J. and Villar-Palasi, C. (1971). In *Topics in Cellular Physiology* (Horrecker, B. and Stadtman, E., editors) **3**, (New York: Academic Press) (In the press)
14. Exton, J. H. and Park, C. R. (1968). II. Effects of glucagon, catecholamines and adenosine 3′,5′-monophosphate on gluconeogenesis in the perfused rat liver. *J. Biol. Chem.*, **244**, 5713
15. Mallette, L. E., Exton, J. H. and Park, C. R. (1969). Control of gluconeogenesis from amino acids in the perfused rat liver. *J. Biol. Chem.*, **244**, 5713
16. Lindsey, C. A. and Madison, L. L. (1972). Is glucagon a gluconeogenic hormone *in vivo*? *Diabetes* (Suppl. 1), **21**, 331 (Abst.)
17. Hepp, K. D. (1971). *Fed. Eur. Biochem. Soc. Lett*, **12**, 263

18. Exton, J. H., Jefferson, L. S., Butcher, R. W. and Park, C. R. (1966). Gluconeogenesis in the perfused liver; the effects of fasting, alloxan diabetes, glucagon, epinephrine, adenosine 3′,5′-monophosphate and insulin. *Amer. J. Med.*, **40**, 709
19. Steinberg, D. M., Shafrir, E. and Vaughan, M. (1959). Direct effect of glucagon on release of esterified fatty acids (U.F.A.) from adipose tissue. *Clin. Res.*, **7**, 250
20. Weinges, K. F. (1961). Der einfluss von glukagon and insulin auf den stoffwechsel der nicht veresterten fettsauren am isolierten, fettgewebe der ratte *in vitro*. *Klin. Wschr.*, **39**, 293
21. Birnbaumer, L. and Rodbell, M. (1969). Adenyl cyclase in fat cells. II. Hormone Receptors. *J. Biol. Chem.*, **244**, 3477
22. Butcher, R. W., Ho., R. J., Meng, H. C. and Sutherland, E. W. (1965). Adenosine, 3′,5′-monophosphate in biological materials. II. The measurement of . . . tissues and the role of the cyclic nucleotide in the lipolytic response of fat to epinephrine. *J. Biol. Chem.*, **240**, 4515
23. Rodbell, M. and Jones, A. B. (1966). Metabolism of isolated fat cells. III. The similar inhibitory action of phospholipase C (Clostridium perfrigens a toxin) and of insulin on lipolysis stimulated by lipolytic hormones and theophylline. *J. Biol. Chem.*, **241**, 140
24. Lefebvre, P. and Luckyx, A. (1969). Physiopathology of adipose tissue (J. Vague, editor), *Excerpta Medica Found.*, Amsterdam, 257
25. Mackrell, D. J. and Sokal, J. E. (1969). Antagonism between the effects of insulin glucagon upon the isolated liver. *Diabetes*, **18**, 724
26. Mallette, L. E., Exton, J. H. and Park, C. A. (1969). Effects of glucagon on amino acid transport and utilization in the perfused rat liver. *J. Biol. Chem.*, **244**, 4724
27. Unger, R. H. (1971). Glucagon and the insulin: glucagon ratio. *Diabetes*, **20**, 834
28. Orci, L., Unger, R. H. and Rend, A. C. (1973). Structural basis for intercellular communications between cells of the islets of Langerhaus. *Experientia*, **29**, 777
29. Rocha, D. M., Santeusanio, F., Faloona, G. R. and Unger, R. H. (1973). Abnormal alpha cell function in bacterial infection. *New Engl. J. Med.*, **288**, 700
30. Aguilar-Parada, E., Eisentraut, A. M. and Unger, R. H. (1969). Effects of starvation on plasma pancreatic glucagon in normal man. *Diabetes*, **18**, 717
31. Cahill, G. F., Jr., Herrera, M. G., Morgan, A. P., Soeldner, J. S., Steinke, J., Levy, P. L. and Reichard, G. A., Jr. (1966). Hormone fuel interrelationships during fasting. *J. Clin. Invest.* **45**, 1751
32. Grey, N., McGuigan, J. E. and Kipnis, D. M. (1970). Neutralization of endogenous glucagon by high titre glucagon antiserum. *Endocrinology*, **86**, 1383
33. Rocha, D. M., Faloona, G. R. and Unger, R. H. (1972). Unpublished observations.
34. Ohneda, A., Aguilar-Parada, E., Eisentraut, A. M. and Unger, R. H. (1969). Control of pancreatic glucagon secretion by glucose, *Diabetes*, **18**, 1
35. Buchanan, K. D., Vance, J. E., Dinstl, K. and Williams, R. H. (1969). Effect of blood glucose on glucagon secretion in anesthetized dogs. *Diabetes*, **18**, 11
36. Unger, R. H., Eisentraut, A. M., McCall, M. S. and Madison, L. L. (1962). Measurements of endogenous glucagon in plasma and the infusion of blood glucose concentration upon its secretion. *J. Clin. Invest.*, **41**, 682
37. Boettger, I., Schlein, E. M., Faloona, G. R., Knochel, J. P. and Unger, R. H. (1972). The effect of exercise on glucagon secretion. *J. Clin. Endocrinol.*, *Metab.*, **35**, 117
38. Von Euler, U. S. and Hellner, S. (1952). Excretion of noradrenaline and adrenaline in muscular work. *Acta Physiol. Scand.*, **26**, 183
39. Vendsalu, A. (1960). Studies on adrenaline and noradrenaline in human plasma. *Acta Physiol. Scand. Suppl.* **49**, 173
40. Iversen, J. (1971). Adrenergic receptors for the secretion of immunoreactive glucagon and insulin from the isolated perfused canine pancreas. *Diabetologia*, **7**, 34
41. Luckyx, A., and Lefebvre, P. J. (1972). Role of catecholamines in exercise-induced glucagon secretion in rats. *Diabetes* Suppl. 1, **21**, 334
42. Harvey. W. D., Faloona, G. R. and Unger, R. H. (1972). Effect of adrenergic blockade on exercise-induced hyperglucagonemia (Abst.) *Clin. Res.*, **20**, 752
43. Unger, R. H., Aguilar-Parada, E., Muller, W. A. and Eisentraut, A. M. (1970). Studies of pancreatic alpha cell function in normal and diabetic subjects. *J. Clin. Invest.*, **49**, 837
44. Müller, W. A., Faloona, G. R., Aguilar-Parada, E. and Unger, R. H. (1970). Abnormal alpha cell function in diabetics: Response to carbohydrate and protein ingestion. *New Engl. J. Med.*, **283**, 109

45. Forster, H., Haslbeck, M. and Mehnert, H. (1972). Metabolic studies following the oral ingestion of different doses of glucose. *Diabetes*, **21**, 1102
46. Unger, R. H. and Eisentraut, A. M. (1969). Entero-insular axis. *Arch. Int. Med.*, **123**, 261
47. Chisholm, D. J., Young, J. D. and Lazarus, R. (1969). The gastrointestinal stimulus to insulin release. I. Secretin. *J. Clin. Invest.*, **48**, 1453
48. Kraegen, E. W., Chisholm, D. J., Young, J. D. and Lazarus, R. (1970). Gastrointestinal stimulus to insulin release. II. A dual action of secretin. *J. Clin. Invest.*, **49**, 524
49. Santeusanio, F., Faloona, G. R. and Unger, R. H. (1973). Inhibition of alanine-stimulated glucagon secretion by secretin. *Hormone and Metabolic Res.* (In press)
50. Muller, W. A., Faloona, G. R. and Unger, R. H. (1971). The effect of experimental insulin deficiency on glucagon secretion. *J. Clin. Invest.*, **50**, 1992
51. Harris, V. and Unger, R. H. (1972). Unpublished observations
52. Edwards, J. C. and Taylor, K. W. (1970). Fatty acids and the release of glucagon from isolated guinea pig islets of Langerhans and incubated *in vitro*. *Biochim. Biophys. Acta*, **215**, 310
53. Seyfert, W. A., Jr. and Madison, L. L. (1967). Physiologic effects of metabolic fuels on carbohydrate metabolism. I. Acute effects of elevation of plasma free fatty acids on hepatic glucose output, peripheral glucose utilization, serum insulin and plasma glucagon levels. *Diabetes*, **16**, 765
54. Luckyx, A. and Lefebvre, P. (1970). Arguments for a regulation of pancreatic glucagon secretion by circulating plasma free fatty acids. *Proc. Soc. Exp. Biol. Med.*, **133**, 524
55. Lefebvre, P. (1972). *Glucagon: Molecular Physiology*. (P. Lefebvre and R. H. Unger, editors). Glucagon and lipid metabolism. Chap. 7, 109. (Pergamon Press: Oxford)
56. Assan, R., Rosselin, G. and Dolais, J. (1967). Effects sur la glucagonémie des perfusions et ingestions d'acides aminés. *Journées Ann. Diabètologie Hôtel Dieu. Editions Médicales*, **7**, 25
57. Levy, L. J., Speigel, G. and Bleicher, S. J. (1970). Glucagon deficient man: Model for the role of glucagon in fasting. *Proc. Endocrinol. Soc.* (Abst.), pp. 134
58. Muller, W. A., Faloona, G. R. and Unger, R. H. (1971). The effect of alanine on glucagon secretion. *J. Clin. Invest.*, **50**, 2218
59. Rocha, D. M., Faloona, G. R. and Unger, R. H. (1972). Glucagon stimulating activity of 20 amino acids in dogs. *J. Clin. Invest.*, **9**, 2356
60. Floyd, J. C., Jr., Fajans, S. S., Conn, J. W., Knopf, R. F. and Rull, J. (1966). Insulin secretion in response to protein ingestion. *J. Clin. Invest.*, **45**, 1487
61. Unger, R. H., Müller, W. A. and Faloona, G. R. Insulin/glucagon (I/G) ratio. (1971). *Trans. Assn. of Am. Phys.*, **84**, 122
62. Muller, W. A., Faloona, G. R. and Unger, R. H. (1971). The influence of the antecedent diet upon glucagon and insulin secretion. *New Engl. J. Med.*, **285**, 1450
63. Dudrick, S. J., Long, J. M. and Steiger, E. (1970). Intravenous hyperalimentation. *Med. Clin. N. Amer.*, **84**, 577
64. Boettger, I., Faloona, G. R. and Unger, R. H. (1973). The effects of triglyceride absorption upon glucagon, insulin and gut glucagon-like immunoreactivity. *J. Clin. Invest.*, **52**, 2532
65. Wang, C. C. and Grossman, M. I. (1951). Physiological determination of release of secretin and pancreozymin from intestine of dogs with transplanted pancreas. *Amer. J. Physiol.*, **164**, 527
66. Go, A. and Summerskill, J. J. (1972). Personal communication
67 Albrink, M. J., Fitzgerald, J. R. and Man, E. B. (1957). Effect of glucagon on alimentary lipemia. *Proc. Soc. Exp. Biol. Med.*, **95**, 778
68. Paloyan, E. and Harper, P. V. (1961). Glucagon as a regulating factor of plasma lipids. *Metabolism*, **11**, 1240
69. De Oya, M., Prigge, W. F., Swenson, D. E. and Grande, F. (1971). Role of glucagon on fatty liver production in birds. *Amer. J. Physiol.*, **221**, 25
70. Lindsey, C. A., Wilmore, D. W., Moylan, J. A., Faloona, G. R. and Unger, R. H. (1972). Glucagon and the insulin: glucagon (I/G) ratio in burns and trauma. *Clin. Res.*, **20**, 802

7
The Hormonal Control of Sodium Excretion

I. A. REID and W. F. GANONG

University of California, San Francisco

7.1   INTRODUCTION

In the vertebrates, regulation of extracellular fluid volume is largely mediated by changes in the renal excretion of sodium. The amount excreted is in turn dependent on the amount filtered in the glomeruli and the amount re-absorbed along the renal tubules (Figure 7.1). Changes in sodium excretion are brought about by changes in the glomerular filtration rate, by changes in the physical factors (hydrostatic and oncotic pressures) governing the movement of solute and water into renal capillaries and by changes in the circulating levels of a number of hormones. (For reviews see Refs. 1–4.) Of this latter group, aldosterone is the most important but a number of other steroids also have significant effects. Aldosterone secretion is regulated primarily by the renin–angiotensin system and ACTH, although other factors including the plasma

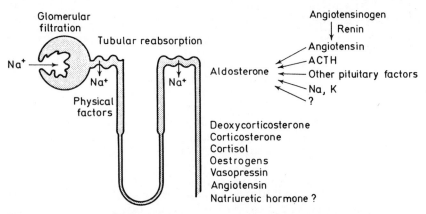

Figure 7.1 Summary of the factors involved in the regulation of renal sodium excretion. Changes in sodium excretion are brought about by changes in glomerular filtration rate or by changes in tubular reabsorption. Changes in the physical factors (hydrostatic and oncotic pressures) are thought to alter sodium reabsorption by the proximal tubule, while the hormones listed at the right of the diagram influence sodium reabsorption at various points along the nephron

concentrations of sodium and potassium also play a role. Angiotensin and vasopressin appear to have direct effects on renal sodium handling in certain situations and, in addition, there is indirect evidence for the existence of an as yet unidentified circulating natriuretic hormone.

In this chapter we have summarised current concepts of the hormonal control of renal sodium excretion, with emphasis on aldosterone and the regulation of its secretion. Some aspects of the subject have been covered in previous reviews. To keep the present chapter concise, we have frequently cited reviews to which the reader is referred for references to original papers. Only work published before November 1972 has been reviewed. In general, we have not included material that has been published only in abstract form.

7.2 ALDOSTERONE

7.2.1 General aspects

Aldosterone is a potent mineralocorticoid steroid hormone which is secreted by the adrenal cortex in a wide variety of species. Although it has been studied most extensively in mammals, it occurs widely throughout the vertebrate kingdom and has been identified in the blood of fish, amphibians, reptiles and birds. In mammals, it appears to be a unique product of the zona glomerulosa, although there are reports that in certain situations, adrenal cortical cells other than those of the zona glomerulosa are capable of producing it (see Ref. 5). It is the most potent naturally occurring mineralocorticoid known, being on a weight basis 25–100 times more potent than deoxycorticosterone. In large doses it also has some glucocorticoid activity. Its structure is shown in Figure 7.2. In normal man on an average diet, plasma aldosterone

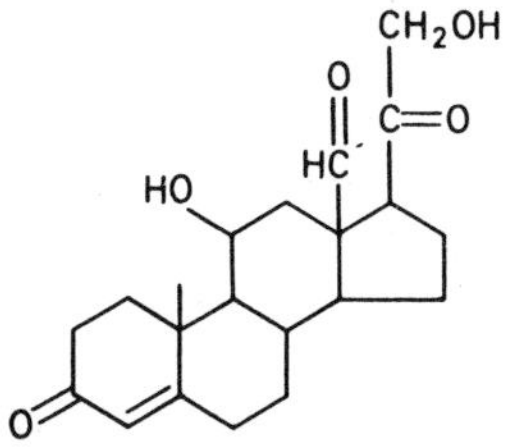

Figure 7.2 Structure of aldosterone

conc. is *ca.* 6 ng 100 ml^{-1}, of which 50–68% is bound to plasma protein. It has a half-life of *ca.* 25 min and is metabolised primarily by the liver[5].

Since its isolation, identification and synthesis early in the 1950s, the biological properties of this steroid hormone have been studied extensively. With other steroids which possess mineralocorticoid activity, aldosterone decreases the excretion of sodium and increases the output of potassium by the kidney and by the salivary, sweat, gastric and intestinal excretory glands.

7.2.2 Renal effects

The most important physiological action of aldosterone is on the renal tubules where it increases the re-absorption of sodium and chloride and decreases the re-absorption of potassium and hydrogen. Although it is often stated that these effects are the consequence of decreased tubular exchange of sodium ions for potassium and hydrogen ions, there is evidence that steroidal regulation of potassium excretion is at least in part independent of steroidal regulation of sodium excretion[5]. There is now general agreement that the major intrarenal site of action is the distal tubule but in addition there is some evidence for a proximal tubular site of action. With regard to the latter possibility, Hierholzer and Stolte[6] have cited the widespread effect of adrenal steroids on transepithelial sodium transport and pointed out that 'proximal sodium re-absorption in the mammalian kidney would constitute a remarkable exception if it were not influenced by mineralocorticosteroids'. They have reviewed a number of micropuncture studies in the rat and concluded that following adrenalectomy, sodium re-absorption is decreased in the proximal as well as in the distal tubule. This deficit is restored to normal at both sites by small doses of d-aldosterone. In studies on the effects of deoxycorticosterone and spironolactone on urine flow in patients during maximal water diuresis, additional evidence has been obtained for an action of aldosterone on sodium re-absorption in the proximal as well as in the distal tubule[7]. On the other hand, other investigators using micropuncture techniques have been unable to demonstrate mineralocorticoid dependent sodium re-absorption in the proximal tubule of dogs[8] or rats[9]. These discrepancies are difficult to resolve and for the present, the question of whether aldosterone acts on the proximal tubule remains unsettled.

7.2.3 Mechanism of action

The mechanism by which aldosterone exerts its effects on sodium re-absorption has been studied extensively and is the subject of a number of recent reviews[10-13]. The initial step involves the interaction of aldosterone with a specific intracellular mineralocorticoid-binding protein. This steroid–protein complex is believed to stimulate an increase in RNA synthesis and the induced messenger RNA directs ribosomal synthesis of proteins which increase the activity of the sodium transport system. Such an increase in activity could be the result of an increase in sodium permeability, an increase in ATP production which would provide more energy for the sodium pump, or a direct action on the sodium pump. To date, it has not been possible to distinguish between these alternatives[13].

7.2.4 Control of aldosterone secretion

The control of aldosterone secretion is complex and involves changes in the renin–angiotensin system, ACTH and the plasma concentrations of sodium and potassium (for reviews see Refs. 14–20). In addition, there is some indirect evidence for the existence of an unidentified humoral factor(s) which may influence aldosterone secretion. Different stimuli to aldosterone secretion appear to exert their effects on at least two different points in the biosynthetic pathway that leads from cholesterol to aldosterone (see Ref. 21). ACTH and potassium act early in the pathway to increase the production of pregnenolone from cholesterol and have no direct effects on the conversion of corticosterone to aldosterone. At least in part, sodium depletion acts late in the pathway, increasing the conversion of corticosterone to aldosterone. Angiotensin may act both early and late. Recent evidence indicates that potassium may play a more important role than was previously thought and it has been suggested that the different stimuli to aldosterone secretion may all act by increasing adrenal cortical potassium uptake[22].

7.2.4.1 The renin—angiotensin system

(a) *Relation to aldosterone*—During the past 15 years a large amount of evidence has accumulated which indicates that, in the mammals, the renin–angiotensin system is the major regulator of aldosterone secretion. This evidence derives from a variety of experiments performed in a number of different species, and much of it has been reviewed elsewhere[14-19]. The earliest evidence has accumulated which indicates that, in the mammals, the renin–secretion was histological. Renin infusions and cellophane wrapping of the kidney were found to produce widening of the adrenal zona glomerulosa[23]. Administration of deoxycorticosterone acetate (DOCA) and salt decreased the granularity of the juxtaglomerular apparatus and the width of the zona glomerulosa, while sodium restriction increased both juxtaglomerular granularity and zona glomerulosa width[24, 25]. More direct evidence for the participation of angiotensin in the control of aldosterone secretion came from studies in which it was shown that intravenous angiotensin infusion stimulated aldosterone secretion. This was shown to be a direct effect since low doses of angiotensin II were more effective when administered into the arterial blood perfusing the adrenal than when administered intravenously[26]. Nephrectomy decreased aldosterone secretion in hypophysectomised dogs[27] and abolished the increment in aldosterone secretion normally produced by haemorrhage[27], constriction of the inferior vena cava[28] or sodium deficiency[28, 29]. The effects of angiotensin on aldosterone production were also studied *in vitro* and it was demonstrated that addition of angiotensin to the medium bathing adrenal slices stimulated aldosterone release[30].

Recent experiments in man have further demonstrated that the renin–angiotensin system plays an important role in the physiological regulation of aldosterone secretion in a variety of situations. There is a good correlation between the circadian rhythms in plasma renin activity and plasma aldosterone concentration[31] and between the changes in plasma renin activity and plasma aldosterone concentration which occur in response to standing[31, 32], sodium and volume depletion[32, 33] and sodium loading[34]. Similar correlations have also been observed during sodium deficiency in dogs[35] and sheep[36]. In marsupials, sodium deficiency increases plasma renin activity[37], juxtaglomerular granulation[37, 38], plasma aldosterone concentration[39] and aldosterone secretion rate[38]. A number of studies in rats suggested that in this species, the renin–angiotensin system has little influence on aldosterone secretion[40, 41]. However, it now seems clear that plasma renin activity in the rat is increased by sodium depletion[19], and that angiotensin does stimulate aldosterone secretion[42]. Further, it has been demonstrated that in the rat[43], as in the dog[44], adrenal sensitivity to angiotensin is increased during sodium deficiency. Taken together, these observations suggest that in this species, as well as the others that have been studied, the renin–angiotensin system plays a role in the regulation of aldosterone secretion.

The renin–angiotensin system is summarised in Figure 7.3. The components of this system have been reviewed elsewhere[18, 45, 46]. In this chapter we have limited ourselves to discussion of recent research on the features of the system which most directly influence the generation of angiotensin II, the peptide which is directly responsible for the stimulation of aldosterone secretion. These include the mechanisms responsible for the control of renin secretion and angiotensinogen production and the kinetics of the reaction between renin and angiotensinogen.

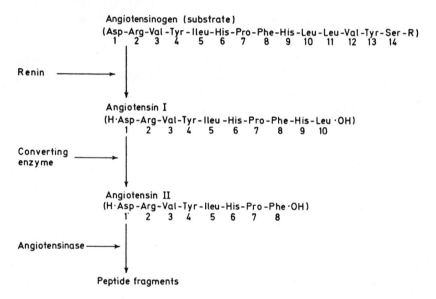

Figure 7.3   The renin–angiotensin system

(b) *Control of renin secretion*

(i) *Intrarenal mechanisms*—The juxtaglomerular cells, the cells which synthesise and secrete renin, are modified smooth muscle cells in the media of the afferent arteriole (Figure 7.4). The juxtaglomerular apparatus also includes the macula densa, an area of modified renal tubular epithelium at the point at which the distal tubule contacts the glomerulus from which the tubule arose. There is considerable evidence that the macula densa is a sodium sensor and that, under certain circumstances, the rate of renin secretion is inversely proportional to the delivery of sodium to, or the rate of transport of sodium across the macula densa. In addition, there appears to be a pressure sensor in the renal vasculature and possibly in the juxtaglomerular cells themselves, which brings about increased renin secretion when the renal perfusion pressure falls. The evidence for the participation of macula densa and baroreceptor mechanisms in the control of renin secretion has been reviewed elsewhere[18, 48, 49].

Until recently it has been difficult to distinguish between effects mediated via the macula densa and effects mediated via the renal baroreceptor since manoeuvres which would affect one of them would also be expected to affect the other. For example, a decrease in renal perfusion pressure which would activate the baroreceptor mechanism would also result in a decrease in glomerular filtration rate so that the delivery of sodium to the macula densa

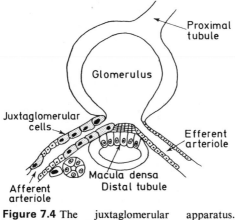

Figure 7.4 The   juxtaglomerular   apparatus. Modified slightly from Cook[47]

would be diminished. However, Blaine *et al.*[50, 51] have produced a non-filtering kidney preparation by using a combination of renal ischaemia and ureteral ligation. Glomerular filtration rate in this model is said to be zero, so no sodium reaches the macula densa. When renal perfusion pressure is reduced in such a preparation, there is a marked increase in renin secretion[50, 51]. Conversely, Humphreys *et al.*[52] have utilised recently a perfused kidney preparation to study the effect of changing the rate of delivery of sodium to the macula densa while maintaining renal perfusion pressure at a constant level. In this study proximal tubular sodium re-absorption was decreased by diluting the blood perfusing the kidney with Ringer's solution. Therefore, delivery of sodium to the distal tubule was presumably increased while renal perfusion pressure was held constant. Renin secretion was consistently reduced by this manoeuvre (Figure 7.5). This effect may be of physiological significance. Blair-West *et al.*[53] observed that renin secretion in sheep increased during dehydration and suggested that this may have been a consequence of decreased delivery of sodium to the macula densa secondary to increased proximal reabsorption resulting from the increase in plasma oncotic pressure. Studies on the effects of ethacrynic acid and chlorothiazide on renin secretion provide evidence that renin release is stimulated when the concentration of sodium at the macula densa is increased[54]. Other lines of evidence supporting a renin-regulating role for the macula densa have been reviewed by Vander[48].

(ii) *Sympathetic nervous system*—In addition to macula densa and baroreceptor mechanisms controlling renin secretion, there is abundant evidence for a role of the autonomic nervous system. This evidence, which has been summarised in a recent review[55], includes the observation that there are sympathetic nerve endings in close proximity to the juxtaglomerular cells[56-58] and the finding that renal denervation reduces granularity of the juxta-glomerular cells[59] and decreases renin secretion[60]. Conversely, direct electrical

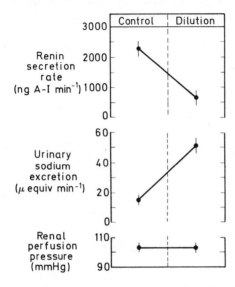

Figure 7.5 The effect of haemodilution with Ringer's solution on sodium excretion and renin secretion in isolated dog kidneys perfused at constant pressure. Data from Humphreys *et al.*[52]

stimulation of the renal nerves increases plasma renin levels[61-64] and a wide variety of manoeuvres which increase sympathetic activity, including carotid occlusion[65-67], non-hypotensive haemorrhage[66], hypoglycaemia[68], brain stem stimulation[69] and may others increase renin secretion. In addition, infusion of catecholamines intravenously[60, 61, 70-74] or directly into the renal artery[62,70,75] stimulates renin release.

It is now clear that a β-adrenergic receptor mechanism is involved in mediating the effects of sympathetic stimuli and circulating catecholamines on the release of renin. For example, the β-adrenergic blocking drug pro-pranolol abolishes the renin responses to brain stem stimulation[76], renal nerve stimulation[63, 64], physostigmine administration[77], hypoglycaemia[73], and infusion of epinephrine[73] or isoproterenol[71]. In all of these studies no blockade was produced by the α-adrenergic blocking drug phenoxybenzamine. In some situations, however, other α-blocking drugs, including dibenamine[78] and phentolamine[64, 79, 80], have been reported to be effective in blocking certain stimuli to renin release. It is therefore possible that some sympathetic effects on renin release involve α- as well as β-adrenergic receptors.

β-Adrenergic effects are mediated via the adenylcyclase–cyclic AMP system[81], and this system also appears to be involved in the regulation of renin secretion. The phosphodiesterase inhibitor theophylline, which inhibits the degradation of cyclic AMP, increases plasma renin activity[79, 82], and the dibutyryl derivtive of cyclic AMP stimulates renin release when infused into the renal artery[83]. Cyclic AMP also increases renin release when added to renal cortical tissue *in vitro*[84]. Taken together, these observations suggest that β-adrenergic stimuli to renin secretion act via the formation of cyclic AMP.

Considerable attention has been focused on the mechanism by which sympathetic stimuli and circulating catecholamines increase renin secretion. The increase in renin release could be a consequence of renal vasoconstriction, which would decrease afferent arteriolar pressure at the level of the proposed baroreceptor and which would also decrease glomerular filtration rate and thereby diminish the delivery of sodium to the macula densa. Such effects may contribute to the increase in renin secretion, especially that produced by infusion of epinephrine[62]. However, there is also evidence that locally released and circulating catecholamines exert a direct effect on the juxtaglomerular cells. For example, in the non-filtering kidney preparation mentioned above, stimulation of the renal nerves produces an increase in renin secretion that is not abolished by infusion of papaverine, a drug which blocks smooth muscle contraction[62]. Intrarenal infusion of norepinephrine has a similar effect. In addition, catecholamines have been reported to increase the release of renin when added to renal cortical tissue *in vitro*[84, 85].

In view of the evidence for the involvement of a β-receptor mechanism in the control of renin secretion, it has been suggested that sympathetic stimuli exert their effects directly on a β-receptor that is located in the membranes of the juxtaglomerular cells[86]. Although most of the evidence is consistent with this hypothesis, the *in vivo* experiments are not conclusive. For example, in the experiments utilising propranolol, the β-adrenergic blockade has not been limited to the kidney. In most experiments in which catecholamines have been infused into the renal artery, the doses used were large enough to produce systemic effects, making it difficult to draw conclusions about selective renal actions. Evidence against the existence of an intrarenal β-adrenergic receptor is provided by the experiments of Reid *et al.*[60, 74], in which the effects on renin secretion of intrarenal and intravenous infusions of the β-agonist isoproterenol were compared. It was found that when small doses were used, renin secretion increased following intravenous but not intrarenal infusion. Resolution of the discrepancy between these and other results awaits detailed *in vitro* studies of the effects of β-agonists and β-blocking drugs.

(iii) *Other factors*—Potassium also affects renin secretion. Potassium administration suppresses renin release[87-90] and potassium deprivation is associated with increased renin secretion[88, 89, 91]. The inhibition of renin secretion by potassium does not occur in the non-filtering kidney[90] and may be a consequence of an increased delivery of sodium to the macula densa secondary to decreased sodium reabsorption in the proximal tubule[92] or in the Loop of Henle[93]. It should be noted that a number of manoeuvres which have been used to manipulate renin secretion alter plasma potassium concentration. These include administration of catecholamines and adrenergic blocking drugs[94-97]. In addition, we have found recently that the suppression of renin secretion produced by clonidine is associated with a rise in plasma potassium concentration[98]. The extent to which potassium participates in the regulation of renin secretion remains to be determined.

Renin secretion is also suppressed by vasopressin. A number of investigators have observed that infusion of exogenous vasopressin inhibits renin release[99-102] and stimulation of the release of endogenous vasopressin by bilateral vagotomy in dogs undergoing a water diuresis also decreases renin secretion[102]. Rats with hereditary diabetes insipidus have higher plasma renin levels than normal rats[103, 104]. Angiotensin II also suppresses renin secretion *in vivo*[105] and *in vitro*[106] and this inhibitory action may provide a negative feedback that tends to stabilise renin secretion.

There may be other humoral substances that influence renin secretion. On the basis of experiments involving acute sodium depletion, Vander[107] suggested that there may be an unidentified hormone which participates in the control of renin secretion. More recently, De Vito *et al.*[108] have reported that dialysed plasma from dogs, which had been subjected to haemorrhage, stimulated renin release when injected into donor dogs. In addition, Nolly *et al.*[109] have presented evidence for a plasma factor which stimulates renin secretion *in vitro*.

(c) *Regulation of angiotensinogen production*—Angiotensinogen, the substrate from which renin releases angiotensin I, is a glycoprotein[110] which occurs in the a-2 globulin fraction of the plasma. The regulation of its secretion is of significance because its availability affects the level of plasma renin activity, and consequently the level of aldosterone secretion. The plasma angiotensinogen level is reduced by hepatectomy[111, 112] suggesting that the liver is the source of this protein. Proof that this conclusion is correct has now come from studies of perfused liver preparations[113, 114]. The methods used to measure plasma substrate concentration vary slightly from laboratory to laboratory but all involve incubating the plasma sample with sufficient renin to produce complete utilisation of the angiotensinogen. The resulting angiotensin is then measured either by bioassay or immunoassay. Plasma angiotensinogen concentration is expressed as the amount of angiotensin formed per ml of plasma under these conditions. No methods are available for the direct measurement of the rate of angiotensinogen production in the intact animal, although production rates have been measured recently in perfused liver preparations[113, 114]. Most investigators concerned with the regulation of angiotensinogen production have relied on measurements of plasma angiotensinogen concentration which obviously may be influenced by changes in the rate of destruction and volume of distribution as well as in the rate of production. Plasma angiotensinogen concentration is altered by nephrectomy, adrenalectomy and hormone treatment.

(i) *Nephrectomy*—Plasma angiotensinogen concentration increases following bilateral nephrectomy in all species that have been studied, although the magnitude and time-course varies from species to species. Because the increase in plasma angiotensinogen occurs in association with a decrease in plasma renin concentration[115, 116] and because there are a number of situations in which there is an inverse correlation between plasma angiotensinogen and plasma renin concentrations[115, 117], it has been suggested that plasma angiotensinogen concentration increases after nephrectomy as a consequence of decreased angiotensinogen consumption by renin. However, the increase in plasma angiotensinogen concentration still occurs after nephrectomy if renin is administered[116] making the increased consumption hypothesis unlikely. Blaine *et al.*[118] have suggested that angiotensinogen production is in some way controlled by changes in glomerular filtration rate or alterations in renal tubular function. This suggestion was based on experiments in which they showed that plasma angiotensinogen increased in dogs following ureteral ligation and renal ischaemia. They were able to eliminate uraemia *per se* as the stimulus to angiotensinogen production. These findings are in agreement with those of Bing and Poulsen[115] who suggested a common mechanism for the increases in plasma angiotensinogen which follow nephrectomy and ureteral ligation. It is unlikely that these changes are simply due to the failure of the kidney to remove angiotensinogen since this glycoprotein has a mol. wt. of 57 000[110] and is therefore probably not filtered in significant amounts.

(ii) *Adrenalectomy*—Plasma angiotensinogen concentration decreases following adrenalectomy[119-123]. This decrease may be prevented[120, 122] or reversed[119, 123] by administration of adrenal steroids. Plasma angiotensinogen concentration also decreases following hypophysectomy[119, 124] and is increased by administration of ACTH[119, 120]. In the dog, these changes appear to be the consequence of changes in circulating glucocorticoids rather than mineralocorticoids because dexamethasone, but not aldosterone, restores plasma angiotensinogen concentration in adrenalectomised animals[123] (Figure 7.6). However, Nasjletti and Masson[122] have reported that in the

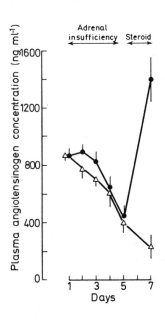

Figue 7.6 The effects of adrenal insufficiency and glucocorticoid (●—●—●) or mineralocorticoid (△—△—△) administration on plasma angiotensinogen concentration in the dog. Following the 5 day period of adrenal insufficiency the dogs were treated either with dexamethasone (0.6 mg i.m. four times a day for 2 days) or with *d*-aldosterone (100 μg i.m. four times a day for 2 days). Data from Reid *et al.*[123]

rat, the decrease in plasma angiotensinogen concentration which follows adrenalectomy is prevented by administration of DOCA or drinking 1% NaCl. They suggested that the maintenance of normal angiotensinogen levels was related to the maintenance of normal fluid and electrolyte balance. It should be pointed out that the doses of DOCA, aldosterone and cortisone used in their study were very high, thereby making it difficult to distinguish between the effects of glucocorticoid and mineralocorticoid activity. In addition, their observations on the effectiveness of saline have not been confirmed by others[119, 125]. It would therefore seem desirable to re-investigate the effects of adrenal steroids on plasma angiotensinogen concentration in the rat using physiological amounts of these agents.

Although it seems clear that adrenal steroids do play a role in the regulation of angiotensinogen production, it has not been established if their role is permissive or if they stimulate angiotensinogen production directly. In this context it should be noted that the increase in plasma angiotensinogen produced by nephrectomy is not prevented by prior adrenalectomy[116].

(iii) *Other factors*—Plasma angiotensinogen concentration is not significantly decreased in a number of situations in which plasma renin and angiotensin concentrations are increased. In these situations there would be increased utilisation of angiotensinogen, but since the blood level stays constant there must be a corresponding increase in angiotensinogen secretion by the liver. Blair-West and his associates reasoned that such an increase might reflect positive feed-back from one of the components of the renin–angiotensin system. To test this possibility they infused angiotensin II intravenously in dogs (J. R. Blair-West, I. A. Reid and W. F. Ganong, unpublished observations). An increase in plasma angiotensinogen concentration was observed beginning 2–3 h after the start of the infusion. This increase did not occur in adrenalectomised dogs, but it was not clear whether the effect of angiotensin infusion was mediated by increased adrenal cortical secretion, or whether adrenal steroids played a permissive role for some more direct effect of angiotensin on angiotensinogen production.

Oestrogens also increase plasma angiotensinogen concentration in a number of species including the rat[126-129] and man[130-132]. This effect appears to be the cause of the increase in plasma angiotensinogen which occurs during pregnancy[133]. Other situations in which plasma angiotensinogen concentration is increased include hypoxia[115] and administration of $HgCl_2$[134].

(iv) *Liver perfusion and liver slice studies*—In general, data obtained from liver perfusion systems or incubated liver slices confirm the observations described above. Nasjletti and Masson[114] perfused rat livers and observed an increased rate of angiotensinogen production in livers from rats which had been subjected previously to bilateral nephrectomy, ureteral ligation, partial hepatectomy and treatment with $HgCl_2$ or stilboestrol. Stilboestrol also increased angiotensinogen production when added to the perfusion fluid. Production was decreased by puromycin. They found that angiotensinogen production was actually increased after adrenalectomy, an observation which is apparently not in accord with the observation that plasma angiotensinogen concentration decreases following adrenalectomy (see earlier). However, Freeman and Rostorfer[135] found that angiotensinogen production by liver slices was reduced when the slices came from adrenalectomised rats. When the slices came from nephrectomised or cortisol-treated donors, angiotensinogen production was increased and these increases were blocked by actinomycin D.

(d) *Renin–angiotensinogen kinetics*—The rate of production of angiotensin is influenced by the concentration of angiotensinogen in the plasma as well as by the concentration of renin. This conclusion is based primarily on the results of *in vitro* studies in which the velocity of angiotensin formation is measured when a fixed amount of renin is incubated with a range of angiotensinogen concentrations. A Lineweaver–Burk plot (1/velocity *v.* 1/angiotensinogen concentration) is usually constructed and from this a Michaelis constant (K_m) can be obtained. When the angiotensinogen concentration is equal to the

K_m, the velocity of the reaction is one half the maximum velocity. Estimates of K_m are available in a number of species[18, 123, 133, 136, 137] and, particularly in man, they vary considerably from laboratory to laboratory[133, 136, 137]. This is not surprising in view of the differences in methodology and the impurity of the renin and angiotensinogen preparations that have been employed. In addition, there is some evidence for the existence of inhibitors of the renin–angiotensinogen reaction[138-140] which would result in erroneous estimates of K_m. Despite these difficulties, it now seems clear that the velocity of formation of angiotensin is limited by the plasma angiotensinogen concentration in man[130, 133, 137], dog[123], and rat[128, 141]. Thus changes in plasma angiotensinogen concentration such as those which occur during pregnancy[133], adrenal insufficiency[123] and a variety of other situations would be expected to influence importantly the rate of angiotensin production.

7.2.4.2 ACTH and other pituitary hormones

Several lines of evidence indicate that the pituitary participates in the regulation of aldosterone secretion. Following hypophysectomy, aldosterone secretion decreases in rats[142] and dogs[143]. Furthermore, patients with pan-hypopituitarism[144], as well as hypophysectomised rats[145, 146], and dogs[147] have a suppressed aldosterone response to sodium restriction. A major cause of these changes in aldosterone secretion appears to be the decrease in ACTH secretion since administration of ACTH increases aldosterone secretion *in vivo*[148, 150] or *in vitro*[21, 30, 151]. In animals and humans on a normal sodium intake, the minimum dose of ACTH that will increase aldosterone secretion is considerably higher than the minimum dose that stimulates 17-hydroxy-corticoid secretion[16]. An interesting feature of the response to ACTH *in vivo* is that the stimulation of aldosterone secretion is transient and does not persist with continued administration[152-154].

In addition to ACTH, other pituitary hormones appear to be involved in the pituitary regulation of aldosterone secretion. The impairment of aldo-sterone secretion in sodium-depleted, hypophysectomised rats is not corrected completely by administration of ACTH[145]. However, if growth hormone is also administered, the aldosterone secretory response to sodium restriction is normalised[155-157]. The mechanism of this effect of growth hormone is unknown, but it does not involve the renin–angiotensin system since growth hormone is effective in nephrectomised animals[158]. In addition, chronic growth hormone treatment does not increase renin secretion in the rat[156] and dog (I. Henderson and W. F. Ganong, unpublished observations). Palmore *et al.*[146] have suggested that pituitary factors other than ACTH and growth hormone may also be involved in the stimulation and maintenance of aldosterone production in sodium depleted rats.

The pituitary can also affect aldosterone secretion via the renin–angiotensin system. As mentioned above, plasma angiotensinogen concentration is decreased by hypophysectomy, and this would be expected to cause a decrease in angiotensin II production. An additional mechanism by which the pituitary could affect circulating angiotensin levels is through the inhibitory effect of vasopressin on renin secretion.

7.2.4.3 Sodium and potassium

Aldosterone secretion by sheep[159, 160] or dog[161] adrenals is increased when the concentration of sodium in the plasma perfusing them is decreased. Conversely, when sheep adrenals are perfused with blood having a high sodium concentration, the aldosterone response to angiotensin is reduced[162]. However, the changes in sodium concentration required for these effects are relatively large (3–10 mequiv l^{-1}) and therefore it seems unlikely that plasma sodium concentration *per se* is an important variable in the physiological regulation of aldosterone secretion. Rather, it appears that the aldosterone responses to changes in sodium balance are mediated primarily via the renin–angiotensin system.

It is now well established that aldosterone secretion is increased by administration of potassium and decreased by potassium deprivation even though administration of potassium inhibits renin secretion. The effects of potassium on aldosterone secretion have been observed in a variety of situations. In man[163] and the rat[164], increased potassium intake or infusion of potassium increases aldosterone secretion. Aldosterone secretion by the transplanted sheep adrenal[165] or the isolated dog adrenal[161] is increased when the concentration of potassium in the fluid circulating through them is increased. Potassium also stimulates aldosterone production *in vitro*[21, 166] indicating that its effect is exerted directly on the gland.

Potassium also modifies the aldosterone responses to other stimuli. Potassium-deficient rats do not respond normally to sodium depletion[164] and, in addition, it has been demonstrated that plasma potassium increases during sodium deficiency[164]. On the basis of these and other findings, Boyd et al.[164] concluded that 'the potassium ion is an important regulator of adrenal function in the rat, playing a significant role in the mediation of the zona glomerulosa response to sodium depletion'. Müller[167, 168] has reported that the aldosterone response of incubated adrenals to serotonin, ACTH, potassium, or angiotensin II does not occur in adrenals taken from potassium-deficient animals. In man, increasing potassium intake increases the aldosterone response to ACTH administration[169], or to potassium infusions[163]. Bayard et al.[170] observed a highly significant correlation between plasma aldosterone concentration and plasma potassium concentration in anephric patients and concluded that in such individuals, the primary regulator of aldosterone secretion is potassium.

The effects of angiotensin II, potassium chloride, ACTH and sodium deficiency on adrenocortical electrolyte content have been studied in the dog[22]. Each of these stimuli to aldosterone secretion produced an increase in adrenocortical potassium content. It was therefore suggested that the effects of these stimuli are mediated by changes in the potassium content of the adrenal cortex. Unfortunately, aldosterone secretion was not measured in these experiments and it was therefore not possible to correlate the rate of aldosterone secretion with adrenocortical potassium content. A discordant note is the report by Szalay[171] that angiotensin inhibits rather than stimulates potassium accumulation by the adrenal cortex. Further evidence in support of a role of adrenocortical potassium in the control of aldosterone production is the demonstration that ouabain decreased potassium uptake by dog adrenal cortical slices and decreased aldosterone production[172]. In addition, the increase in aldosterone production produced by potassium administration or prior sodium depletion was reduced greatly by ouabain[172]. Boyd et al.[173] have confirmed and extended these observations in the rat and have shown that the aldosterone, but not the corticosterone, response to ACTH is blocked by ouabain.

7.2.4.4   Other factors which influence aldosterone secretion

There may be factors in addition to those described above which influence the secretion of aldosterone. Indirect evidence for such factors has been derived from a variety of experiments in humans, sheep and rats. Best et al.[174] studied the effect of dietary sodium restriction for 5 days on plasma angiotensin II concentration and plasma aldosterone in normal volunteers. Although plasma angiotensin concentration did not increase, plasma aldosterone rose. Plasma sodium and cortisol concentrations did not change significantly, but there was a small increase in plasma potassium concentration. Boyd et al.[175] compared the aldosterone response to sodium restriction with that to exogenous angiotensin II in normal male subjects. Angiotensin infusion resulted in plasma angiotensin concentrations equal to or greater than those produced by salt restriction, but there was a greater increase in plasma aldosterone associated with salt restriction than with angiotensin infusion. They argued that this difference could not be explained by changes in plasma ACTH or electrolytes and they were unable to demonstrate differences in adrenal sensitivity which could account for the discrepancy. They therefore suggested that an unknown factor was involved in the aldosterone response to sodium restriction.

A number of investigators have studied aldosterone secretion in nephrectomised patients. McCaa et al.[176] reported an increase in plasma aldosterone concentration when sodium and volume were depleted by dialysis in anephric patients. They were able to exclude a role of plasma potassium in this response and, since plasma cortisol did not increase, changes in ACTH output were probably not responsible for the changes in aldosterone secretion. However, there was a decrease in plasma sodium concentration averaging 5 mequiv l^{-1}. On the other hand, Boyd et al.[177] failed to observe an increase in plasma aldosterone concentration when sodium depletion was induced by peritoneal dialysis in three nephrectomised patients. However, these results were complicated by the finding of decreased adrenal sensitivity to exogenous angiotensin[177]. Mitra et al.[178] observed that plasma aldosterone concentration in anephric patients was not significantly different from the concentration in normal subjects. They also observed an increased concentration after 2 h in the standing position. This increase was apparently unrelated to plasma sodium and potassium concentration and, at least in some patients, was probably not due to increased ACTH secretion. On the other hand, Bayard et al.[170] reported that anephric patients showed less consistent changes in plasma aldosterone due to changes in posture than normal subjects. They observed a highly significant correlation between plasma aldosterone and potassium concentrations and suggested that potassium is the primary regulator of aldosterone secretion in the absence of the kidney. In the experiments cited above, the metabolic clearance rate of aldosterone was not measured and therefore a possibility that cannot be excluded is that the changes in plasma aldosterone which were observed were secondary to changes in the metabolism of aldosterone, rather than to changes in its secretion[179]. Thus, there are discrepancies and problems, but these experiments at least raise the possibility that an unknown factor or factors participates in the control of aldosterone secretion in man.

When sheep were depleted of sodium via the loss of parotid saliva, plasma renin concentration, plasma angiotensin concentration, and plasma aldosterone concentration increased in parallel[36]. However, when the sodium deficit was corrected, plasma angiotensin II and aldosterone levels became dissociated and plasma aldosterone concentration fell more rapidly than plasma angiotensin[36]. Cortisol and corticosterone concentrations remained within the normal range, suggesting that changes in ACTH secretion were not involved. The changes in plasma sodium and potassium which occurred during sodium repletion may have contributed to the decrease in aldosterone secretion. However, when similar changes in adrenal arterial electrolyte concentrations were produced by infusing hypertonic sodium bicarbonate into the arterial blood supplying the adrenal gland, plasma aldosterone did not fall to the same extent as during sodium repletion[180]. In another series of experiments, it was observed that if plasma angiotensin II concentration was maintained at a constant level by infusion of exogenous angiotensin II, plasma aldosterone still fell following sodium repletion[181]. These and other experiments which point toward the involvement of an unidentified factor which influences aldosterone secretion in the sheep have recently been reviewed[181].

Plasma aldosterone concentration has been reported to remain constant following nephrectomy in rats and to be increased by sodium depletion in the absence of the kidneys[182]. These results did not appear to be a consequence of changes in plasma electrolytes or ACTH.

Thus, it seems possible that some unidentified factor participates in the regulation of aldosterone secretion. However, it is difficult to rule out the effects of pituitary factors, plasma and adrenal electrolytes, and changes in the metabolic clearance rate of aldosterone. More direct approaches to the problem would be of value. In the meantime, it should be pointed out that while these various lines of evidence suggest the existence of unidentified factors in the control of aldosterone secretion, they do not diminish the importance of the established mechanisms by which the secretion of this steroid is known to be regulated.

7.2.4.5 *Sites at which various stimuli act to increase aldosterone secretion*

The generally-accepted pathway for aldosterone biosynthesis is summarised in Figure 7.7. In a recent monograph, Müller[21] summarised data on the site of action of the various stimuli which influence the secretion of aldosterone. Most of this evidence indicates that angiotensin II, ACTH and potassium act early in the pathway to increase the formation of pregnenolone from cholesterol. When body sodium is depleted, the conversion of corticosterone to aldosterone is also increased. Since the publication of Müller's review a number of additional studies have been reported. Aguilera and Marusic[183] administered angiotensin II or renin, either acutely or chronically, to dogs and then compared the effects of these treatments on the conversion of corticosterone to aldosterone. Acute administration of angiotensin or renin had no effect on the conversion of corticosterone to aldosterone. However, chronic administration of renin to either intact or hypophysectomised dogs on a normal sodium intake stimulated the conversion of corticosterone to aldosterone. On the basis of these results, it was suggested that the conversion

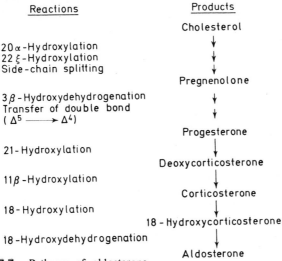

Figure 7.7. Pathway of aldosterone synthesis (Modified from Müller[21].)

of corticosterone to aldosterone in sodium deficient animals may also be regulated by the renin–angiotensin system[183]. It was also suggested that an action of angiotensin late in the biosynthetic pathway, together with its action early in the pathway, could explain the increased adrenal sensitivity to angiotensin or ACTH which has been observed during sodium deficiency[43, 184-186].

In a recent *in vitro* study utilising rat adrenal glomerulosa tissue, various stimuli to aldosterone production including ACTH, potassium and serotonin were found by Williams and his associates to increase the conversion of [^{3}H]corticosterone to [^{3}H]aldosterone but not of [^{3}H]corticosterone to [^{3}H]18-hydroxycorticosterone[187]. Addition of corticosterone also increased the [^{3}H]corticosterone to [^{3}H]aldosterone conversion. The results of other experiments[187] suggested that this effect on the late pathway was not secondary to enzyme induction by substrate. It was postulated therefore that the effect was due to enzyme activation by substrate, resulting either from increased coenzyme concentration or from an allosteric effect. It seems unlikely that this effect can explain the findings of Aguilera and Marusic[183]; the enzyme activation by corticosterone occurred within 15 min[187], while chronic renin treatment was required to increase the conversion of corticosterone to aldosterone[183].

Baumann and Müller[188] have studied the effects of potassium deficiency and repletion on the final steps of the aldosterone biosynthetic pathway in rat zona glomerulosa tissue and mitochondria. They observed a decreased conversion of corticosterone to 18-hydroxycorticosterone and aldosterone after potassium depletion, an effect which was reversed by potassium repletion. This study confirms and extends an earlier report by Boyd et al.[164] that mitochondria from rats which had been subjected to oral potassium loading converted more corticosterone to aldosterone than control animals. Although the findings of Bauman and Müller[188] are in part consistent with those of Williams et al.[187] described above, the time-course of the effect of potassium was different in the two studies. Furthermore, Williams et al.[187] failed to observe any effects of potassium on the conversion of corticosterone to 18-hydroxycorticosterone. The 11β-hydroxylase activity of the zona glomerulosa may also be affected by potassium intake[189].

Saruta et al.[190] have studied the effects of ACTH, angiotensin I and II, sodium and potassium on steroidogenesis in beef adrenal slices. ACTH and potassium increased aldosterone synthesis in association with increased formation of cyclic AMP. The effects on steroidogenesis and cyclic AMP were abolished by puromycin. Angiotensin did not stimulate cyclic AMP but its effect on aldosterone was blocked by puromycin. In common with ACTH, angiotensin required calcium to stimulate steroidogenesis. Angiotensin I as well as angiotensin II was effective in stimulating aldosterone production and the effectiveness of angiotensin I did not appear to be a consequence of its partial conversion to angiotensin II. The effects of ACTH, angiotensin and potassium were accompanied by increases in corticosterone production, while decreases in sodium concentration in the incubation medium increased aldosterone production in association with a decrease in corticosterone production. These observations are consistent with earlier proposals that ACTH, angiotensin and potassium stimulate aldosterone production by an action early in the biosynthetic pathway, while a decrease in sodium concentration increases the conversion of corticosterone to aldosterone.

The effects of angiotensin and potassium on the early portion of the aldosterone biosynthetic pathway have also been studied in normal human subjects[191]. ACTH-dependent steroid production was suppressed using dexamethasone and metyrapone was used to block corticosterone production. Plasma deoxycorticosterone concentration was used as an index of the activity of the zona glomerulosa while plasma deoxycortisol concentration indicated changes in zona fasiculata activity. Under these conditions, administration of potassium or angiotensin increased plasma deoxycorticosterone without increasing plasma deoxycortisol. ACTH administration produced small increases in deoxycorticosterone and large increases in deoxycortisol concentration. These findings indicate that angiotensin and potassium stimulate the aldosterone biosynthetic pathway at some point before deoxycorticosterone formation.

In summary, it seems clear that angiotensin, ACTH and potassium increase aldosterone production through actions early in the biosynthetic pathway, while alterations in sodium balance affect the conversion of corticosterone to aldosterone. However, it now appears that angiotensin, potassium and possibly ACTH, also increase the conversion of corticosterone to aldosterone and, in addition, there is evidence that potassium may increase 11β-hydroxylase activity. More experiments are required before the relative importance of these different actions can be established.

7.3 OTHER STEROIDS WITH MINERALOCORTICOID ACTIVITY

Although aldosterone is the most potent naturally occurring mineralocorticoid, a number of other steroids have significant sodium retaining activity. Of these, the most important are deoxycorticosterone, corticosterone, cortisol and oestrogens.

7.3.1 Deoxycorticosterone

Next to aldosterone, deoxycorticosterone is the most potent adrenal mineralocorticoid. In man, its plasma concentration is similar to that of aldosterone[192], but since its sodium retaining potency is only 3% that of aldosterone, it is thought to be of little physiological significance. However, in the dog the secretion rate of deoxycorticosterone is 7–9 times that of aldosterone[193], and it may therefore contribute to sodium homeostasis in this species. In both man and dog, deoxycorticosterone secretion is primarily under anterior pituitary control. Its secretion is increased following ACTH administration in man[192, 194] and the dog[193] and decreased when ACTH secretion is decreased by hypophysectomy in the dog[193] or by dexamethasone administration in man[194]. Deoxycorticosterone secretion is not increased following subpressor[192] or pressor[194] infusions of angiotensin II or sodium restriction in normal man[192, 194]; however, Schambelan and Biglieri[194] reported an increase in tetrahydrodeoxycorticosterone excretion following angiotensin II infusion in two patients with panhypopituitarism. In hypophysectomised dogs, deoxycorticosterone secretion was increased by pressor doses of angiotensin II but not by administration of potassium or sodium depletion[193].

7.3.2 Corticosterone

In birds, rodents and the rabbit, corticosterone is the major secretory product of the adrenal cortex; in most other species, cortisol is secreted in greater amounts. The mineralocorticoid activity of corticosterone is considerably less than aldosterone or deoxycorticosterone but it is secreted in greater amounts and has important effects on electrolyte metabolism. The secretion of corticosterone is predominantly under the control of ACTH.

7.3.3 Cortisol

Cortisol is the major steroid product of the adrenal cortex in nearly all mammals. Its secretion is under the control of ACTH. Cortisol is predominantly a glucocorticoid, but some mineralocorticoid activity has been demonstrated. In some situations, especially sodium loading, cortisol may actually be natriuretic, probably because of its capacity to increase glomerular filtration rate[195]. Previous studies suggested that glucocorticoids rather than mineralocorticoids correct the impaired water excretion which occurs in adrenal insufficiency[196]. However, more recent data suggest that both gluco- and mineralo-corticoids are required to correct the impaired water excretion[197]. In addition, Ufferman and Shrier[198] have reported recently that there is a diluting deficit in adrenalectomised dogs which is related to negative sodium balance and may be corrected by either administration of DOCA or a high intake of sodium.

7.3.4 Oestrogens

It is now well established that oestrogens cause sodium retention[199], but the exact mechanism by which this effect is produced is not known. It has been reported that oestrogens increase plasma renin activity[200] and aldosterone secretion[201], effects which are possibly secondary to an increase in plasma angiotensinogen concentration[130]. Aldosterone may contribute to the sodium retention but other factors must be involved since oestradiol produces sodium retention in adrenalectomised dogs[202]. This latter finding suggests that oestrogens may have a direct action on the renal tubule. Evidence in support of this possibility is provided by the recent demonstration of oestradiol receptor sites in the cytosol fraction of rat kidney homogenates[203]. It seems unlikely that the sodium retention which occurs during pregnancy is a direct consequence of increased plasma levels of oestradiol[204].

7.4 EFFECTS OF ANGIOTENSIN AND VASOPRESSIN ON SODIUM EXCRETION

7.4.1 Angiotensin

Numerous reports indicate that angiotensin influences the renal excretion of sodium by mechanisms other than stimulation of aldosterone secretion. This subject has been reviewed in detail elsewhere[18]. Both increases and decreases in sodium excretion have been observed following infusion of angiotensin II. The nature of the response (i.e. an increase or a decrease) appears to depend on the dose of angiotensin and on a number of other factors. Large pressor doses are frequently accompanied by natriuresis and diuresis while subpressor or mildly pressor doses generally cause sodium retention. The pressor response to the larger doses of angiotensin undoubtedly contributes to the natriuresis and diuresis, but changes in renal function also accompany the administration of both pressor and subpressor doses. These changes include alterations in glomerular filtration rate and tubular function. For example, the antinatriuretic response to angiotensin is usually accompanied by a decrease in glomerular filtration rate. Angiotensin also appears to decrease tubular reabsorption of sodium and it has been suggested that the natriuretic effect of angiotensin is in part mediated by a decrease in proximal tubular sodium reabsorption. For example, infusion of a mildly pressor dose of angiotensin in rats undergoing a furosemide diuresis decreased fractional sodium reabsorption and increased sodium excretion[205]. Conversely, blockade of endogenous angiotensin by infusion of antibodies to angiotensin II increased fractional sodium reabsorption and decreased sodium excretion without changing blood pressure[205].

7.4.2 Vasopressin

In addition to its important role in the regulation of renal water excretion, vasopressin may influence sodium reabsorption and excretion. Several investigators have reported that infusion of vasopressin during a water diuresis increases sodium excretion[206-210]. This effect, which has been observed in the dog and man, is not due to decreased aldosterone secretion since it occurs even when exogenous sodium-retaining steroids are administered and is not prevented by adrenalectomy[210]. In addition, this effect does not appear to be the consequence of an increase in glomerular filtration rate, blood volume, or blood pressure since it occurs when haemorrhage is used as the stimulus to vasopressin secretion, a situation in which glomerular filtration rate, blood volume and pressure are all decreased[209]. There is evidence that vasopressin depresses tubular sodium reabsorption at a site proximal to the distal convoluted tubule. Martinez-Maldonado[211] argued that vasopressin decreases proximal tubular sodium reabsorption because the natriuresis accompanying vasopressin infusion was associated with increased phosphate excretion. However, micropuncture studies[212, 213] indicate that vasopressin has no effect on proximal sodium reabsorption. Humphreys et al.[209] suggested that the natriuresis might be a consequence of decreased sodium reabsorption by the Loop of Henle secondary to increased reabsorption of water by the collecting duct. Further studies are required to delineate the mechanism and physiological role of this natriuretic effect of vasopressin.

7.4.3 Interaction of vasopressin and angiotensin

Intraventricular[214], intracarotid[215] and intravenous[216] administration of angiotensin have been reported to increase vasopressin secretion. It has therefore been suggested that angiotensin stimulates vasopressin secretion at some central site[215]. Since vasopressin inhibits renin release (see earlier) it has been proposed that the vasopressin secreted in response to an increase in circulating angiotensin feeds back to inhibit further renin secretion[101]. The plasma concentration of vasopressin which inhibits renin release is said to be within the physiological range[101]. However, Claybaugh et al.[217] have been unable to confirm the earlier reports that intravenous or intracarotid infusion of angiotensin increases plasma vasopressin concentration in anaesthetised dogs. These investigators also studied the effect of haemorrhage on vasopressin release in dogs in which renin release was prevented by temporary occlusion of the renal vessels[218]. They observed a greater increase in plasma vasopressin concentration in these 'nephrectomised' animals than in control animals in which plasma renin increased. It is therefore difficult to believe that angiotensin released *in vivo* plays a significant role in the control of vasopressin secretion in dogs.

7.5 NATRIURETIC HORMONE

During the past 20 years, various investigators have proposed that an, as yet, unisolated natriuretic hormone or 'third factor' is involved in the regulation of renal sodium excretion. Much of the evidence for this hormone is indirect and inconclusive and in many instances there are remarkable discrepancies between the results obtained in different laboratories. Nevertheless, the general consensus is in favour of the possibility that such a hormone exists. The subject has been reviewed elsewhere[3, 4, 219-222]. Recent evidence for a natriuretic hormone includes the observations that volume expansion of donor animals increases sodium excretion in recipient animals in cross-circulation experiments[223, 224] and in isolated kidneys in perfusion studies[225, 226]. Extracts of plasma and urine from volume expanded animals have been reported to increase sodium excretion when administered to assay rats[227] or to inhibit sodium transport *in vitro*[228-230]. These effects are difficult to explain on the basis of known mechanisms regulating sodium excretion. However, other investigators using similar techniques to those used in the above studies have not found evidence for a natriuretic hormone[52, 231, 232].

Other suggestive evidence for a natriuretic hormone includes the finding that intraventricular administration of hypertonic saline induces a natriuresis in dogs[233] and goats[234] while ventriculocisternal perfusion with hypotonic saline solutions decreases sodium excretion[235]. The changes in sodium excretion in these experiments do not appear to be a consequence of changes in renal blood flow or glomerular filtration rate, but a possible role of the renal nerves has not been eliminated. Another situation in which the participation of a natriuretic humoral factor has been invoked is the phenomenon of 'escape' from mineralocorticoids[236].

Attempts to determine the source and chemical nature of the proposed natriuretic hormone have not been successful. Organs that have been considered as possible sources include the liver, brain, kidneys and adrenals, but the data does not permit definite conclusions[219, 227]. Known substances that have been considered as possible natriuetic hormones include prostaglandins, calcitonin, and a-MSH[222]. Estimates of molecular weight range from < 3000[229] to 50 000[227]. The site of action of the proposed hormone is also a subject of debate with arguments being advanced for both proximal and distal tubular sites[221].

Thus, although there is indirect evidence for the existence of a natriuretic hormone, conclusive evidence that it exists is not at hand.

7.6 CONCLUSIONS

Although it is difficult to summarise a review article which is itself a summary of a large body of information, the following conclusions seem warranted:

(a) Several hormones participate in the regulation of renal sodium excretion. These include the adrenal corticosteroids, oestrogens, vasopressin and angiotensin. In addition, there is considerable evidence for the existence of a natriuretic hormone.

(b) The most important adrenal steroid is aldosterone, a hormone secreted primarily by the zona glomerulosa. Its secretion is regulated mainly by the renin–angiotensin system, but ACTH, growth hormone, potassium and, to a lesser extent, sodium also play important roles. There is also some indirect evidence that aldosterone secretion may be influenced by an, as yet, unidentified humoral factor.

(c) The activity of the renin–angiotensin system is influenced primarily by the rate of renin secretion and by the plasma concentration of angiotensinogen. Renin secretion varies in response to changes in renal perfusion pressure, macula densa sodium transport and the activity of the sympathetic nervous system. In addition, renin secretion is suppressed by vasopressin, angiotensin and potassium. The regulation of plasma angiotensinogen concentration is not well understood, but current evidence indicates that angiotensinogen production is influenced by changes in the secretion of pituitary and adrenal hormones and by alterations in renal function.

(d) Stimulation of aldosterone secretion by angiotensin, ACTH, or potassium is associated with increased conversion of cholesterol to pregnenolone and, at least in some situations, of corticosterone to aldosterone. Alterations in sodium balance affect the conversion of corticosterone to aldosterone. It is possible that these stimuli also affect other steps in the biosynthetic pathway.

(e) Other adrenal steroids which influence renal sodium excretion include deoxycorticosterone, corticosterone and cortisol. The secretion of these compounds is regulated primarily by ACTH.

(f) Administration of oestrogens produces sodium retention: this appears to be the result of activation of the renin–angiotensin system and of a direct effect of oestrogens on the renal tubule.

(g) The peptides vasopressin and angiotensin also alter sodium excretion by direct and indirect mechanisms. They both have actions on the renal tubule but, in addition, they decrease the activity of the renin–angiotensin system through the inhibition of renin secretion.

(h) There is considerable evidence for the existence of a natriuretic hormone, but conclusive proof of its existence is not at hand.

Acknowledgements

This chapter includes previously unpublished results of experiments supported by USPHS grant AM06704 and the L. J. and Mary C. Skaggs Foundation. Support from the Bay Area Heart Research Committee for Dr. Reid is gratefully acknowledged.

References

1. Mills, I. H. (1970). Renal regulation of sodium excretion. *Annu. Rev. Physiol.*, **32**, 75
2. Earley, L. E. and Daugharty, T. M. (1969). Sodium metabolism. *N. Engl. J. Med.*, **281**, 72

3. Schrier, R. W. and de Wardener, H. E. (1972). Tubular reabsorption of sodium ion: influence of factors other than aldosterone and glomerular filtration rate. *N. Engl. J. Med.*, **285**, 1231

4. Schrier, R. W. and de Wardener, H. E. (1972). Tubular reabsorption of sodium ion: influence of factors other than aldosterone and glomerular filtration rate. *N. Engl. J. Med.*, **285**, 1292

5. Gláz, E. and Vecsei, P. (1971). *Aldosterone* (Braunschweig: Pergamon)

6. Hierholzer, K. and Stolte, H. (1969). The proximal and distal tubular action of adrenal steroids on Na reabsorption. *Nephron*, **6**, 188

7. Gill, J. R., Delea, C. S. and Bartter, F. C. (1972). A role for sodium-retaining steroids in the regulation of proximal tubular sodium reabsorption in man. *Clin. Sci.*, **42**, 423

8. Lynch, R. E., Schneider, E. G., Willis, L. R. and Knox, F. G. (1972). Absence of mineralocorticoid-dependent sodium reabsorption in dog proximal tubule. *Amer. J. Physiol.*, **223**, 40

9. Martin, D. G. and Berliner, R. W. (1969). The effect of aldosterone on proximal tubular sodium reabsorption in the rat. *Proc. Annu. Meet Amer. Soc. Nephrol.*, **3**, 45

10. Sharp, G. W. G. and Leaf, A. (1966). Studies on the mode of action of aldosterone. *Recent. Progr. Horm. Res.*, **22**, 431

11. Fanestil, D. D. (1969). Mechanism of action of aldosterone. *Annu. Rev. Med.*, **20**, 223

12. Edelman, I. S. and Fanestil, D. D. (1970). Mineralocorticoids. In: *Biochemical Actions of Hormones*, Vol. 1, 321 (G. Litwack, editor) (New York: Academic Press)

13. Pelletier, M., Ludens, J. H. and Fanestil, D. D. (1972). The role of aldosterone in active sodium transport. *Arch. Intern. Med.*, **129**, 248

14. Ganong, W. F., Biglieri, E. G. and Mulrow, P. J. (1966). Mechanisms regulating adrenocortical secretion of aldosterone and glucocorticoids. *Recent Progr. Horm. Res.*, **22**, 381

15. Mulrow, P. J. (1966). Neural and other mechanisms regulating aldosterone secretion. In: *Neuroendocrinology*, Vol. 1, 407 (L. Martini and W. F. Ganong, editors) (New York: Academic Press)

16. Ganong, W. F. and Van Brunt, E. E. (1968). Control of aldosterone secretion. In: *Handbook of Experimental Pharmacology*, Vol. 14, (3), 1 (H. W. Deane and B. L. Rubin, editors) (Berlin: Springer-Verlag)

17. Gross, F. (1968). Control of aldosterone secretion by the renin-angiotensin system and by corticotropin. *Advan. Intern. Med.*, **14**, 281

18. Page, I. H. and McCubbin, J. W. (1968). *Renal Hypertension* (Chicago: Year Book Medical Publishers)

19. Davis, J. O. (1971). The renin-angiotensin system in the control of aldosterone secretion. In: *Kidney Hormones*, 173. (J. W. Fisher, editor) (London: Academic Press)

20. Mulrow, P. J. (1972). The adrenal cortex. *Annu. Rev. Physiol.*, **34**, 409

21. Müller, J. (1971). *Regulation of Aldosterone Biosynthesis* (Berlin: Springer-Verlag)

22. Baumber, J. S., Davis, J. O., Johnson, J. A. and Witty, R. T. (1971). Increased adrenocortical potassium in association with increased biosynthesis of aldosterone. *Amer. J. Physiol.*, **220**, 1094

23. Deane, H. G. and Masson, G. M. C. (1951). Adrenal cortical changes in rats with various types of experimental hypertension. *J. Clin. Endocrinol. Metab.*, **11**, 193

24. Hartroft, P. M. and Hartroft, W. S. (1953). Studies on renal juxtaglomerular cells. I. Variations produced by sodium chloride and DOCA. *J. Exp. Med.*, **97**, 415

25. Hartroft, P. M. and Hartroft, W. S. (1955). Studies on renal juxtaglomerular cells. II. Correlation of the degree of granulation of juxtaglomerular cells with width of the zona glomerulosa of the adrenal cortex. *J. Exp. Med.*, **102**, 205

26. Ganong, W. F., Mulrow, P. J., Boryczka, A. and Cera, G. (1962). Evidence for a direct effect of angiotensin II on adrenal cortex of the dog. *Proc. Soc. Exp. Biol. Med.*, **109**, 381

27. Ganong, W. F. and Mulrow, P. J. (1962). Role of the kidney in adrenocortical response to hemorrhage in hypophysectomized dogs. *Endocrinology*, **70**, 182

28. Davis, J. O., Ayers, C. R. and Carpenter, C. C. J. (1961). Renal origin of an aldosterone-stimulating hormone in dogs with thoracic caval constriction and in sodium-depleted dogs. *J. Clin. Invest.*, **40**, 1466

29. Davis, J. O., Binnion, P. F., Brown, T. C. and Johnston, C. I. (1966). Mechanisms involved in the hypersecretion of aldosterone during sodium depletion. *Circulat. Res.*, **18–19** (Suppl. I), 143

30. Kaplan, N. and Bartter, F. (1962). The effect of ACTH, renin, angiotensin II and various precursors on biosynthesis of aldosterone by adrenal slices. *J. Clin. Invest.*, **41**, 715
31. Michelakis, A. M. and Horton, R. (1970). The relationship between plasma renin and aldosterone in normal man. *Circulat. Res.*, **26–27** (Suppl. I), 185
32. Williams, G. H., Cain, J. P., Dluhy, R. G. and Underwood, R. H. (1972). Studies of the control of plasma aldosterone concentration in normal man. I. Response to posture, acute and chronic volume depletion, and sodium loading. *J. Clin. Invest.*, **51**, 1731
33. Bull, M. B., Hillman, R. S., Cannon, P. J. and Laragh, J. H. (1970). Renin and aldosterone secretion in man as influenced by changes in electrolyte balance and blood volume. *Circulat. Res.*, **27**, 953
34. Williams, G. H., Tuck, M. L., Rose, L. I., Dluhy, R. G. and Underwood, R. H. (1972). Studies of the control of plasma aldosterone concentration in normal man. III. Response to sodium chloride infusion. *J. Clin. Invest.*, **51**, 2645
35. Brown, T. C., Davis, J. O. and Johnston, C. I. (1966). Acute response in plasma renin and aldosterone secretion to diuretics. *Amer. J. Physiol.*, **211**, 437
36. Blair-West, J. R., Cain, M. D., Catt, K. J., Coghlan, J. P., Denton, D. A., Funder, J. W., Scoggins, B. A. and Wright, R. D. (1971). The dissociation of aldosterone secretion and systemic renin and angiotensin II levels during the correction of sodium deficiency. *Acta Endocrinol.*, **66**, 229
57. Reid, I. A. and McDonald, I. R. (1969). The renin–angiotensin system in a marsupial (*Trichosurus vulpecula*). *J. Endocrinol.*, **44**, 231
38. Johnston, C. I., Davis, J. O. and Hartroft, P. M. (1967). Renin–angiotensin system, adrenal steroids and sodium depletion in a primitive mammal, the American opposum. *Endocrinology*, **81**, 633
39. Blair-West, J. R., Coghlan, J. P., Denton, D. A., Nelson, J. F., Orchard, E., Scoggins, B. A., Wright, R. D., Myers, K. and Junqueira, C. L. (1968). Physiological, morphological, and behavioural adaptation to a sodium deficient diet by wild native Australian and introduced species of animals. *Nature (London)*, **217**, 922
40. Cade, R. and Perenich, T. (1965). Secretion of aldosterone by rats. *Amer. J. Physiol.*, **208**, 1026
41. Marieb, N. J. and Mulrow, P. J. (1965). Role of the renin–angiotensin system in the regulation of aldosterone secretion in the rat. *Endocrinology*, **76**, 657
42. Dufau, M. L. and Kliman, B. (1968). Pharmacologic effects of angiotensin-II-amide on aldosterone and corticosterone secretion by the intact anesthetized rat. *Endocrinology*, **82**, 29
43. Kinson, G. A. and Singer, B. (1968). Sensitivity to angiotensin and ACTH in the sodium deficient rat. *Endocrinology*, **83**, 1108
44. Ganong, W. F. and Boryczka, A. T. (1967). Effect of low sodium diet on aldosterone stimulating activity of angiotensin II in dogs. *Proc. Soc. Exp. Biol. Med.*, **124**, 1230
45. Peart, W. S. (1965). The renin–angiotensin system. *Pharmacol. Rev.*, **17**, 143
46. Helmer, O. M. (1971). Purification, standardization and assay of renin and angiotensin. In: *Kidney Hormones*, 59 (J. W. Fisher, editor) (London: Academic Press)
47. Cook, W. F. (1963). Renin and the juxtaglomerular apparatus. In: *Hormones and the Kidney*, 247 (P. C. Williams, editor) (London: Academic Press)
48. Vander, A. J. (1967). Control of renin secretion. *Physiol. Rev.*, **47**, 359
49. Davis, J. O. (1971). What signals the kidney to release renin? *Circulat. Res.*, **28**, 301
50. Blaine, E. H., Davis, J. O. and Witty, R. T. (1970). Renin release after hemorrhage and after suprarenal aortic constriction in dogs without sodium delivery to the macula densa. *Circulat. Res.*, **27**, 1081
51. Blaine, E. H., Davis, J. O. and Prewitt, R. L. (1971). Evidence for a renal vascular receptor in control of renin secretion. *Amer. J. Physiol.*, **220**, 1593
52. Humphreys, M. H., Reid, I. A., Ufferman, R. C. and Earley, L. E. (1971). Relationship between intrarenal control of sodium reabsorption and renin secretory activity. *J. Clin. Invest.*, **50**, 47a
53. Blair-West, J. R., Brook, A. H. and Simpson, P. A. (1972). Renin responses to water restriction and rehydration. *J. Physiol. (London)*, **226**, 1
54. Cooke, C. R., Brown, T. C., Zacherle, B. J. and Walker, W. G. (1970). The effect of altered sodium concentration in the distal nephron segments on renin release. *J. Clin. Invest.*, **49**, 1630

55. Assaykeen, T. A. and Ganong, W. F. (1971). The sympathetic nervous system and renin secretion. In: *Frontiers in Neuroendocrinology, 1971*, 67 (L. Martini and W. F. Ganong, editors) (New York: Oxford University Press)
56. DeMuylder, C. G. (1952). *The "Neurility" of the Kidney* (Springfield: Charles C. Thomas)
57. Barajas, L. (1964). The innervation of the juxtaglomerular apparatus. *Lab. Invest.*, **13**, 916
58. Wågermark, J., Ungerstedt, U. and Ljungqvist, A. (1968). Sympathetic innervation of the juxtaglomerular cells of the kidney. *Circulat. Res.*, **22**, 149
59. Tobian, L., Braden, M. and Maney, J. (1965). The effect of unilateral renal denervation on the secretion of renin. *Fed. Proc. (Fed. Amer. Soc. Exp. Biol.)*, **24**, 405
60. Reid, I. A., Schrier, R. W. and Earley, L. E. (1972). An effect of extrarenal beta adrenergic stimulation on the release of renin. *J. Clin. Invest.*, **51**, 1861
61. Vander, A. J. (1965). Effect of catecholamines and the renal nerves on renin secretion in anesthetized dogs. *Amer. J. Physiol.*, **209**, 659
62. Johnson, J. A., Davis, J. O. and Witty, R. T. (1971). Effects of catecholamines and renal nerve stimulation on renin release in the nonfiltering kidney. *Circulat. Res.*, **29**, 646
63. Loeffler, J. R., Stockigt, J. R. and Ganong, W. F. (1972). Effect of alpha- and beta-adrenergic blocking agents on the increase in renin secretion produced by stimulation of the renal nerves. *Neuroendocrinology*, **10**, 129
64. Coote, J. H., Johns, E. J., Macleod, V. H. and Singer, B. (1972). Effect of renal nerve stimulation, renal blood flow and adrenergic blockade on plasma renin activity in the cat. *J. Physiol. (London)*, **226**, 15
65. Hodge, R. L., Lowe, R. D. and Vane, J. R. (1966). Increased angiotensin formation in response to carotid occlusion in dog. *Nature (London)*, **221**, 491
66. Bunag, R. D., Page, I. H. and McCubbin, J. W. (1966). Neural stimulation of release of renin. *Circulat. Res.*, **19**, 851
67. McPhee, M. S. and Lakey, W. H. (1971). Neurologic release of renin in mongrel dogs. *Can. J. Surg.*, **14**, 142
68. Otsuka, K., Assaykeen, T. A., Goldfien, A. and Ganong, W. F. (1970). Effect of hypoglycemia on plasma renin activity in dogs. *Endocrinology*, **87**, 1306
69. Passo, S. S., Assaykeen, T. A., Otsuka, K., Wise, B. L., Goldfien, A. and Ganong, W. F. (1971). Effect of stimulation of the medulla oblongata on renin secretion in dogs. *Neuroendocrinology*, **7**, 1
70. Ayers, C. R., Harris, R. H. and Lefer, L. G. (1969). Control of renin release in experimental hypertension. *Circulat. Res.*, **24–25** (Suppl. I), 103
71. Allison, D. J., Clayton, P. L., Passo, S. S. and Assaykeen, T. A. (1970). The effect of isoproterenol and adrenergic blocking agents on plasma renin activity and renal function in anesthetized dogs. *Fed. Proc. (Fed. Amer. Soc. Exp. Biol.)*, **29**, 782
72. Ueda, H., Yasuda, H., Takabatake, Y., Iizuka, M., Iizuka, T., Ihori, M. and Sakamoto, Y. (1970). Observations on the mechanism of renin release by catecholamines. *Circulat. Res.*, **26–27** (Suppl. II), 195
73. Assaykeen, T. A., Clayton, P. L., Goldfien, A. and Ganong, W. F. (1970). Effect of alpha- and beta-adrenergic blocking agents on the renin response to hypoglycemia and epinephrine in dogs. *Endocrinology*, **87**, 1318
74. Reid, I. A., Schrier, R. W. and Earley, L. E. (1972). Effect of beta-adrenergic stimulation on renin release. In: *Control of Renin Secretion*, 49 (T. A. Assaykeen, editor) (New York: Plenum)
75. Wathen, R. L., Kingsbury, W. S., Stouder, D. A., Schneider, E. G. and Rostorfer H. H. (1965). Effects of infusion of catecholamines and angiotensin II on renin release in anesthetized dogs. *Amer. J. Physiol.*, **209**, 1012
76. Passo, S. S., Assaykeen, T. A., Goldfien, A. and Ganong, W. F. (1971). Effect of alpha- and beta-adrenergic blocking agents on the increase in renin secretion produced by stimulation of the medulla oblongata in dogs. *Neuroendocrinology*, **7**, 97
77. Alexandre, J. M., Menard, J., Chevillard, C. and Schmitt, H. (1970). Increased plasma renin activity induced in rats by physostigmine and effects of alpha- and beta- receptor blocking drugs thereon. *Europ. J. Pharmacol.*, **12**, 127
78. Birbari, A. (1971). Effect of sympathetic nervous system on renin release. *Amer. J. Physiol.*, **220**, 16

79. Winer, N., Chokshi, D. S., Yoon, M. S. and Freedman, A. D. (1969). Adrenergic receptor mediation of renin secretion. *J. Clin. Endocrinol. Metab.*, **29,** 1168
80. Winer, N., Chokshi, D. S. and Walkenhorst, W. G. (1971). Effects of cyclic AMP. sympathomimetic amines, and adrenergic receptor antagonists on renin secretion. *Circulat. Res.*, **29,** 239
81. Robison, G. A. and Sutherland, E. W. (1970). Sympathin E, Sympathin I and the intracellular level of cyclic AMP. *Circulat. Res.*, **26–27** (Suppl. I), 147
82. Reid, I. A., Stockigt, J. R., Goldfien, A. and Ganong, W. F. (1972). Stimulation of renin secretion in dogs by theophylline. *Europ. J. Pharmacol.*, **17,** 325
83. Allison, D. J., Tanigawa, H. and Assaykeen, T. A. (1972). The effects of cyclic nucleotides on plasma renin activity and renal function in dogs. In: *Control of Renin Secretion*, 33 (T. A. Assaykeen, editor) (New York: Plenum)
84 Michelakis, A. M., Caudle, J. and Liddle, G. W. (1969). *In vitro* stimulation of renin production by epinephrine, norepinephrine and cyclic AMP. *Proc. Soc. Exp. Biol. Med.*, **130,** 748
85. Veyrat, R. and Rosset, E. (1972). *In vitro* renin release by human kidney slices: effect of norepinephrine, angiotensin II and I, and aldosterone. In: *Hypertension '72*, 44 (J. Genest and E. Koiw, editors) (Berlin: Springer-Verlag)
86. Ganong, W. F. (1972). Sympathetic effects on renin secretion: mechanism and physiological role. In: *Control of Renin Secretion*, 17 (T. A. Assaykeen, editor) (New York: Plenum)
87. Vander, A. J. (1970). Direct effects of potassium on renin secretion and renal function. *Amer. J. Physiol.*, **219,** 455
88. Sealey, J. E., Clark, I., Bull, M. B. and Laragh, J. H. (1970). Potassium balance and the control of renin secretion. *J. Clin. Invest.*, **49,** 2119
89. Brunner, H. R., Baer, L., Sealey, J. E., Ledingham, J. G. G. and Laragh, J. H. (1970). The influence of potassium administration and of potassium deprivation on plasma renin in normal and hypertensive subjects. *J. Clin. Invest.*, **49,** 2128
90. Shade, R. E., Davis, J. O., Johnson, J. A. and Witty, R. T. (1972). Effects of renal arterial infusion of sodium and potassium on renin secretion in the dog. *Circulat. Res.*, **31,** 719
91. Abbrecht, P. H. and Vander, A. J. (1970). Effects of chronic potassium depletion on plasma renin activity. *J. Clin. Invest.*, **49,** 1510
92. Brandis, M., Keyes, J. and Windhager, E. E. (1972). Potassium-induced inhibition of proximal tubular fluid reabsorption in rats. *Amer. J. Physiol.*, **222,** 421
93. Schneider, E. G., Lynch, R. E., Willis, L. R. and Knox, F. G. (1972). The effect of potassium infusion on proximal sodium reabsorption and renin release in the dog. *Kidney International*, **2,** 197
94. Vick, R. L. and Todd, E. P. (1969). Effects of autonomic blocking agents on plasma potassium concentration. *Proc. West. Pharmacol. Soc.*, **12,** 124
95. Todd, E. P. and Vick, R. L. (1971). Kalemotropic effect of epinephrine: analysis with adrenergic agonists and antagonists. *Amer. J. Physiol.*, **220,** 1964
96. Grassi, A. O., De Lew, M. F., Cingolani, H. E. and Blessa, E. S. (1971). Adrenergic beta blockade and changes in plasma potassium following epinephrine administration. *Europ. J. Pharmacol.*, **15,** 209
97. Castro-Tavares, J. (1971). The effects of noradrenaline infusions on dog plasma potassium levels. *Europ. J. Pharmacol.*, **15,** 252
98. Reid, I. A., MacDonald, D. M. and Ganong, W. F. (1973). Suppression of renin secretion by clonidine. *Fed. Proc. (Fed. Amer. Soc. Exp. Biol.)*, **32,** 765
99. Bunag, R. D., Page, I. H. and McCubbin, J. W. (1967). Inhibition of renin release by vasopressin and angiotensin. *Cardiovasc. Res.*, **1,** 67
100. Vander, A. J. (1968). Inhibition of renin release in the dog by vasopressin and vasotocin. *Circulat. Res.*, **23,** 605
101. Tagawa, H., Vander, A. J., Bonjour, J. -P. and Malvin, R. L. (1971). Inhibition of renin secretion by vasopressin in unanesthetized sodium-deprived dogs. *Amer. J. Physiol.*, **220,** 949
102. Schrier, R. W., Berl, T., Reid, I. A. and Earley, L. E. (1972). Suppression of renin secretion by interruption of parasympathetic pathways. *Clin. Res.*, **20,** 637
103. Gutman, Y. and Benzakein, F. (1971). Effect of an increase and of lack of antidiuretic hormone on plasma renin activity in the rat. *Life Sci.*, **10** (Part I), 1081

104. Gross, F., Dauda, G., Kazda, S., Kynčl, J., Möhring, J. and Orth, H. (1972). Increased fluid turnover and the activity of the renin-angiotensin system under various experimental conditions. *Circulat. Res.*, **30–31** (Suppl. II), 173
105. Blair-West, J. R., Coghlan, J. P., Denton, D. A., Funder, J. W., Scoggins, B. A. and Wright, R. D. (1971). Inhibition of renin secretion by systemic and intrarenal angiotensin infusion. *Amer. J. Physiol.*, **220**, 1309
106. Michelakis, A. M. (1971). The effect of angiotensin on renin production and release *in vitro*. *Proc. Soc. Exp. Biol. Med.*, **138**, 1106
107. Vander, A. J. and Luciano, J. R. (1967). Neural and humoral control of renin release in salt depletion. *Circulat. Res.*, **20–21** (Suppl. II), 69
108. De Vito, E., Wilson, C., Shipley, R. E., Miller, R. P. and Martz, B. L. (1971). A plasma humoral factor of extrarenal origin causing release of renin-like activity in hypotensive dogs. *Circulat. Res.*, **29**, 446
109. Nolly, H. L., Cabrera, R. A. and Fasciolo, J. C. (1972). Renin releasing activity of a blood plasma fraction. *Experientia*, **28**, 418
110. Skeggs, L. T., Lentz, K. E., Hochstrasser, H. and Kahn, J. R. (1964). The chemistry of renin substrate. *Can. Med. Ass. J.*, **90**, 185
111. Page, I. H., McSwain, B., Knapp, G. M. and Andrus, W. D. (1941). Origin of renin activator. *Amer. J. Physiol.*, **135**, 214
112. Tateishi, H. and Masson, G. M. C. (1972). Role of the liver in the regulation of plasma angiotensinogen and renin levels. *Proc. Soc. Exp. Biol. Med.*, **139**, 304
113. Nasjletti, A. and Masson, G. M. C. (1971). Hepatic origin of renin substrate. *Can. J. Physiol. Pharmacol.*, **49**, 931
114. Nasjletti, A. and Masson, G. M. C. (1972). Studies on angiotensinogen formation in a liver perfusion system. *Circulat. Res.*, **30–31** (Suppl. II), 187
115. Bing, J. and Poulsen, K. (1969). Experimentally induced changes in plasma angiotensinogen and plasma renin. *Acta Pathol. Microbiol. Scand.*, **77**, 389
116. Tateishi, H., Nasjletti, A. and Masson, G. M. C. (1971). Role of renin in the regulation of angiotensinogen levels in plasma. *Proc. Soc. Exp. Biol. Med.*, **137**, 1424
117. Rosset, E. and Veyrat, R. (1971). Inverse variations of plasma renin activity and renin substrate in normal man. *Europ. J. Clin. Invest.*, **1**, 328
118. Blaine, E. H., Davis, J. O. and Baumber, J. S. (1971). Plasma renin substrate changes in experimental uremia. *Proc. Soc. Exp. Biol. Med.*, **136**, 21
119. Helmer, O. M. and Griffith, R. S. (1951). Biological activity of steroids as determined by assay of renin-substrate (angiotensinogen). *Endocrinology*, **49**, 154
120. Haynes, F. W., Forsham, P. H. and Hume, D. M. (1953). Effects of ACTH, cortisone, deoxycorticosterone and epinephrine on the plasma hypertensinogen and renin concentration of dogs. *Amer. J. Physiol.*, **172**, 265
121. Carretero, O. and Gross, F. (1967). Renin substrate in plasma under various experimental conditions in the rat. *Amer. J. Physiol.*, **213**, 695
122. Nasjletti, A. and Masson, G. M. C. (1969). Effects of corticosteroids on plasma angiotensinogen and renin activity. *Amer. J. Physiol.*, **217**, 1396
123. Reid, I. A., Tu, W. H., Otsuka, K., Assaykeen, T. A. and Ganong, W. F. (1973). Studies concerning the regulation and importance of plasma angiotensinogen in the dog. *Endocrinology*, **93**, 107
124. Goodwin, F. J., Kirshman, J. D., Sealey, J. E. and Laragh, J. H. (1970). Influence of the pituitary gland on sodium conservation, plasma renin and renin substrate concentrations in the rat. *Endocrinology*, **86**, 824
125. Dauda, G. and Dévényi, I. (1971). Interrelation of adrenocortical function and angiotensinogen production. *Acta Physiol. Acad. Sci. Hung.*, **39**, 329
126. Nasjletti, A., Matsunaga, M. and Masson, G. M. C. (1969). Effects of estrogens on plasma angiotensinogen and renin activity in nephrectomized rats. *Endocrinology*, **85**, 967
127. Menard, J., Malmejac, A. and Milliez, P. (1970). Influence of diethylstilbestrol on the renin-angiotensin system of male rats. *Endocrinology*, **86**, 774
128. Nasjletti, A., Matsunaga, M. and Masson, G. M. C. (1971). Effects of sex hormones on the renal pressor system. *Can. J. Physiol. Pharmacol.*, **49**, 292
129. Nasjletti, A., Matsunaga, M., Tateishi, H. and Masson, G. M. C. (1971). Effects of stilbestrol on the renal pressor system as modified by adrenalectomy and secondary aldosteronism. *J. Lab. Clin. Med.*, **78**, 30

130. Newton, M. A., Sealey, J. E., Ledingham, J. G. G. and Laragh, J. H. (1968). High blood pressure and oral contraceptives. *Amer. J. Obstet. Gynecol.*, **101**, 1037

131. Skinner, S. L., Lumbers, E. R. and Symonds, E. M. (1969). Alterations by oral contraceptives of normal menstrual changes in plasma renin activity, concentration and substrate. *Clin. Sci.*, **36**, 67

132. Beckerhoff, R., Luetscher, J. A., Wilkinson, R., Gonzales, C. and Nokes, G. W. (1972). Plasma renin concentration, activity and substrate in hypertension induced by oral contraceptives. *J. Clin. Endocrinol. Metab.*, **34**, 1067

133. Skinner, S. L., Lumbers, E. R. and Symonds, E. M. (1972). Analysis of changes in the renin-angiotensin system during pregnancy. *Clin. Sci.*, **42**, 479

134. Sen, S., Smeby, R. R. and Bumpus, F. M. (1972). Effect of mercuric chloride on plasma renin substrate level in rats. *Amer. J. Physiol.*, **222**, 38

135. Freeman, R. H. and Rostorfer, H. H. (1972). Hepatic changes in renin substrate biosynthesis and alkaline phosphatase activity in the rat. *Amer. J. Physiol.*, **223**, 364

136. Rosenthal, J., Wolff, H. P., Weber, P. and Dahlheim, H. (1971). Enzyme kinetic studies on human renin and its purified homologous substrate. *Amer. J. Physiol.*, **221**, 1292

137. Gould, A. B. and Green, D. (1971). Kinetics of the human renin and human substrate reaction. *Cardiovasc. Res.*, **5**, 86

138. Smeby, R. R., Sen, S. and Bumpus F. M. (1967). A naturally occurring renin inhibitor. *Circulat. Res.*, **20–21** (Suppl. II), 129

139. Smeby, R. R. and Bumpus, F. M. (1971). Renin inhibitors. In: *Kidney Hormones*, 207 (J. W. Fisher, editor) (London: Academic Press)

140. Kotchen, T. A., Rice, T. W. and Walters, D. R. (1972). Renin reactivity in normal, hypertensive and uraemic plasma. *J. Clin. Endocrinol. Metab.*, **34**, 928

141. Menard, J. and Catt, K. J. (1972). Measurement of renin activity, concentration and substrate in rat plasma by radioimmunoassay of angiotensin I. *Endocrinology*, **90**, 422

142. Singer, B. and Stack-Dunne, M. P. (1955). Secretion of aldosterone and corticosterone by the rat adrenal. *J. Endocrinol.*, **12**, 130

143. Ganong, W. F., Lieberman, A. H., Daily, W. J. R., Yuen, V. S., Mulrow, P. J., Luetscher, J. A. and Bailey, R. E. (1959). Aldosterone secretion in dogs with hypothalamic lesions. *Endocrinology*, **65**, 18

144. Williams, G. H., Rose, L. I., Dluhy, R. G., Dingman, J. F. and Lauler, D. P. (1971). Aldosterone response to sodium restriction and ACTH stimulation in panhypopituitarism. *J. Clin. Endocrinol. Metab.*, **32**, 27

145. Lee, T. C., van der Wal, B. and de Wied, D. (1968). Influence of the anterior pituitary on the aldosterone secretory response to dietary sodium restriction in the rat. *J. Endocrinol.*, **42**, 465

146. Palmore, W. P., Anderson, R. and Mulrow, P. J. (1970). Role of the pituitary in controlling aldosterone production in sodium-depleted rats. *Endocrinology*, **86**, 728

147. Binnion, P. F., Davis, J. O., Brown, T. C. and Olichney, M. J. (1965). Mechanisms regulating aldosterone secretion during sodium depletion. *Amer. J. Physiol.*, **208**, 655

148. Mulrow, P. J. and Ganong, W. F. (1961). The effect of hemorrhage upon aldosterone secretion in normal and hypophysectomized dogs. *J. Clin. Invest.*, **40**, 579

149. Holzbauer, M. (1964). The part played by ACTH in determining the rate of aldosterone secretion during operative stress. *J. Physiol. (London)*, **172**, 138

150. Rayyis, S. S. and Horton, R. (1971). Effect of angiotensin II on adrenal and pituitary function in man. *J. Clin. Endocrinol. Metab.*, **32**, 539

151. Dyrenfurth, I., Lucis, O., Beck, J. C. and Venning, E. H. (1960). Studies in patients with adrenocortical hyperfunction. III. *In vitro* secretion of steroids by human adrenal glands. *J. Clin. Endocrinol. Metab.*, **20**, 765

152. Venning, E. H., Dyrenfurth, I. and Beck, J. C. (1956). Effect of corticotropin and prednisone on the excretion of aldosterone in man. J. *Clin. Endocrinol. Metab.*, **16**, 1541

153. Newton, M. A. and Laragh, J. H. (1968). Effect of corticotropin on aldosterone excretion and plasma renin in normal subjects, in essential hypertension and in primary aldosteronism. *J. Clin. Endocrinol. Metab.*, **28**, 1006

154. Benraad, T. J. and Kloppenborg, P. W. C. (1970). Plasma renin activity and aldosterone secretory rate in man during chronic ACTH administration. *J. Clin. Endocrinol. Metab.*, **31**, 581

155. Lee, T. C. and de Wied, D. (1968). Somatotropin as the non-ACTH factor of anterior pituitary origin for the maintenance of enhanced aldosterone secretory responsiveness of dietary sodium restriction in chronically hypophysectomized rats. *Life Sci.*, **7** (Part I), 35

156. Palkovits, M., de Jong, W., van der Wal, B. and de Wied, D. (1970). Effect of adreno-corticotrophic and growth hormones on aldosterone production and plasma renin activity in chronically hypophysectomized sodium-deficient rats. *J. Endocrinol.*, **47**, 243

157. Palkovits, M., de Jong, W., van der Wal, B. and de Wied, D. (1971). The aldosterone secretory response to sodium restriction in chronically hypophysectomized cortico-trophin-maintained rats as a function of duration and amount of growth hormone treatment. *J. Endocrinol.*, **50**, 407

158. Palkovits, M., Strik, J. J. T. W. A., de Jong, W. and de Wied, D. (1971). Effect of growth hormone on the aldosterone secretory response to sodium restriction in corticotrophin-maintained hypophysectomized nephrectomized rats. *J. Endocrinol.*, **51**, 369

159. Blair-West, J. R., Coghlan, J. P., Denton, D. A., Goding, J. R., Wintour, M. and Wright, R. D. (1963). The action of electrolyte changes and some naturally-occurring pharmacological substances on the adrenal cortex. In: *Hormones and the Kidney*, 341 (P. C. Williams, editor) (London: Academic Press)

160. Blair-West, J. R., Coghlan, J. P., Denton, D. A., Goding, J. R., Wintour, M. and Wright, R. D. (1963). The control of aldosterone secretion. *Recent Progr. Horm. Res.*, **19**, 311

161. Davis, J. O., Urquhart, J. and Higgins, J. T. (1963). The effects of alterations of plasma sodium and potassium concentration on aldosterone secretion. *J. Clin. Invest.*, **42**, 597

162. Blair-West, J. R., Coghlan, J. P., Denton, D. A., Goding, J. R., Wintour, M. and Wright, R. D. (1965). Effect of variations of plasma sodium concentration on the adrenal response to angiotensin II. *Circulat. Res.*, **17**, 386

163. Dluhy, R. G., Axelrod, L., Underwood, R. H. and Williams, G. H. (1972). Studies of the control of plasma aldosterone concentration in normal man. II. Effect of dietary potassium and acute potassium infusion. *J. Clin. Invest.*, **51**, 1950

164. Boyd, J. E., Palmore, W. P. and Mulrow, P. J. (1971). Role of potassium in the control of aldosterone secretion in the rat. *Endocrinology*, **88**, 556

165. Funder, J. W., Blair-West, J. R., Coghlan, J. P., Denton, D. A., Scoggins, B. A. and Wright, R. D. (1969). Effect of plasma potassium concentration on the secretion of aldosterone. *Endocrinology*, **85**, 381

166. Boyd, J. E. and Mulrow, P. J. (1972). Further studies of the influence of potassium upon aldosterone production in the rat. *Endocrinology*, **90**, 299

167. Müller, J. (1970). Steroidogenic effect of stimulators of aldosterone biosynthesis upon separate zones of the rat adrenal cortex. *Europ. J. Clin. Invest.*, **1**, 180

168. Müller, J. and Huber, R. (1969). Effects of sodium deficiency, potassium deficiency and uremia upon the steroidogenic response of rat adrenal tissue to serotonin, potassium ions and adrenocorticotropin. *Endocrinology*, **85**, 43

169. Williams, G. H., Dluhy, R. G. and Underwood, R. H. (1970). The relationship of dietary potassium intake to the aldosterone stimulating properties of ACTH. *Clin. Sci.*, **39**, 489

170. Bayard, F., Cooke, C. R., Tiller, D. J., Beitins, I. Z., Kowarski, A., Walker, W. G. and Migeon, C. J. (1971). The regulation of aldosterone secretion in anephric man. *J. Clin. Invest.*, **50**, 1585

171. Szalay, K. S. (1969). Inhibiting effect of angiotensin on potassium accumulation of adrenal cortex. *Biochem. Pharmacol.*, **18**, 962

172. Cushman, P. (1969). Inhibition of aldosterone secretion by ouabain in dog adrenal cortical tissue. *Endocrinology*, **84**, 808

173. Boyd, J. E., Mulrow, P. J., Palmore, W. P. and Silva, P. (1973). Importance of potassium in the regulation of aldosterone production. *Circulat. Res.*, **32–33**, (Suppl. I), 39

174. Best, J. B., Bett, J. H. N., Coghlan, J. P., Cran, E. J. and Scoggins, B. A. (1971). Circulating angiotensin-II and aldosterone levels during dietary sodium restriction. *Lancet*, **1**, 1353

175. Boyd, G. W., Adamson, A. R., Arnold, M., James, V. H. T. and Peart, W. S. (1972). The role of angiotensin II in the control of aldosterone in man. *Clin. Sci.*, **42**, 91

176. McCaa, R. E., McCaa, C. S., Read, D. G., Bower, J. D. and Guyton, A. C. (1972). Increased plasma aldosterone concentration in response to hemodialysis in nephrectomized man. *Circulat. Res.*, **31**, 473

177. Boyd, G. W., Adamson, A. R., James, V. H. T. and Peart, W. S. (1969). The role of the renin-angiotensin system in the control of aldosterone in man. *Proc. Roy. Soc. Med.* **62**, 1253

178. Mitra, S., Genuth, S. M., Berman, L. B. and Vertes, V. (1972). Aldosterone secretion in anephric patients. *N. Engl. J. Med.*, **286**, 61

179. Davis, J. O. (1972). Are there unidentified factors in the control of aldosterone secretion? *N. Engl. J. Med.*, **286**, 100

180. Blair-West, J. R., Coghlan, J. P., Denton, D. A., Funder, J. W., Scoggins, B. A. and Wright, R. D. (1971). The effects of adrenal arterial infusion of hypertonic $NaHCO_3$ solution on aldosterone secretion in sodium deficient sheep. *Acta Endocrinol.*, **66**, 448

181. Blair-West, J. R., Coghlan, J. P., Denton, D. A., Funder, J. W. and Scoggins, B. A. (1972). The role of the renin-angiotensin system in control of aldosterone secretion. In: *Control of Renin Secretion*, 167 (T. A. Assaykeen, editor) (New York: Plenum)

182. Palmore, W. P., Marieb, N. J. and Mulrow, P. J. (1969). Stimulation of aldosterone secretion by sodium depletion in nephrectomized rats. *Endocrinology*, **84**, 1342

183. Aguilera, G. and Marusic, E. T. (1971). Role of the renin–angiotensin system in the biosynthesis of aldosterone. *Endocrinology*, **89**, 1524

184. Ganong, W. F., Boryczka, A. T. and Shackelford, R. (1967). Effect of renin on adrenocortical sensitivity to ACTH and angiotensin II in dogs. *Endocrinology*, **80**, 703

185. Ganong, W. F., Boryczka, A. T., Shackelford, R., Clark, R. M. and Converse, R. P. (1965). Effect of dietary sodium restriction on adrenal cortical response to ACTH. *Proc. Soc. Exp. Biol. Med.*, **118**, 792

186. Fraser, R., Brown, J. J., Chinn, R., Lever, A. F. and Robertson, J. I. S. (1969). The control of aldosterone secretion and its relationship to the diagnosis of hyperaldosteronism. *Scot. Med. J.*, **14**, 420

187. Williams, G. H., McDonnell, L. M., Tait, S. A. S. and Tait, J. F. (1972). The effect of medium composition and *in vitro* stimuli on the conversion of corticosterone to aldosterone in rat glomerulosa tissue. *Endocrinology*, **91**, 948

188. Baumann, K. and Müller, J. (1972). Effect of potassium intake on the final steps of aldosterone biosynthesis in the rat. I. 18-hydroxylation and 18-hydroxydehydrogenation. *Acta Endocrinol.*, **69**, 701

189. Baumann, K. and Müller, J. (1972). Effect of potassium intake on the final steps of aldosterone biosynthesis in the rat. II. 11β-hydroxylation. *Acta Endocrinol.*, **69**, 718

190. Saruta, T., Cook, R. and Kaplan, N. M. (1972). Adrenocortical steroidogenesis: studies on the mechanism of action of angiotensin and electrolytes. *J. Clin. Invest.*, **51** 2239

191. Brown, R. D., Strott, C. A. and Liddle, G. W. (1972). Site of stimulation of aldosterone biosynthesis by angiotensin and potassium. *J. Clin. Invest.*, **51**, 1413

192. Oddie, C. J., Coghlan, J. P. and Scoggins, B. A. (1972). Plasma deoxycorticosterone levels in man with simultaneous measurement of aldosterone, corticosterone, cortisol and 11-deoxycortisol. *J. Clin. Endocrinol. Metab.*, **34**, 1039

193. Taylor, A. A., Davis, J. O. and Johnson, J. A. (1972). Control of deoxycorticosterone secretion in the dog. *Amer. J. Physiol.*, **223**, 466

194. Schambelan, M. and Biglieri, E. G. (1972). Deoxycorticosterone production and regulation in man. *J. Clin. Endocrinol. Metab.*, **34**, 695

195. Goodman, L. S. and Gilman, A. (1970). *The Pharmacological Basis of Therapeutics*, 1619 (New York: MacMillan)

196. Gaunt, R. and Chart, J. J. (1962). Mineralocorticoid action of adrenocortical hormones. In: *Handbook of Experimental Pharmacology* Vol. 14, (1), 514 (H. W. Deane, editor) (Berlin: Springer-Verlag)

197. Green, H. H., Harrington, A. R. and Valtin, H. (1970). On the role of antidiuretic hormone in the inhibition of acute water diuresis in adrenal insufficiency and the effects of gluco- and mineralo-corticoids in reversing the inhibition. *J. Clin. Invest.*, **49**, 1724

198. Ufferman, R. C. and Schrier, R. W. (1972). Importance of sodium intake and mineralocorticoid hormone in the impaired water excretion in adrenal insufficiency. *J. Clin. Invest.*, **51**, 1639

199. Johnson, J. A., Davis, J. O., Baumber, J. S. and Schneider, E. G. (1970). Effects of estrogens and progesterone on electrolyte balances in normal dogs. *Amer. J. Physiol.*, **219**, 1691

200. Crane, M. G. and Harris, J. J. (1969). Plasma renin activity and aldosterone excretion rate in normal subjects. I. Effect of ethinyl estradiol and medroxyprogesterone acetate. *J. Clin. Endocrinol. Metab.*, **29**, 550

201. Katz, F. H. and Kappas, A. (1967). The effects of estradiol and estriol on plasma levels of cortisol and thyroid hormone-binding globulins and on aldosterone and cortisol secretion rates in man. *J. Clin. Invest.*, **46**, 1768

202. Johnson, J. A., Davis, J. O., Brown, P. R., Wheeler, P. D. and Witty, R. T. (1972). Effects of estradiol on sodium and potassium balances in adrenalectomized dogs. *Amer. J. Physiol.*, **223**, 194

203. Devries, J. R., Ludens, J. H. and Fanestil, D. D. (1972). Estradiol renal receptor molecules and estradiol-dependent antinatriuresis. *Kidney International*, **2**, 95

204. Johnson, J. A., Davis, J. O. and Hotchkiss, J. (1972). Plasma levels of estrogens in pregnant dogs in relation to sodium retention. *Endocrinology*, **90**, 322

205. Worcel, M. and Meyer, P. (1970). Inhibitory effect of angiotensin on renal sodium reabsorption. *Pflügers Arch.*, **317**, 124

206. Ali, M. N. (1958). A comparison of some activities of arginine vasopressin and lysine vasopressin on kidney function in conscious dogs. *Brit. J. Pharmacol.*, **13**, 131

207. Chan, W. Y. and Sawyer, W. H. (1961). Saluretic actions of neurohypophyseal peptides in conscious dogs. *Amer. J. Physiol.*, **201**, 799

208. Chan, W. Y. and Sawyer, W. H. (1962). Natriuresis in conscious dogs during arginine vasopressin infusion and after oxytocin injection. *Proc. Soc. Exp. Biol. Med.*, **110**, 697

209. Humphreys, M. H., Friedler, R. M. and Earley, L. E. (1970). Natriuresis produced by vasopressin or hemorrhage during water diuresis in the dog. *Amer. J. Physiol.*, **219**, 658

210. Jones, N. F., Barraclough, M. A. and Mills, I. H. (1963). The mechanism of increased sodium excretion during water loading with 2.5% dextrose and vasopressin. *Clin. Sci.*, **25**, 449

211. Martinez-Maldonado, M., Eknoyan, G. and Suki, W. N. (1971). Natriuretic effects of vasopressin and cyclic AMP: possible site of action in the nephron. *Amer. J. Physiol.*, **220**, 2013

212. Davis, B. B., Knox, F. G. and Berliner, R. W. (1967). Effect of vasopressin on proximal tubule sodium reabsorption in the dog. *Amer. J. Physiol.*, **212**, 1361

213. Schnermann, J., Valtin, H., Thurau, K., Nagel, W., Horster, M., Fishbach, H., Wahl, M. and Liebau, G. (1969). Micropuncture studies on the influence of antidiuretic hormone on tubular fluid reabsorption in rats with hereditary hypothalamic diabetes insipidus. *Pflügers Arch.*, **306**, 103

214. Severs, W. B., Summy-Long, J., Taylor, J. S. and Connor, J. D. (1970). A central effect of angiotensin: release of pituitary pressor material. *J. Pharmacol. Exp. Ther.*, **174**, 27

215. Mouw, D., Bonjour, J.-P., Malvin, R. L. and Vander, A. J. (1971). Central action of angiotensin in stimulating ADH release. *Amer. J. Physiol.*, **220**, 239

216. Bonjour, J.-P. and Malvin, R. L. (1970). Stimulation of ADH release by the renin-angiotensin system. *Amer. J. Physiol.*, **218**, 1555

217. Claybaugh, J. R., Share, L. and Shimizu, K. (1972). The inability of infusions of angiotensin to elevate the plasma vasopressin concentration in the anesthetized dog. *Endocrinology*, **90**, 1647

218. Claybaugh, J. R. and Share, L. (1972). Role of the renin-angiotensin system in the vasopressin response to hemorrhage. *Endocrinology*, **90**, 453

219. de Wardener, H. E. (1969). Control of sodium reabsorption. *Brit. Med. J.*, **3**, 676

220. Orloff, J. and Burg, M. (1971). Kidney. *Annu. Rev. Physiol.*, **33**, 83

221. Howards, S. S. (1971). Regulation of sodium excretion with special emphasis on the current status of natriuretic hormone. *J. Urol.*, **105**, 749

222. Share, L. and Claybaugh, J. R. (1972). Regulation of body fluids. *Annu. Rev. Physiol.*, **34**, 235

223. Blythe, W. B., D'Avila, D., Gitelman, H. J. and Welt, L. G. (1971). Further evidence for a humoral natriuretic factor. *Circulat. Res.*, **28–29** (Suppl. II), 21

224. Sonnenberg, H., Veress, A. T. and Pearce, J. W. (1972). A humoral component of the natriuretic mechanism in sustained blood volume expansion. *J. Clin. Invest.*, **51**, 2631

225. Kaloyanides, G. J. and Azer, M. (1971). Evidence for a humoral mechanism in volume expansion natriuresis. *J. Clin. Invest.*, **50**, 1603

226. Bengele, H. H., Houttuin, E. and Pearce, J. W. (1972). Volume natriuresis without renal nerves and renal vascular pressure rise in the dog. *Amer. J. Physiol.*, **223**, 68

227. Sealey, J. E. and Laragh, J. H. (1971). Further studies of a natriuretic substance occurring in human urine and plasma. *Circulat. Res.*, **28–29** (Suppl. II), 32

228. Clarkson, E. M., Talner, L. B. and de Wardener, H. E. (1970). The effect of plasma from blood volume expanded dogs on sodium, potassium and PAH transport of renal tubule fragments. *Clin. Sci.*, **38**, 617

229. Buckalew, V. M., Martinez, F. J. and Green, W. E. (1970). Effect of dialysates and ultrafiltrates of plasma of saline-loaded dogs on toad bladder sodium transport. *J. Clin. Invest.*, **49**, 926

230. Clarkson, E. M. and de Wardener, H. E. (1972). Inhibition of sodium and potassium transport in separated renal tubule fragments incubated in extracts of urine obtained from salt-loaded individuals. *Clin. Sci.*, **42**, 607

231. Wright, F. S., Brenner, B. M., Bennett, C. M., Keimowitz, R. I., Berliner, R. W., Schrier, R. W., Verroust, P. J., de Wardner, H. E. and Holzgreve, H. (1969). Failure to demonstrate a hormonal inhibitor of proximal sodium reabsorption. *J. Clin. Invest.*, **48**, 1107

232. Bonjour, J.-P. and Peters, G. (1970). Non-occurrence of a natriuretic factor in circulating blood of rats after expansion of the extracellular or the intravascular space. *Pflügers Arch.*, **318**, 21

233. Dorn, J. B., Levine, N., Kaley, G. and Rothballer, A. B. (1969). Natriuresis induced by injection of hypertonic saline into the third cerebral ventricle of dogs. *Proc. Soc. Exp. Biol. Med.*, **131**, 240

234. Anderson, B., Dallman, M. F. and Olsson, K. (1969). Evidence for a hypothalamic control of renal sodium excretion. *Acta Physiol. Scand.*, **75**, 496

235. Mouw, D. R. and Vander, A. J. (1970). Evidence for brain Na receptors controlling renal Na excretion and plasma renin activity. *Amer. J. Physiol.*, **219**, 822

236. Buckalew, V. M. and Lancaster, C. D. (1972). The association of a humoral sodium transport inhibitory activity with renal escape from chronic mineralocorticoid administration in the dog. *Clin. Sci.*, **42**, 69

8
Parathyroid Hormone, Thyrocalcitonin and the Control of Mineral Metabolism

T. K. GRAY, C. W. COOPER and P. L. MUNSON
University of North Carolina

8.1 INTRODUCTION. PARATHYROID HORMONE AND THYROCALCITONIN

The discovery of thyrocalcitonin (TCT) a decade ago initiated a period of intensive research on this hormone, particularly with respect to its chemistry, mode of action and physiological function in concert with parathyroid hormone (PTH) and vitamin D in the regulation of calcium homeostasis and skeletal metabolism. TCT is produced and secreted by the C cells of the mammalian thyroid gland and the ultimobranchial body of lower vertebrates. The characteristic hypocalcaemia and hypophosphataemia associated with administration of the hormone is due to an inhibitory action on bone metabolism. Extraskeletal actions also may contribute to the changes in plasma calcium and phosphate produced by TCT. In the short space of the past 5 years, five different forms of TCT have been sequenced and synthesised. Synthetic analogues and specific fragments of the whole molecule are being produced and tested for biological and immunological activity, and radioimmunoassays are being used to study the secretion and metabolism of the hormone in several species.

Dramatic and stimulating findings concerning PTH also have recently appeared. Our knowledge about PTH has advanced rapidly particularly with regard to its basic molecular structure, the chemical nature of the stored, secreted and circulating forms of the hormone, its mechanism of action, and the control of its secretion.

Attempts to identify the roles and relative importance of PTH and TCT in the regulation of calcium homeostasis are of special interest. The exact physiological function of TCT remains somewhat elusive despite a decade of vigorous investigation. However, a considerable body of information is being accumulated to suggest that PTH and TCT act in concert to prevent wide fluctuations in the blood calcium level and to provide optimal conditions for normal skeletal growth and remodelling.

The progress which has occurred so rapidly in this area stimulated the recent convening of several international conferences[1-4] dealing wholly or in part with these hormones and their effects on mineral metabolism. In addition, a recent authoritative review of PTH and its actions has appeared[5]. The recent findings concerning PTH, TCT, and their actions on mineral metabolism in the context of our understanding and interpretation of them form the substance of this review.

8.2 PARATHYROID HORMONE (PTH)

8.2.1 Chemistry

Within the past few years major advances have been made in the elucidation of the detailed chemical nature of PTH and in the identification of a discrete region of the molecule responsible for most of the biological activity. Furthermore, it has been possible, by solid-phase synthesis of the active region of the molecule, to produce marketable quantities of a biologically-active peptide only about one-third as large as the native hormone.

8.2.1.1 *Structures*

The amino acid sequence of bovine PTH (Figure 8.1), comprised of a single chain of 84 amino acid residues, was reported independently in 1970 by Niall, Potts and associates and by Brewer and Ronan (cited in Refs. 1 and 2). Subsequently, the predominant form of extracted bovine hormone was termed 'BPTH-I' (for Bovine PTH-I) to distinguish it from two other biologically active peptides thought to represent isohormones and termed 'BPTH-II' and 'BPTH-III'[6-8]. Brewer[9] has reported a preliminary study of the conformation of the predominant form (I) of bovine PTH, and Aloj and Edelhoch[10] have examined the tertiary structures of both bovine and porcine PTH. Both studies suggest that the molecular properties of PTH in solution are intermediate between those of a fully-organised helical protein and those of a random coil polypeptide.

The amino acid sequence of porcine PTH, deduced by Woodhead *et al.*[11], differs from BPTH-I in only seven out of the 84 residues[5,6,11] (Figure 8.1). The biological and immunological activities of porcine PTH are similar to those of bovine PTH[12].

The chemistry of human PTH has been studied, but the limited amounts of material available for chemical studies have hampered elucidation of the entire amino acid sequence. Studies of the amino acid composition, molecular size and charge properties of the human hormone extracted from parathyroid adenomas indicate that human PTH closely resembles bovine PTH and porcine PTH although clear differences in amino acid composition exist[13]. Recently, Brewer *et al.*[14] and Potts and associates[15] independently have determined the amino acid sequence of the first *N*-terminal 30 or more amino acids of human PTH. Both groups isolated the biologically-active fragment of the human hormone from extracts of human parathyroid tissue removed at surgery. At present the two independent reports do not agree completely on the precise amino acid sequence of the *N*-terminal 34 amino acids of human

242

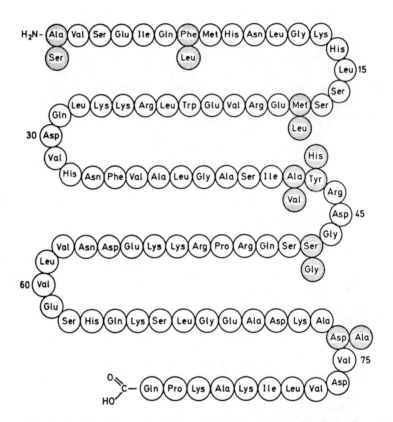

Figure 8.1 Amino acid sequences of bovine PTH-I and porcine PTH. The backbone structure represents bovine PTH-I. Porcine PTH differs from bovine PTH-I at 7 sequence positions shown as shaded circles beside the bovine residues. (From Potts *et al.*[6] by courtesy of Heinemann.)

Human parathyroid hormone

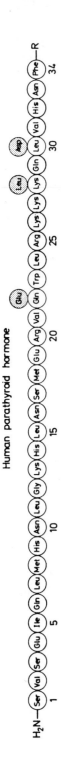

Bovine parathyroid hormone

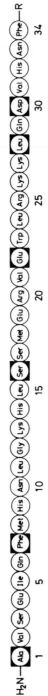

Porcine parathyroid hormone

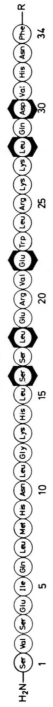

Figure 8.2 Amino acid sequence of the amino-terminal 34 amino acids of human PTH. The 1–34 sequences of bovine and porcine PTH also are shown, blackened residues indicating differences in sequence from the human structure reported. (From Brewer *et al.*[14], by courtesy of U.S. Nat. Acad. Sci.). The three shaded residues shown alongside the human structure show the structure reported for human 1–34 PTH by Jacobs *et al.*[15]; if this structure is correct the three residues in question would be identical for all three species.

PTH, three specific residues are in question. However, it is clear that the 1–34 *N*-terminal biologically-active region of human PTH will prove to be similar, but not identical to, corresponding regions of bovine and porcine PTH, differing from the porcine 1–34 structure by at least two residues and from the bovine 1–34 structure by at least three residues (Figure 8.2).

8.2.1.2 Active fragments

Determination of the complete amino acid sequence of bovine PTH has enabled detailed study of structure–activity relationships. It has been known for some time that the amino-terminal portion of the PTH molecule represents the most important region for expression of biological activity. More recently, fragments of the amino-terminal portion of the molecule varying in length from 13 to 35 amino acids were prepared. Synthetic 1–34 PTH* was found to be biologically active[16,17] both *in vivo* to produce hypercalcaemia and phosphaturia and *in vitro* to activate adenyl cyclase and elevate levels of cyclic 3′,5′-adenosine monophosphate (cyclic-AMP) in appropriate preparations of renal cortical tissue. PTH fragments shorter than 1–34 retain some biological activity. However, fragments less than 1–20 are completely inactive, and alterations of the initial amino terminal residue (either extension or deletion) also abolish biological activity[6]. The minimal length of PTH peptide required for substantial biological activity has not been established with certainty but appears to fall between 1–20 and 1–29 amino acids in length

8.2.1.3 Proparathyroid hormone (pro-PTH)

Recent evidence indicates that bovine and human PTH are synthesised by the parathyroid gland as larger peptide moieties than the 1–84 PTH molecules actually released by the gland into the circulation. Hamilton, Cohn and associates[18-20] first provided clear evidence for the existence of a pro-PTH in bovine parathyroid glands. The material, designated 'calcaemic fraction-A', was identified by its behaviour during column purification of gland extracts. Additional studies of bovine glands in tissue culture involving labelled amino acid incorporation and pulse-chase experiments indicated a precursor–product relationship between calcaemic fraction-A and native PTH[20]. The precursor was shown to be larger in size (mol. wt. *ca.* 12 000 dalton) than native PTH (mol. wt. 9563 dalton) but present in the gland in only small concentrations. The precursor possessed both immunological and biological activities but both activities were lower than those of native 1–84 PTH. Formation of the precursor fraction *in vitro* was inversely related to calcium concentration[19] and immunological activity of samples increased as precursor was converted to PTH[20].

Kemper *et al.*[21] confirmed the findings of Cohn and co-workers using similar methods to study bovine glands in culture. Pro PTH was determined

---

* The *N*-terminal 1–34 synthetic peptide can be obtained from Beckman Instruments Inc., Palo Alto, Calif., U.S.A. The potency of this product, determined by bioassay *in vitro*, is reported to be 1500–2100 Units mg^{-1}.

(a) to have a molecular weight of *ca.* 11 500 dalton; (b) to be characterised by the presence of 15–20 amino acid residues more than 1–84 PTH and (c) to be converted to 1–84 PTH during appropriate incubation studies[21]. More recent studies by Habener *et al.*[22] and Martin[23] have demonstrated the presence of pro-PTH in cultured human parathyroid adenomas. Experiments revealed that human pro-PTH, like bovine pro-PTH, is a basic protein with a molecular weight of *ca.* 11 500 dalton and that it could be synthesised and converted by cultured adenomas to 1–84 PTH[22]. The precursor may be biologically inactive because the additional amino acids present in pro-PTH are attached to the *N*-terminal portion of PTH, a site known to be critical for expression of biological activity. The biological significance of pro-PTH remains to be clarified.

8.2.1.4 *Secreted, circulating and active molecular species*

The major secreted form of PTH appears to be the native 1–84 polypeptide formed by cleavage of pro-PTH prior to release[5-7,22]. This conclusion is based on studies by Potts and associates, who have utilised gel filtration of plasma, selective venous catheterisation of human thyroid veins and sequence-specific antisera to study parathyroid hormone newly released into the circulation and its subsequent fate[6,7,24].

Although the principal form of PTH secreted into the blood appears to be the intact 84-amino acid hormone, measurements using different antisera to PTH to evaluate immunochemical behaviour of peripheral plasma subjected to gel filtration clearly showed that major portions of the circulating immunoreactive peptide were not standard 1–84 PTH but rather were smaller fragments of the original molecule[6,7]. Recent findings using sequence-specific antisera[24,25] indicate that secretion of 1–84 PTH from the parathyroid gland is followed by rapid cleavage in extravascular tissue beds. One of the major circulating products is a biologically inactive peptide mol. wt. *ca.* 7500 dalton, which probably comprises the carboxyl terminal portion of PTH. These molecular cleavages may act to control the amounts of biologically active hormone available in the circulation for interaction with target tissues. A practical consideration is the fact that measurement of immunoreactive PTH using antisera that react with biologically-inactive circulating *C*-terminal fragments could be unrepresentative of biologically-active PTH in peripheral blood. Parsons and Potts[5] have observed that 'The heterogeneity of circulating PTH at present makes it impossible to measure absolute concentrations of hormone in the plasma. Absolute measurements must await further studies of the peripheral metabolism of PTH to determine the . . . significance of the fragments . . . measured, and will require provision of appropriate standards and thorough characterisation of antisera to guard against misleading cross-reactivity'.

8.2.2 Biological and radioimmunological assays

A variety of *in vitro* and *in vivo* bioassay methods has been developed. No bioassay method developed has had sufficient sensitivity to detect the small quantities of PTH present in the circulation, but bioassay methods offer the clear advantage of measuring biologically-active hormone or hormonal fragments. Radioimmunoassays possess distinct advantages in terms of their greater sensitivity and specificity, but measurement of immunoreactive PTH may not necessarily reflect levels of biologically-active peptide.

8.2.2.1 Biological assays

Both *in vivo* and *in vitro* methods for biological assay of PTH have been reviewed recently and the procedures, advantages and disadvantages of the various methods have been outlined[5,26]. Probably the most widely used method is that developed by Munson, which depends on the ability of PTH to prevent the hypocalcaemia occurring in young rats 5–6 h after parathyroidectomy by cautery[26]. Various modifications of this basic procedure account for the majority of bioassays developed.

The recent development of *in vivo* avian bioassays for PTH offers possible distinct advantages compared to bioassays using rodents. Parsons and associates[5] have described a bioassay employing young chicks while Dacke and Kenny[27] have developed one in chicks or quail using the hypercalcaemic response at 1 h after i.v. injection of test materials in a calcium-containing diluent. Injection of small amounts of calcium chloride together with PTH enhances the hypercalcaemic response and improves the slope of the dose-response curve. The reported index of precision (λ) is about 0.25, and the advantages are no requirement for surgery, good sensitivity (1–10 Units), ease of performance, and a short interval (1 h) between injection and blood collection.

In vitro bioassay methods for PTH also have been developed. Generally, they depend on the ability of PTH either to resorb bone in tissue culture or to promote formation of cyclic-AMP in preparations of rat renal or skeletal tissues.

In the past, the standard preparation used for all bioassays for PTH was Parathyroid Injection, USP (Eli Lilly & Co.), a preparation standardised in terms of 'animal units' by evaluation of hypercalcaemic activity in the dog. More recently, through international collaborative assays, an international reference standard (partially purified bovine PTH) with an assigned potency of 200 Units ampoule^{-1} has been made available to investigators*.

8.2.2.2 Radioimmunoassays

Over the past 10 years several laboratories have developed immunoassays capable of measuring levels of PTH circulating in the plasma of man and certain other species[28-32].

For the most part, currently used immunoassays are of the standard type employing purified radioiodinated bovine or porcine PTH. Most of the

---

* Division of Biological Standards, National Institute for Medical Research, Mill Hill, London, England.

assay methods employ antisera raised against either bovine porcine or PTH and either homologous animal reference standards or crude heterologous reference material, e.g. human hyperparathyroid plasma. Measurement of human plasma PTH has been possible by selecting antisera raised against bovine or porcine PTH which cross-react to a certain extent with human PTH. Because of multiple problems already mentioned involving assay methodology, the apparent presence of fragments of secreted 1–84 PTH in the circulation, and lack of availability of purified human PTH in adequate quantities, it is not possible at present to establish the absolute amounts of PTH circulating in the blood of man or animals.

8.2.3   Sites and modes of action

PTH is a dominant factor in the maintenance of normal levels of blood calcium and phosphate, acting concurrently to raise calcium and lower phosphate. The major target organs for the hormone are bone and kidney; the intestine also responds to PTH. The actions of PTH on these target tissues lead to a net movement of calcium into extracellular fluid. The ability of the hormone to lower blood phosphate via its phosphaturic effect counterbalances the phosphate released from bone and helps to ensure that the level of blood calcium maintained by PTH normally will not be accompanied by undesirable and dangerous precipitation of calcium phosphate salts in susceptible soft tissues.

8.2.3.1   Bone

Classically, the action of PTH on bone to supply calcium to the blood has been viewed as achieved by 'resorption' or demineralisation of bone. Bone resorption indeed can elevate blood calcium by the cellular actions of both osteocytes (osteolysis) and osteoclasts (osteoclasis). Recent elegant studies by Raisz and associates[33-35] and Reynolds[36] using bone in tissue culture have clearly extended our knowledge of the more subtle aspects of PTH-promoted bone resorption (see Section 8.3.4.1).

Some workers have suggested that bone resorptive responses to PTH represent a relatively slow response not directly responsible for minute-to-minute maintenance of blood calcium levels. Talmage[37] and Neuman[38] agree in suggesting that rapid transcellular fluxes in calcium across bone cells are subject to the influence of PTH and provide for rapid, acute changes in blood calcium. They contend that calcium movement from a 'bone fluid' compartment to extracellular fluid, rather than classical bone mineral 'resorption', constitutes the important mechanism by which PTH can rapidly provide calcium to blood. Recent studies also suggest that a primary and early action of PTH is to promote movement of calcium into bone cells[37, 39, 40]. Evidence for this action has been provided by both *in vitro*[39] and *in vivo* studies[37, 41-43]. *In vivo* studies by Parsons and co-workers in both rats and dogs[41-43] have shown that at very early time intervals (a few minutes to 1 h) after i.v. PTH a small (4%) but demonstrable fall in serum calcium occurs accompanied by a calcium shift into bone. The classic hypercalcaemic action of PTH follows this earlier transient hypocalcaemic effect. These new findings support earlier proposals that PTH action is initiated and mediated by elevations in calcium intracellularly in bone cells.

8.2.3.2 Kidney

It has long been established that PTH promotes phosphate excretion by inhibiting phosphate reabsorption by the proximal tubule of the kidney. More recent research continues to support this view and provides further insight into the mechanisms involved. Micropuncture studies in the dog by Goldberg and co-workers[44, 45] have established that PTH inhibits reabsorption of both sodium and phosphate in the proximal tubule, sodium reabsorption being affected to an even greater extent than phosphate reabsorption. It is hypothesised that the primary action of PTH may be via cyclic-AMP to inhibit sodium reabsorption, phosphate effects being secondary to this action. Increased amounts of sodium are not excreted after injection of PTH because the sodium is reabsorbed distally; phosphate, not being reabsorbed distally to any significant extent, is excreted in increased amounts.

Another renal action of PTH is to promote calcium reabsorption and thus decrease calcium excretion. The mechanism by which PTH produces this effect and the renal site involved have not been clarified. Nordin et al.[46], examining alterations in urinary calcium excretion in persons with hypo- or hyper-parathyroidism, have suggested that regulation of plasma calcium levels is more dependent on the influence of PTH on renal handling of calcium than on skeletal actions of PTH. Undoubtedly the renal action of PTH is an important factor in maintaining calcium homeostasis, especially in certain species. Biddulph[47] has shown that in the hamster maintenance of the normal blood calcium level is more dependent on the response of the kidney to PTH than on mobilisation of skeletal calcium by PTH.

At present it would be difficult to assess the relative importance of bone and kidney in mediating the hypercalcaemic action of PTH. Undoubtedly both mechanisms operate to help regulate plasma calcium and whether one or the other is dominant may depend on a variety of factors, including species, diet, age, and the particular situation in which calcium homeostasis is examined.

8.2.3.3 Intestine

Studies over the past 15 years have produced evidence that PTH enhances absorption of dietary calcium across the small intestine, being especially effective when dietary calcium is low. However, the fact that vitamin D metabolites act more rapidly and are more effective than PTH in promoting calcium absorption has tended to draw attention away from this action of PTH. The picture has become even more complicated because recent reports suggest that PTH may influence the renal conversion of hydroxylated vitamin D to a dihydroxylated metabolite which is very potent in promoting intestinal calcium absorption (see Section 8.4.3.).

The most recent evidence for a direct and specific effect of PTH on intestinal absorption of calcium was provided by Olson *et al.*[48]. Using an *in vitro* isolated vascularly-perfused rat intestinal preparation, these workers evaluated calcium transport by measuring ^{45}Ca fluxes between intestinal lumen and perfusate. Enhanced transport was observed within 30 min after a brief infusion of 100 USP Units of highly purified PTH, reaching a peak 30 min later and then rapidly declining. This response to PTH suggested a direct, specific action of the hormone to promote calcium absorption, but the high dose of hormone employed raises some doubt as to whether the effect represents a physiological response.

Other possible means by which PTH may enhance calcium absorption have been explored. Using preparations of rat intestinal mucosal cells from parathyroidectomised rats injected 4 h earlier with PTH, Birge and Gilbert[49] demonstrated an enhanced efflux of calcium out of the cells which was associated with alterations in Ca and Na-dependent ATPase. It was suggested that this enzyme might mediate a PTH-influenced active transport of calcium across the intestinal mucosa.

The possible important action of PTH to promote intestinal absorption of calcium requires further study. Equally important unresolved questions involve possible effects of PTH on absorption of other ions, e.g. magnesium and phosphate[50]. The exciting new findings implicating PTH and calcium in the regulation of vitamin D metabolism should promote great interest in this area of research.

8.2.3.4 *Other tissues*

Recently, PTH has been reported to produce effects in tissues not normally considered to be targets for its action. The physiological importance of such effects and their possible influences on calcium homeostasis, if any, remain unknown. However, Chausmer *et al.*[51] have reported an acute *in vitro* effect of PTH to promote influx of calcium into liver cells, which appeared not to be explained by non-hormonal contaminants of the crude PTH preparation used. MacManus *et al.*[52] found that partially purified PTH (*ca.* 1000 U mg^{-1}) increased both cyclic-AMP levels and cell proliferation in rat thymocytes maintained *in vitro;* it was contended that this action reflects a general property of PTH to promote calcium entry into cells which, in turn, can mediate subsequent biological events.

There is evidence both from clinical and animal studies to show that high levels of PTH may promote soft-tissue calcification in vital organs such as kidney, heart, arteries and lung. The mechanism by which this occurs has not yet been clarified, and it is not certain that the effect can be attributed solely to hypercalcaemia. Recent studies in rats by Peng and Munson[53] demonstrate that a single injection of a moderate dose of PTH is sufficient to induce soft-tissue calcification in thryoidectomised but not in intact rats, indicating a protective effect of thyrocalcitonin.

8.2.3.5   Mechanism of action

It is likely that most, if not all, physiological actions of PTH on various target tissues are mediated by an increase in intracellular levels of cyclic-AMP through activation of adenyl cyclase. The ability of PTH to increase cyclic-AMP in renal, cortical and bone cells is 'well documented[54]. The exact mechanisms by which cyclic-AMP induces target cells to perform their various functions is unknown, but models have been proposed[40] in an attempt to interpret reported findings in the light of current knowledge about the biochemical events produced in a variety of cells by cyclic-AMP. It is likely that both enhanced entry of calcium into the cell and concurrent elevation in cyclic-AMP following activation of adenyl cyclase by PTH probably constitute the important early events of PTH action.

8.2.4   Regulation of secretion

Current findings support the well established concept that the level of secretion of PTH is inversely related to the concentration of ionised calcium in the blood, being increased during hypocalcaemia; calcium inhibits secretion of PTH. Hyperphosphataemia does not stimulate PTH except indirectly when it is sufficiently severe to lower blood calcium. Ions other than calcium, especially magnesium, may influence the secretion of PTH; Sherwood and his co-workers[29] have suggested that the total concentration of circulating divalent cations (calcium and magnesium together) may be the important determinant of the rate of PTH secretion. Some evidence suggests that cyclic-AMP may mediate secretion of PTH since (a) there are appreciable levels of adenyl cyclase[55] and cyclic-AMP[56] in the gland, (b) dibutyryl cyclic-AMP can promote PTH secretion *in vitro*[29, 56]; and (c) parathyroid gland cyclic-AMP levels increase in response to hypocalcaemic challenge and decrease during hypercalcaemia[56].

   One would expect thyrocalcitonin (TCT) to stimulate PTH secretion if the action of TCT produces hypocalcaemia. Administration of TCT to cows has been shown to elevate circulating levels of PTH during the hormone-induced hypocalcaemia[57]. Reitz *et al.*[57] employed a series of experimental manoeuvres to show that the secretion of PTH was not responsive to the amount of TCT administered but rather to the extent and duration of the ensuing hypocalcaemia. These findings were of special interest in view of the report by Fischer *et al.*[58] that salmon calcitonin and porcine TCT could increase secretion of PTH from porcine parathyroid tissue *in vitro* even when calcium concentrations were normal or high (2.75 mM Ca^{2+}). It was suggested that TCT directly stimulated PTH secretion by reducing the concentration of intracellular calcium within parathyroid cells. However, in view of the high doses of calcitonins used by Fischer *et al.*[58] and the *in vivo* studies of Reitz *et al.*[57], it seems unlikely that PTH secretion normally is influenced directly by TCT.

8.2.5   Metabolism

A variety of earlier studies has indicated that PTH is cleared rapidly from the circulation. Current evidence favours the view that both the liver and the kidney play important roles in metabolising PTH. Recent studies by Fujita *et al.*[59] support their earlier findings that bovine PTH is inactivated by rat renal tissue. Fang and Tashjian[60] have provided recent evidence that the liver also may play an important role in metabolising PTH. The disappearance of injected bovine PTH was followed in normal rats and rats subjected to nephrectomy or partial hepatectomy. Both surgical procedures produced a decrease in the PTH disappearance rate. Additional *in vitro* studies suggested that the PTH-inactivating activity of renal tissue was five to six times greater than that of hepatic tissue on the basis of tissue protein, but since the total liver mass is six times that of the kidneys, the authors suggested that the total capacity of the liver to inactive circulating PTH rivals that of the kidney.

8.3 THYROCALCITONIN (TCT)

8.3.1 Cellular and embryonic origin

The C cell of the mammalian thyroid gland or the ultimobranchial body of lower vertebrates synthesises and stores TCT[61]. The C cell, so named by Pearse to distinguish it from follicular cells and vascular endothelial cells[62], has the structural and histochemical features of an endocrine secretory cell. The C cells of the thyroid gland and ultimobranchial body possess the ability to take up and decarboxylate amine precursors, the so-called 'APUD' (Amine Precursor Uptake and Decarboxylation) phenomenon. In the thyroid glands of most mammals C cells generally are sparse in number, but in certain hibernators like the bat large numbers of C cells are present and contain both TCT and serotonin. These cells vary in number and ultrastructure throughout the annual cycle[63]. In 1967, Pearse and Carvalheira showed that the C cells of the embryonic rat thyroid are derived from the ultimobranchial pouch; subsequently Copp, Tauber and others demonstrated hypocalcaemic activity in extracts of the ultimobranchial glands of the chicken and dogfish (cited in Ref. 61). Other studies examining the early embryonic life in rats demonstrated that the ultimobranchial C cells originate from the embryonic neural crest[64].

The neural origin of C cells also was demonstrated by the ingenious method of grafting quail neural tubes to chick embryonic hosts[65]. The nuclear chromatin pattern of the cells from the two avian species were distinguishable when subjected to a Feulgen reaction. This difference, serving as a biological marker, allowed the identification of the transplanted quail cells in the chick host. Grafting of neural anlage from a quail embryo to a chick host produced an ultimobranchial gland composed of a mixture of quail and chick C cells. Removal of the chick neural anlage without the subsequent graft of the quail neural tube led to deformities of the ultimobranchial gland and the absence of recognisable C cells. These elegant experiments provided convincing evidence that C cells originate from neural crest tissue.

The use of fluorogenic amine markers has identified cells with APUD characteristics in many tissues[64]. Pearse has suggested that all APUD polypeptide-producing cells are derivatives of embryonic neural crest cells and, therefore, are modified neurosecretory cells with specialised amine metabolism[62]. The hypothetical relationships between different cells of neural crest origin is given some credence by the fact that immunoreactive TCT has been detected in several extrathyroidal tissues of neural crest origin in the pig[66] and in several extrathyroidal neoplasms in man[67,68].

Histochemical studies have revealed that C cells contain arylethylamines, particularly dopamine, and that the amine content of the C cells can be altered by reserpine or monoamine oxidase inhibitors or by stimulating the release of TCT by hypercalcaemia[69]. The numbers of fluorogenic cells (i.e. C cells) of the thyroid or ultimobranchial gland correlated positively with amine decarboxylase activity[70]. High levels of dopa decarboxylase activity have been reported both in tumour tissue of human medullary carcinoma of the thyroid gland and in another human tumour of embryonic neural crest origin, pheochromocytoma[71].

8.3.2 Chemistry and structure–activity relationships

The hormones from five species (porcine, bovine, ovine, salmon and human) have been isolated and characterised with respect to amino acid composition and sequence[72,73]. The general peptide structure is similar in all five species, consisting of a single-chain polypeptide of 32 amino acids with prolinamide at the C-terminus and a 1,7-disulphide bridge at the N-terminus. However, a comparison of the amino acid sequences of the five hormones reveals many amino acid differences, especially in the central part of the molecule (Figure 8.3). Only nine of the 32 amino acids are homologous for all five calcitonins,

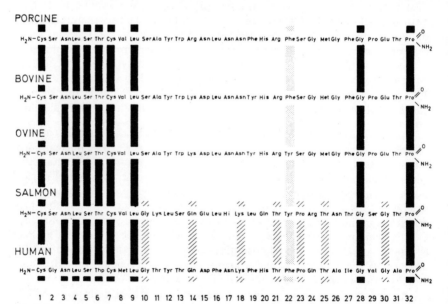

Figure 8.3 Comparison of amino acid sequences of porcine, ovine, salmon I and human calcitonins. Solid bars show sequence homologies among all five molecules; cross-hatched bars show homologies between human and salmon. (From Potts *et al.*[72], by courtesy of Excerpta Medica.)

but seven of the nine *N*-terminal amino acids are identical, suggesting that preservation of this part of the molecule is important for biological activity. Porcine, bovine and ovine TCT are very similar, but the human and salmon forms differ markedly from these three species and from one another. Some seemingly minor changes in amino acid sequence, such as removal of the terminal prolinamide, usually reduce or abolish biological activity.

Isohormones of TCT have been described[72,73]. Porcine TCT has been isolated in two biologically-active forms, differing only in the presence of either methionine sulphoxide or methionine at position 25. Human TCT has a methionine at position 8, adjacent to the disulphide bridge. The sulphoxide derivative of human TCT or salmon CT is not biologically active. The influence of minor variations in amino acid sequence on biological activity is well demonstrated in the case of the three salmon isohormones[73]. The amino acid sequences and the biological potencies of the three salmon forms have been confirmed by synthesis[74]. Salmon CT I and II have specific activities of 2400–2700 MRC Units mg^{-1}, 20–50-fold higher than any form of hormone studied except that recently isolated from the Japanese eel[75]. The potency of salmon CT III is 600 MRC Units mg^{-1}, less than that of I or II but still high compared to the TCT of other species[73]. Form I is the major circulating form in all species of salmon studied thus far. Three types of salmon exhibit form II as a minor plasma component, while only the Coho salmon has form III as a minor circulating component. Whether the three forms of salmon CT are the result of the secretion of three distinct forms from the ultimobranchial gland or are the result of peripheral alterations of a single secreted precursor is not known. Attempts to correlate biological and immunological activity of the TCT molecule with its tertiary structure are still in the preliminary stage[76,77].

Two laboratories have synthesised a biologically and immunologically active human TCT by solid-phase methods[78,79]. The biological potencies of these synthetic products are about one-third to one-half that of the native human TCT (100 MRC Units mg^{-1}). A synthetic fragment of human TCT lacking an intact disulphide loop, prepared by Ontjes *et al.*[78], had limited biological activity (0.3 MRC Units mg^{-1}), being less than 1% as active as native human TCT. The amino terminal portion of the synthetic human TCT was not required for immunological activity with antisera raised against the entire molecule.

Hormones with potencies of 3000–5000 MRC Units mg^{-1} have been extracted recently from ultimobranchial glands of the chicken[80] and Japanese eel[75]. The amino acid sequences of these hormones have not yet been resolved. Their high biological activity suggests that their structures might be similar to the salmon hormone.

8.3.3 Biological and radioimmunological assays

8.3.3.1 Biological assays

Biological assays for TCT have been reviewed recently[81]. A variety of assay techniques based on the ability of TCT to produce hypocalcaemia in rodents has been developed. Various manoeuvres have been employed to improve sensitivity or lower the dose requirements. In general, *in vivo* bioassay techniques are more popular than *in vitro* methods because the former are simpler to perform and require less specialised equipment and skills.

The *in vivo* bioassay of TCT remains the standard procedure for evaluating potencies of the native hormones and of synthetic materials including fragments and analogues, and it has been used to compare biological and immunological activities of TCT in biological fluids. However, the bioassay has been replaced by the radioimmunoassay for the sensitive and specific measurement of circulating TCT in several species. TCT is still measured by bioassay in the blood of birds because a radioimmunoassay for avian TCT is not yet available[82]. Plasma TCT levels range from 100 to 1500 MRC μ Units ml^{-1} in several avian species. These levels are the highest circulating TCT values found in normal animals, an apparent paradox since exogenous TCT has not yet been shown to produce a biological effect in birds[83, 84].

In vitro methods for the bioassay of TCT involve tissue culture of foetal or embryonic bones[36, 85]. These methods depend on the inhibition by TCT of the release of ^{45}Ca previously incorporated into the cultured bones. Resorption, or release of the ^{45}Ca, is stimulated by the addition of PTH or vitamins A or D to the culture media. As little as 0.0001 MRC Unit ml^{-1} of TCT can be detected by these methods. Since TCT has been shown to increase the levels of cyclic-AMP in bone cells in *vitro*[86], the measurement of cyclic-AMP before and after the addition of TCT to incubation medium may prove to be a sensitive method for measuring TCT.

8.3.3.2 Radioimmunoassays

Sensitive and specific radioimmunoassays have been developed for the five sequenced peptides[28, 87] and applied to other species such as the rabbit and rat[88] in which cross-reactivity occurs. Antisera raised against either porcine, ovine or bovine TCT cross-react with the other two, probably because of the similarities in amino acid sequence. In contrast, human and salmon TCT usually bind poorly to antisera raised against the hormones from other species. However, salmon and porcine hormones have been observed to cross-react in a system using guinea-pig antisera to porcine TCT[89]. Porcine and salmon hormones are structurally similar only in the 1–9 portion of the amino acid sequence, suggesting that such antisera may react primarily with the N-terminal portion of the molecule.

Immunoassays for porcine and bovine TCT were the first to be described[28]. The porcine assay has been applied extensively to the measurement of TCT in the venous effluent blood from the isolated pig thyroid gland[90, 91]. The concentration of TCT in porcine thyroid venous blood, undiluted by the systemic circulation, usually is in the range of 10–30 ng ml^{-1}, considerably higher than circulating peripheral levels (<1 ng ml^{-1}). Hypercalcaemia produced by calcium infusion elevates the TCT concentration in thyroid venous blood to levels of 300–1000 ng ml^{-1} [90, 92]. This unique experimental system has been used extensively to study regulation of TCT secretion (see Section 8.3.5).

Deftos and associates[28] have developed an extremely sensitive immunoassay for bovine TCT with a lower limit of detection of 1 pg ml^{-1}. Peripheral plasma TCT levels in normal cows or bulls have been measured and shown to increase four- to seven-fold after intravenous administration of calcium.

The measurement of human TCT by immunoassay was first applied to the study of patients with medullary carcinoma of the thyroid gland[93-97]. The high level of circulating TCT in these patients 500–100 000 pg ml^{-1}, can be detected readily by antisera against human TCT. Attempts to measure TCT in normal human plasma have been less successful. Tashjian and associates[93, 94] originally reported a range of 20–400 pg ml^{-1} in normal human plasma but the possibility that plasma constituents other than human TCT reacted non-specifically in their assay system was suggested by apparent activity in the sera of some thyroidectomised patients. Deftos and his co-workers[95-97] have not detected TCT in normal human sera either under basal conditions or after attempted stimulation by infusion of calcium even though the lower limit of detection for their assay was 100 pg ml^{-1}. Deftos has emphasised the problems posed by interference in the assay systems when large amounts of plasma proteins are present, but the radioimmunoassay still has been used successfully to study patients with medullary carcinoma of the thyroid gland and hypocalcaemic patients who store or secrete unusually large quantities of TCT[97]. Huefner and Hesch[98], using a sensitive human immunoassay, reported TCT levels of 50–150 pg ml^{-1} in the peripheral plasma of five normal subjects. In our laboratory, Hennessy has not been able to detect human TCT in normal human sera with a method capable of measuring as little as 100 pg ml^{-1}. Low blood levels of TCT in normal subjects and possible assay interference from plasma proteins continue to pose serious problems.

The level of immunoreactive CT in the plasma of male salmon is *ca.* 2000 pg ml^{-1}, while the levels in the non-spawning females are in the range of 6000–12 000 pg ml^{-1}. The significance of these high plasma levels in the salmon and of the sex difference is unknown. There is an opposite sex difference in the bovine species where plasma TCT levels in the male (303 pg ml^{-1}) are higher than those in the female (165 pg ml^{-1})[28].

TCT levels in the plasma of normal rats, previously undetectable by bioassay, have been reported by Milhaud *et al.*[88] to be approximately 0.00003 MRC Unit ml^{-1}. Immunisation of rats with extracts of human medullary thyroid carcinomas resulted in antisera reacting with both human TCT and rat TCT and allowed them to measure TCT in a species where the chemical structure of the hormone has not been elucidated. They reported that circulating rat TCT increased during hypercalcaemia and became undetectable after thyroidectomy. The level of 0.0003 Unit ml^{-1} estimated for hypercalcaemic rat plasma by immunoassay is comparable to that (0.0005–0.001 Unit ml^{-1}) reported for the sera of hypercalcaemic rats based on the *in vitro* bone culture bioassay (cited in Ref. 61), showing good agreement between immunoassay and bioassay values, and despite possible differences in assay specificity.

8.3.4   Sites and modes of action

Originally, the characteristic hypocalcaemic, hypophosphataemic effect of TCT seemed adequately explained by its ability to inhibit the resorption of bone mineral[61]. Talmage and his co-workers[99,100] recently have reported that the hypophosphataemic effect of TCT may precede the fall in the blood calcium and point out that the degree of the hypocalcaemic response is dependent on the level of the blood phosphate under a variety of experimental circumstances. They have proposed that changes in phosphate transport rates in osteocytes and other cells may represent the primary effect of TCT. In the renal tubule, phosphate fluxes appear to be dependent on active transport of sodium and water. Goldberg et al.[45] have demonstrated that the phosphaturia induced by PTH is dependent on the proximal tubular inhibition of sodium reabsorption (see Section 8.2.3.2). However, the apparent dependence of phosphate transport on sodium movement in the kidney need not also be true for bone cells, and a rapid change in phosphate transport in bone cells might be produced directly by TCT.

The early observations that TCT can produce hypocalcaemia and hypophosphataemia in the absence of the kidneys or the gastrointestinal tract tended to minimise the possible importance of these organs as target tissues for TCT. However, recent reports that TCT acts on the kidney in man and experimental animals (see Section 8.3.4.2) and on the small intestine (see Section 8.3.4.3) require that these organs not be overlooked in consideration of the overall physiology and pharmacology of TCT.

8.3.4.1 Bone

Evidence obtained from both in vivo and in vitro studies has established that TCT inhibits the movement of calcium from bone to blood and can lead to inhibition of bone resorption[61]. The evidence for effects of TCT to promote calcium movement into bone mineral is not as convincing. In a recent series of experiments, the long-term administration of high doses of TCT to intact, parathyroidectomised and thyroparathyroidectomised rats did not alter the amounts of calcium, magnesium or hydroxyproline in the clavicles and tibiae[101]. However, TCT can diminish or block completely the histological changes of excessive bone resorption produced by high doses of vitamin A[102].

The inhibition of resorption by TCT is a transient event in cultured foetal rat bones stimulated to resorb with PTH or vitamin D metabolites[33]. The loss of activity of TCT despite its continued presence has been termed an 'escape' phenomenon. The mechanisms of 'escape' are unclear; 'escape' appears dependent on the agent used to stimulate bone resorption and on calcium and phosphate concentrations of the culture media. 'Escape' occurs only if resorption is stimulated, and a variety of other weak stimulators of resorption do not lead to TCT 'escape'. The 'induction' of bone resorption in cultured bones is a related phenomenon, where bone resorption persists even after PTH is withdrawn. Exposing the 'induced' foetal bones to antisera to PTH abolished the resorptive activity, indicating that bound PTH continues to stimulate bone cells until it is displaced or removed. Cyclic-AMP did not seem to mediate this phenomenon, since the PTH effect was not enhanced by the addition of dibutyryl cyclic-AMP or theophylline. In earlier work from the Raisz laboratory[103], it was reported that theophylline potentiated PTH-stimulated resorption and that there was a resorptive response to dibutyryl cyclic-AMP at low doses of the nucleotide but loss of the effect at high doses. It was suggested that there are two cyclic-AMP-dependent systems in bone, one sensitive to PTH and one sensitive to TCT[103]. However, localisation of two such systems either within different bone cells or within different compartments of a single bone cell has not been achieved.

Bone structure, evaluated by light and electron microscopy, can be altered by TCT. Bélanger and Copp[104] reported that prolonged administration of TCT to young birds reduced both osteocytic and osteoclastic resorption, causing more dense bones. In contrast, laying-hens on a calcium-enriched diet, paradoxically, developed osteoporosis of cortical bone in response to administered TCT, presumably due to compensatory secretion of PTH. Osteoclasts have been reported to lose their ruffled border within 15 min after TCT injection[105,106], and changes in osteocytic size have been observed by Matthews et al. after TCT injections[107].

8.3.4.2 Kidney

Increases in the urinary excretion of inorganic phosphate, calcium, magnesium, sodium and potassium after the injection of TCT have been described[61]. Superphysiological doses of porcine TCT given to intact or parathyroidectomised rats acutely elevated the urinary excretion of sodium and potassium while the urinary excretion of calcium and magnesium fell[108]. Multiple injections of porcine TCT given every 3 h to intact rats led to hypercalciuria, phosphaturia, and natriuresis[109]. The acute fall in the urinary calcium excretion was explained by the TCT-induced hypocalcaemia while subsequent hypercalciuria may represent a direct effect of TCT on the renal tubule after PTH had restored the blood calcium to normal. The hypercalciuria cannot be attributed to a secondary increase in PTH secretion since PTH would be expected to lower the urinary excretion of calcium in the absence of hypercalcaemia[108].

Phosphaturia has been observed after administration of TCT to intact rats, but not consistently in parathyroidectomised rats[109]. These differences may be due to a phosphaturic effect of PTH, secreted in increased amounts in the intact rat in response to TCT-induced hypocalcaemia. This interpretation would be consistent with the finding that porcine TCT given to intact and thyroparathyroidectomised dogs produced phosphaturia only in the intact dogs[110]. However, Barlet[111], reported that infusion of purified porcine and human TCT and salmon CT (20 MRC m Units $kg^{-1} h^{-1}$ for 96 h) produced enhanced excretion of phosphate, sodium, potassium and calcium in both intact and thyroparathyroidectomised sheep and he suggested that these renal effects of TCT represented a physiological response to the hormone. Salt loading alone in dogs produces phosphaturia, indicating that the renal effects of TCT or PTH may be due to alterations in the tubular handling of sodium[45].

Studies in man using purified hormones have clarified some of the conflicting results obtained in the early studies with less purified preparations. Haas and his associates[112] administered TCT (porcine, human and salmon) to hypoparathyroid patients without altering endogenous creatinine clearance or serum electrolytes. However, urinary excretion of phosphorus, sodium, potassium, calcium and magnesium increased after the i.v. infusion of 150 MRC Units of any of the three hormones. PTH (500 Units) given to the same subjects increased the urinary excretion of phosphorus, sodium and potassium, but the excretion of calcium and magnesium fell. Similar studies from another laboratory using synthetic salmon CT[113] revealed that CT produced an early increase in the urinary excretion of calcium, magnesium, sodium and phosphorus in normal subjects followed 2 h later by a fall in the urinary excretion of calcium and magnesium. The delayed fall in the urinary excretion of calcium and magnesium, observed in the normal subjects but not in hypoparathyroid subjects, was attributed to the release of PTH in response to TCT-induced hypocalcaemia.

The natriuretic effect of TCT in man has been described by Bijvoet and his colleagues[114]. Infusion of porcine TCT or synthetic human TCT for periods of 6–39 days was associated with transient increases in the urinary excretion of sodium and water along with a phosphaturia which persisted for the duration of the infusion. Weight losses of 0.5–1.6 kg occurred during the first 48 h. Thereafter, the urinary sodium and water excretion returned to normal, the reduced body weight was maintained and both plasma renin activity and aldosterone secretion rates increased, presumably in response to the initial natriuresis. Cessation of the TCT infusion reversed these effects. The fact that urinary excretion of cyclic-AMP did not rise in response to TCT suggested that the renal effects observed were not caused by secondary stimulation of PTH secretion. Others also have reported acute increases in urinary sodium excretion in normocalcaemic or hypercalcaemic patients given porcine TCT[115], and high doses of porcine TCT (100 MRC Units) produced three- to seven-fold increases in the urinary sodium excretion when given to hypoparathyroid patients[116].

Despite the numerous studies showing renal effects of TCT administration, whether or not endogenous TCT has an important direct effect on the kidney under normal physiological conditions remains to be clarified.

8.3.4.3 GI tract and related structures

The first convincing evidence for a direct effect of TCT on the small intestine was reported by Olson[48, 117] (see Section 8.2.3.3), who studied the calcium transport ratio in an isolated, vascularly perfused preparation of rat small intestine from vitamin D-deficient or vitamin D-supplemented young rats. Small (10 MRC m Units) doses of porcine TCT lowered the transport ratio and higher doses (500 MRC m Units) increased it with D-supplementation but not in D-deficiency. These *in vitro* effects of TCT cannot be explained by an action on the renal conversion of vitamin D in the kidney to its active metabolites which is now thought to be a major factor regulating the intestinal absorption of calcium (see Section 8.4.3).

Superphysiological doses of TCT in man appear to increase the intestinal absorption of calcium[118]. Milhaud *et al.*[119], using radiocalcium kinetics, observed increases in calcium absorption in patients given TCT injections for 3 days, but they attributed this alteration to an increased release of PTH induced by hypocalcaemia. Pak *et al.*[120] observed increased intestinal absorption of ^{45}Ca in patients with idiopathic osteoporosis given infusions of calcium, a finding which was attributed to the release of endogenous TCT. They also observed that the injection of PTH increased the intestinal absorption of ^{45}Ca in hypoparathyroid patients with intact thyroid glands but was ineffective in thyroidectomised, hypoparathyroid subjects, suggesting again that the release of endogenous TCT may have been responsible for the intestinal effect[121].

Gray and Juan[122] have observed increases in the net jejunal transport of calcium *in vivo* after administration of salmon hormone (100–500 MRC m Units kg^{-1} min^{-1}) to anaesthetised dogs. Net jejunal transport of calcium was measured by perfusing isolated jejunal loops. These *in vivo* observations are in harmony with the *in vitro* effects seen in the rat by Olson with high doses of TCT.

Other gastrointestinal functions in addition to the absorption of calcium may be influenced by TCT. Hesch *et al.*[123] and Orimo *et al.*[124] recently reported that high doses of TCT inhibited pentagastrin-stimulated gastric acid production in man. Despite the large doses of TCT used, no significant changes in the total serum calcium were seen. In related studies, Orimo reported a decreased incidence of gastric ulcers and gastric-acid secretion in rats with the pylorus ligated and treated with TCT[124]. Large doses of porcine and human TCT also have been shown to inhibit the increased pancreatic enzyme and fluid secretion produced in man by infusion of secretin and pancreozymin/cholecystokinin[125]. Hypercalcaemia, produced by calcium infusion, stimulated gastric and pancreatic secretion while EGTA-induced hypocalcaemia inhibited both gastric and pancreatic secretions[126]. However, gastric acid secretion stimulated by intragastric calcium was inhibited by administration of porcine TCT given in amounts too small to lower the plasma calcium, suggesting a direct effect of TCT on the gastric parietal cell[127].

8.3.4.4 Mechanism of action

The mechanisms responsible for the diverse effects of TCT have not been established. The most likely explanation is that TCT activates adenylcyclase which increases intracellular levels of cyclic-AMP. An increase in cyclic-AMP after TCT administration has been demonstrated in bone and renal tissue[128]. However, the maximal levels of cyclic-AMP attained in both tissues after TCT were significantly less than those achieved with PTH (see Section 8.2.3). The combined effect of PTH and TCT produced additive effects on the cyclic-AMP level in bone tissue, suggesting separate receptors for the two peptides. The role of cyclic-AMP as a mediator of TCT effects is consistent with other reports showing (a) the effects of dibutyryl cyclic-AMP, theophylline, catecholamines and imidazole on calcium homeostasis in normal and thyroparathyroidectomised animals[61]; (b) an inhibition by TCT of the epinephrine-stimulated rise in cyclic-AMP in cultured thymocytes[52]; (c) the stimulation of TCT secretion *in vivo* from the pig thyroid gland by dibutyryl-cyclic AMP (see Section 8.3.5).

Several investigators have proposed direct effects of TCT on the membrane function of its target cells. Borle concludes from his studies of calcium kinetics in cultured renal cells that TCT inhibits the efflux of calcium from cells[39]. This inhibition of calcium efflux may be regulated by changes in the activity of a membrane-bound Ca^{2+} and Mg^{2+}-dependent ATPase. A reduction in osteocyte cell size has been observed in rats after the injection of large amounts of TCT[107]. These striking morphological changes may reflect sudden shifts in transport of cellular water and electrolytes and suggest that TCT may cause rapid changes in membrane transport.

Other changes in intracellular enzyme activity have been proposed as a primary TCT effect. The inhibition of lysosomal enzymes by TCT in cultured osteocytes has been described[129]. Increases in skeletal pyrophosphatase activity after the administration of TCT to animals with intact parathyroid glands have been observed[130].

8.3.5 Regulation of secretion

Studies of the secretion of TCT have been facilitated greatly by the development and application of radioimmunoassay for the measurement of TCT[28]. The blood calcium level has a direct effect on the isolated pig thyroid gland, stimulating secretion of TCT at levels of calcium above 10 mg per 100 ml[90]. Cultured foetal rat thyroids secrete TCT in direct proportion to the calcium concentration of the medium over a range of 1–2.5 mM[131]. The addition of calcium to the ambient water causes abrupt increases in the concentration of plasma CT in Sockeye salmon[132]. However, the fact that the blood calcium level can regulate TCT secretion does not eliminate the possibility that other factors may play a role in the regulation of TCT secretion. Experiments showing that the presence of calcium in the gastrointestinal tract increased TCT secretion in pigs without detectable changes in the blood calcium level suggested that the thyroid gland is responsive to very small changes in the blood calcium level such as might occur during the intestinal absorption of calcium[92].

The observation that gastrointestinal calcium stimulated TCT secretion without detectable hypercalcaemia suggested that some other factor, perhaps an intestinal hormone, could be released and act to signal the thyroid gland to release TCT. Care reported that the infusion of pancreozymin at concentrations of 5×10^{-9} M into the pig thyroid artery evoked fourfold increases in TCT secretion[134]. In our laboratory, preliminary experiments of a similar nature showed that glucagon-like material of gastrointestinal origin, secretin and crude intestinal extracts had no effect on TCT secretion[92], while gastrin and its synthetic analogues, pentagastrin and tetragastrin, produced equally marked elevations in TCT concentrations in the venous effluent of the isolated pig thyroid gland (Figure 8.4)[92,135,136]. Systemic doses of pentagastrin covering a wide range (26–2600 ng kg^{-1}) produced 10–40-fold increases in TCT secretion[135]. The stimulatory effect of pentagastrin on TCT secretion also was demonstrated by the production of hypocalcaemia and hypophosphataemia in both pigs[135,137] and rats[138] given pentagastrin provided that the thyroid gland was present. In more recent studies in man, intravenous

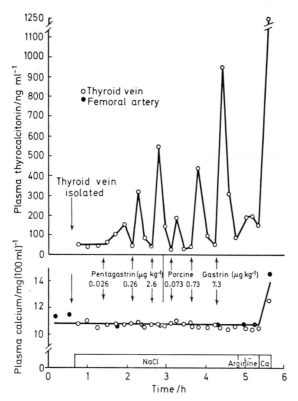

Figure 8.4 Stimulation of secretion of TCT in pig thyroid venous blood by pentagastrin and porcine gastrin. Arrows (↕) show times at which various doses of the hormones were administered systemically (femoral vein). Blocks along the abscissa show durations of i.v. infusions into the femoral vein. (From Cooper et al.[136], by courtesy of *Endocrinology*.)

infusion of physiological amounts (0.15 μg kg^{-1} h^{-1}) of gastrin over a 3 h period lowered the blood calcium by 0.6–0.8 mg per 100 ml[139].

Administration of pentagastrin into the thyroid artery at doses so low that they are ineffective systemically have produced transient two- to six-fold increases in TCT secretion[136]. The increased TCT secretion occurred despite the fact that the blood calcium level perfusing the thyroid gland was low, being diluted by the injection fluid. From experiments in the pig, Care et al.[140] reported that pancreozymin, the *C*-terminal octapeptide of pancreozymin (but not the *N*-terminal hexapeptide) and caerulin all are TCT secretagogues but are less potent than gastrin. In our laboratory, pancreatic glucagon and the histamine analogue, betazole, in large doses were shown to have little or no effect on TCT secretion from the pig thyroid gland although large doses of pancreatic glucagon have been reported to increase TCT secretion in some species[141].

Solutions of calcium or acetylcholine delivered intragastrically to the pig are associated with concurrent increases in immunoreactive gastrin and TCT in the thyroid venous blood[142]. A high positive correlation between the concentrations of TCT and gastrin at levels of plasma gastrin only slightly above the normal range (50–100 pg^{-1} ml^{-1}) has been observed suggesting a previously unappreciated relationship between these two hormones. These findings support the idea that gastrointestinal hormones play a part in the regulation of TCT secretion.

Gastrointestinal handling of dietary calcium has been proposed to be important in regulating the blood levels of bovine TCT[143]. The mean concentration of TCT in bulls is significantly higher than the mean concentration in cows (see Section 8.3.3.2). Both bulls and cows ingest large amounts of dietary calcium, but the lactating cow loses a large portion of the absorbed calcium in the milk. Medullary carcinoma of the thyroid gland, a neoplasm of C cell origin, recently has been described in bulls[28], and it has been suggested that the ingestion and absorption of large amounts of calcium may lead to chronic C cell stimulation and eventual neoplasia. The role of dietary calcium in the regulation of TCT secretion in man remains unsettled. Slight increases in circulating TCT were observed in two of four patients with medullary thyroid carcinoma given oral calcium[94]. Normal subjects have been reported to increase their TCT levels after ingesting large amounts of calcium even without detectable elevations in the blood calcium level[144].

Cations other than calcium may influence TCT secretion. High concentrations of magnesium, 4.4–12.7 mequiv l^{-1} stimulated TCT release when the blood calcium was held in the normal range but lower concentrations of magnesium were ineffective[145]. Changes in the magnesium concentrations in the medium of cultured foetal rat thyroid glands from 0.4–3.2 mM were reported not to influence TCT release[131]. In studies in the pig, potassium, strontium and barium stimulated TCT secretion when given in large doses, but infusions of sodium or inorganic phosphate were ineffective[142].

Changes in intracellular concentrations of cyclic-AMP within the thyroid gland C cells may regulate secretion of TCT[146, 147]. Theophylline potentiates the stimulation of TCT secretion in pigs by pancreozymin and other stimuli of TCT secretion[140]. Dibutyryl cyclic-AMP stimulates the secretion of TCT *in vitro* from cultured foetal rat thyroids[131] or porcine thyroid tissue[146] and *in vivo* from the pig thyroid gland[147].

In patients with medullary carcinoma of the thyroid, TCT release has been stimulated by infusion of calcium and suppressed by EDTA infusion[94, 97]. Calcium infusions also have produced increased TCT levels in patients with pseudohypoparathyroidism[148, 149]. Injections of pancreatic glucagon have produced a variable effect on the TCT levels of patients with medullary carcinoma or pseudohypoparathyroidism, occasionally but not always causing an increase. Recently, we have shown that pentagastrin also can stimulate the release of TCT in patients with medullary thyroid carcinoma[150].

Oestrogen and progesterone also may have unappreciated effects on TCT secretion. Progesterone in large doses reduced both the TCT content of the thyroid gland and the TCT secretion rate in ewes[151]. Plasma osmotic pressure could be another factor influencing TCT secretion, based on preliminary studies in the salmon[152] and Japanese eel[153].

8.3.6 Metabolism

Species-related differences in the metabolism of TCT were first revealed by the finding that salmon CT was more potent that TCT from other mammalian species in the rat bioassay[152] and the observation that immunoreactive salmon CT, administered to dogs, was cleared more slowly from the blood than mammalian TCT[154]. Using two separate immunoassays, the volumes of distribution and the metabolic clearance rates for salmon CT and porcine TCT have been studied over a wide range of equilibrium concentrations in anaesthetised dogs[154]. The distribution volumes for both hormones were similar to the extracellular fluid volume, but the clearance rate of porcine TCT was tenfold faster than that of salmon CT. The clearance rate for porcine TCT in the dog is approximately four- to five-fold higher than the glomerular filtration rate, indicating that mechanisms other than glomerular filtration are responsible for its disappearance from the blood. Two components of the plasma disappearance curves of the hormones, one rapid and one slow, were seen. The rapid component, due to the fall in free (unbound) hormone, was tenfold less for salmon CT than for porcine TCT. The slow component, attributable to protein binding of the hormones, was similar for the two molecules. The binding characteristics of these peptides are unknown. Other studies showed that salmon CT resisted inactivation when incubated *in vitro* with dog plasma, while porcine TCT lost 80% of its initial activity under the same conditions. Supernatants from homogenised liver and renal tissues of rats can rapidly inactivate porcine TCT but homogenates from other tissues do not. Plasma disappearance rates of chick and salmon CT in the rat are nearly identical with a half-life of *ca.* 10 min. Nephrectomy in the rat delays the disappearance rate of chick and salmon CT[155].

Liver, muscle, and bone are organs which can clear porcine TCT and salmon CT from the blood of the dog. Arteriovenous (A–V) differences of three hormones (salmon, porcine and human) across the lung, kidney, liver and musculoskeletal compartment have been examined[156]. Salmon CT was unaltered by hepatic and musculoskeletal passage, while the porcine and human TCT showed a 30% fall in concentration. The A–V differences across the lung and kidney were similar for all three hormones. Less than 1% of the total doses of the hormones was detected in the urine. In addition to hepatic A–V differences, renal A–V differences in levels of immunoreactive human TCT were observed in anaesthetised dogs[157]. The urinary excretion of the total dose of TCT infused was less than 1%, confirming the results obtained with porcine TCT and salmon CT[156]. Nephrectomy in dogs led to higher serum levels of TCT and a prolonged disappearance rate. These findings and the recovery of TCT-like biologically active material from the urine of patients with medullary carcinoma[158] may be explained by the binding of TCT to renal receptors with subsequent urinary excretion of an altered immunologically-unreactive fragment. A highly specific renal receptor for TCT has been described recently by Marx and Aurbach[159], who report that salmon CT binds to membrane fractions from rat renal cortex which also are capable of inactivating the CT.

Preliminary studies in man indicate that the metabolic clearance rate and the distribution volume for porcine TCT follow the pattern observed in the dog[160]. The plasma disappearance curve of porcine TCT after a single intravenous injection or a continuous infusion revealed two components with half-lives of 2.4 and 40.9 min, respectively. In contrast, the clearance rate (ml min^{-1}) of porcine TCT by the pig is 13 in the intact animals and 16 in the isolated perfused pig liver[161]. Human TCT and salmon CT are not degraded to a significant extent by the isolated perfused pig liver.

It appears that porcine TCT, and possibly ovine and bovine TCT, because of their structural similarities, are rapidly metabolised in heterologous species by hepatic inactivation. However, renal binding and degradation seem to be more important in the metabolism of the salmon and human hormones.

8.3.7 Pregnancy and lactation

The possible importance of TCT in pregnancy and lactation is beginning to be explored. The net calcium loss in these conditions can be attributed to the foetal uptake of calcium and the excretion of calcium in the milk. Increased intestinal absorption of calcium is thought to accompany both pregnancy and lactation. Although the increased intestinal absorption of calcium has been attributed to increased parathyroid activity. Heaney and Skillman[162] have demonstrated increased intestinal absorption of calcium in pregnant women as early as the second trimester, a time when immunoreactive PTH levels in the blood are within the normal range. They suggested that hormones other than PTH may be involved in intestinal calcium absorption. Cushard and associates[31] have reported increases in the immunoreactive PTH levels of pregnant women during the third trimester, but they were unable to identify the signal for the release of PTH since the diffusible calcium levels did not change during pregnancy. Furthermore, the mean PTH levels of 14 lactating women were normal, indicating that factors other than PTH may be responsible for the increased intestinal absorption of calcium accompanying lactation.

Recent experiments in lactating rats by Harper et al.[163] suggest a function for TCT in this special situation. Injected TCT produced a greater hypocalcaemic response in lactating rats than in non-lactating rats of the same age, a finding consistent with a more active bone metabolism in lactation. Intragastric administration of a calcium salt produced hypercalcaemia in lactating rats deprived of their thyroid glands but not in sham-operated lactating rats, reminiscent of the earlier experiences of Gray and Munson[164] in young male rats. Fasting, 4–5 h in duration, produced marked hypocalcaemia in lactating rats. The authors concluded that during lactation TCT was important for prevention of hypercalcaemia during the intestinal absorption of calcium, and that even maximal parathyroid activity was unable to prevent a fall in the blood calcium when dietary calcium was not available as long as calcium was excreted in the milk.

The observations of Harper et al.[163] in the rat are consistent with the concept, initially proposed by Gray and Munson[164] and advanced by Munson and his co-workers[165-169], that TCT is important for the prevention of hypercalcaemia during the intestinal absorption of calcium and that this role is the principal physiological function of TCT. Other studies provide support for this concept. Milhaud *et al.*[170] observed elevations of the blood calcium in rats after thyroidectomy only when the thyroid was removed during a period of feeding. These experiments by Milhaud *et al.*, performed on rats adapted to a 12 h dark (fed) and light (unfed) diurnal cycle, suggested that a diurnal rhythm exists for both endogenous TCT secretion and responsiveness to TCT in the rat. Swaminathan *et al.*[171] reported small but significant increases in blood calcium levels of young pigs after thyroidectomy even though the animals were fasted, suggesting that in some species TCT may help regulate the blood calcium level during periods of fasting as well as of feeding.

8.4 CONTROL OF MINERAL METABOLISM

8.4.1 Parathyroid hormone (PTH)

The principal physiological function of PTH is to help maintain normocalcaemia by raising the concentration of calcium in blood and extracellular fluid. In addition, the action of the hormone on bone permits extensive 'turnover' or 'remodelling' while normocalcaemia is being maintained. The action of the hormone protects vertebrates against a life-threatening hypocalcaemia which ensues rapidly in the absence of PTH, especially if exogenous sources of calcium are lacking. Indirectly, the parathyroid glands also serve to help TCT restrict hypercalcaemia since hypercalcaemia suppresses secretion of PTH.

Although normally PTH effectively helps maintain normocalcaemia, numerous recent studies have uncovered situations where the parathyroid glands appear unable to counteract even a modest fall in blood calcium. For example, in our own laboratory Peng *et al.*[172,173] observed that ethanol and urethane both produce a modest hypocalcaemia in animals which persists for several (5–12 or more) hours before the parathyroid glands can restore the blood calcium level to normal. Heath *et al.*[174] recently reported that colchicine also can cause hypocalcaemia. These recently reported agents join a lengthy list of other drugs (e.g. protamine, diphosphonates, 2-thiophenecarboxylic acid) which previously have been shown to be able to affect bone and/or produce hypocalcaemia despite the presence of the parathyroid glands.

All actions of PTH raise blood calcium and concurrently lower blood phosphate. However, the hormone also may exert important influences on other ions, e.g. magnesium and sodium. Although bone, kidney, and intestine are currently regarded as the primary target tissues for PTH, other important actions of PTH may exist. Earlier evidence for effects of the hormone on salivary and mammary glands requires further study. More recent suggestions that PTH may act on liver[51] or promote renal and hepatic blood flow by causing arterial vasodilatation[175] are difficult to incorporate into our present general picture of the action of PTH. Recent studies indicate that a newly discovered role of PTH may be to help control renal conversion of vitamin D to its active metabolites, but the importance of this action for the maintenance of calcium homeostasis remains to be fully clarified (see Section 8.4.3).

8.4.2 Thyrocalcitonin (TCT)

The principal physiological function of TCT appears to be to protect mammals against hypercalcaemia especially during periods of intestinal absorption of calcium after feeding. Until recently, this role of TCT was difficult to appreciate because dramatic elevations in blood calcium normally do not occur in thyroidectomised mammals; and skeletal defects with long term deficiency of TCT are difficult to demonstrate. Neverthelesss, several lines of experimental evidence now favour the idea that TCT protects against hypercalcaemia (see Section 8.3.4). The importance of this action of the hormone may lie with the possibility that episodic bouts of even moderate hypercalcaemia may predispose the organism to calcification of susceptible vital soft tissues[53]. Other possible roles for the hormone have been suggested, e.g. in lactation or in controlling renal conversion of vitamin D to its active metabolites (see Section 8.4.3), but remain to be proved.

A most challenging task for the future is to identifiy the actions of this hormone in man and in submammalian vertebrates. TCT is not present in large quantities in human thyroid glands and its secretion in normal man has not yet been evaluated. While the hormone is secreted in considerable quantities even in fishes, an action in submammalian species other than the frog[176] has not been well documented.

8.4.3 Interrelationships among PTH, TCT, vitamin D and bone

Vitamin D is no less important in calcium homeostasis and in skeletal growth and remodelling than PTH and TCT. The recent elucidation of the steps involved in the metabolism of vitamin D has greatly clarified our understanding of its physiology. The availability of radiolabelled vitamin D of high specific activity was a critical factor in the identification of active metabolites in a variety of tissues from D-deficient animals. The first important metabolite to be isolated was 25-hydroxycholecalciferol (25-(OH)D_3) which stimulates the intestinal transport of calcium in D-deficient rats more rapidly than its precursor, vitamin D_3. The metabolite is formed by the hydroxylation of the parent D_3 by hepatic mitochondrial hydroxylases[177]. Later, metabolites more polar than 25-(OH)D_3, 1,25-dihydroxycholecalciferol (1,25-(OH)$_2D_3$), 21,25-(OH)$_2D_3$* and 25,26-(OH)$_2D_3$ were identified, and the 1,25-derivative was shown to be more active than 25-(OH)D_3 in promoting the intestinal transport of calcium and the mobilisation of skeletal mineral. 1,25-(OH)$_2D_3$ was the predominant metabolite isolated from the intestinal mucosa of D-deficient animals injected with [^{3}H]-25-(OH)D_3. Actinomycin D or cycloheximide can block the stimulation of intestinal calcium transport produced by the administration of 25-(OH)D_3 to D-deficient animals but these cytotoxic agents are without effect when 1,25-(OH)$_2D_3$ is administered, indicating that action of the dihydroxy-metabolite does not require DNA–RNA transcription or new RNA synthesis[177]. Wong et al.[178] found 1,25(OH)$_2D_3$ to be

* The metabolite originally identified as 21,25-(OH)$_3D_3$ recently has been found by the DeLuca group to be 24,25-(OH)$_2D_3$.

5.5 times more effective than cholecalciferol, and 3.6 times more effective than 25-(OH)D_3 in stimulating bone calcium mobilisation in chicks and rats; in addition the 1,25-derivative acted more rapidly than the other forms of vitamin D_3.

Fraser and Kodicek demonstrated that 1,25-(OH)$_2D_3$ is produced in renal tissue from 25-(OH)D_3 and that calcium concentrations of 10^{-4} to 10^{-5} M inhibited the hydroxylation of 25-(OH)D_3 by incubated kidney slices[179]. Boyle et al.[180] reported an inverse relationship between the formation of 1,25-(OH)$_2D_3$ from 25-(OH)D_3 and the blood calcium level. At blood calcium levels above 9.6 mg per 100 ml, the conversion to 1,25-(OH)$_2D_3$ was repressed and increased amounts of 21,25-(OH)$_2D_3$ were detected. At blood calcium levels below 9.6 mg per 100 ml, the conversion to 1,25-(OH)$_2D_3$ was stimulated and decreased amounts of 21,25-(OH)$_2D_3$ were found. Based on these observations, Boyle et al.[180] suggested that either the blood calcium level or the hormones regulating blood calcium (PTH and TCT) could control the rate of conversion of 25-(OH)D_3 to 1,25-(OH)$_2D_3$ and that this feedback system represented the 'endogenous factor' proposed by Nicolaysen over two decades ago.

The possibility that PTH and TCT might directly regulate the conversion of vitamin D to its biologically-active metabolites stimulated additional studies by several groups of investigators. At first there was disagreement; Galante et al.[181] concluded that PTH inhibits renal conversion of 25-(OH)D_3 to 1,25-(OH)$_2D_3$, while Garabedian et al.[182] found that it stimulated the conversion. The latter conclusion appears to be the correct one since other laboratories have confirmed Garabedian et al.[182]. Garabedian et al.[182] postulated that PTH increased the cellular level of cyclic-AMP which, in turn, led to activation of a hydroxylase responsible for the conversion of 25-(OH)D_3 to 1,25-(OH)$_2D_3$. In addition to demonstrating the PTH-stimulated conversion during hypocalcaemia, they showed that the conversion was not dependent on an elevation of the blood calcium above normal. Rasmussen et al.[183] also reported that PTH enhances the renal conversion to 1,25-(OH)$_2D_3$ by isolated chick renal tubules. Both PTH and cyclic-AMP stimulated the renal conversion of 25-(OH)D_3 to 1,25-(OH)$_2D_3$ while TCT inhibited it. Kodicek has confirmed the stimulatory effect of PTH on the renal conversion of 25-(OH)D_3 to 1,25-(OH)$_2D_3$. The stimulation of this renal conversion, attributed to TCT in the experiments of Galante et al.[184], may have been due to PTH released in response to the TCT-induced hypocalcaemia.

Intestinal calcium binding proteins, first demonstrated by Wasserman and his colleagues, are dependent on vitamin D for their formation. The mucosal concentration of calcium binding proteins increases after vitamin D is given to D-deficient chicks, and there is a positive correlation between the increase in calcium transport and the concentration of the calcium binding proteins. DeLuca and his co-workers have identified a calcium-dependent ATPase which they detect before the appearance of calcium binding proteins and which they feel correlates better than calcium-binding protein with increased intestinal calcium transport. The Wisconsin group proposes that 1,25-(OH)$_2D_3$ converts a precursor protein to calcium binding proteins which interact in some unknown way with the membrane bound ATPase to increase calcium transport[177]. The precursor protein, detectable in the mucosal cells of D-deficient animals, may be cleaved by a peptidase activated directly by $1,25\text{-}(OH)_2D_3$. The differences between the Wasserman group and the De-Luca group have not yet been resolved.

Acknowledgements

The authors express appreciation to Mrs. Martha Byrd for assistance in the preparation of the manuscript. The preparation of this review was assisted by a research grant from the National Institute of Arthritis and Metabolic Diseases (AM-10558) and by a USPHS General Research Support Grant (FR-5406). Cary W. Cooper is the recipient of a Career Development Award from the National Institute of Arthritis and Metabolic Diseases (AM-50293) and a Merck Grant for Faculty Development.

References

1. Talmage, R. V. and Munson, P. L. (editors) (1972). *Calcium, Parathyroid Hormone and the Calcitonins*, (Amsterdam: Excerpta Medica)
2. Taylor, S. (editor) (1972). *Endocrinology 1971* (London: Heinemann)
3. Nichols, G. Jr. and Wasserman, R. H. (editors) (1971). *Cellular Mechanisms for Calcium Transfer and Homeostasis*, (New York: Academic Press)
4. Scow, R. O. (editor) (in the press), *Proceedings IV International Congress of Endocrinology*, 1972, (Amsterdam: Excerpta Medica)
5. Parsons, J. A. and Potts, J. T. Jr. (1972). *Clinics in Endocrinology and Metabolism*, Vol. 1, No. 1, (I. MacIntyre, editor) (Philadelphia: Saunders)
6. Potts, J. T. Jr., Keutmann, H. T., Niall, H. D., Tregear, G. W., Habener, J. F., O'Riordan, J. L. H., Murray, T. M., Powell, D. and Aurbach, G. D. (1972). Parathyroid hormone: Chemical and immunochemical studies of the active molecular species. In Ref. 2, p. 333
7. Potts, J. T. Jr., Keutmann, H. T., Niall, H. D., Habener, J. F., Tregear, G. W., Deftos, L. J., O'Riordan, J. L. H. and Aurbach, G. D. (1972). Chemistry of the parathyroid hormones: clinical and physiological implications. In Ref. 1, p. 159
8. Keutmann, H. T., Aurbach, G. D., Dawson, B. F., Niall, H. D., Deftos, L. J. and Potts, J. T. Jr. (1971). Isolation and characterization of the bovine parathyroid iso-hormones. *Biochemistry*, **10**, 2779
9. Brewer, H. B. Jr. (1972). Chemistry and conformation of the bovine parathyroid hormone. In Ref. 2, p. 324
10. Aloj, S. and Edelhoch, H. (1972). Structural studies on polypeptide hormones. II. Parathyroid hormone. *Arch. Biochem. Biophys.*, **150**, 782
11. Woodhead, J. S., O'Riordan, J. L. H., Keutmann, H. T., Stoltz, M. L., Dawson, B. F., Niall, H. D., Robinson, C. J. and Potts, J. T. Jr. (1971). Isolation and chemical properties of porcine parathyroid hormone. *Biochemistry*, **10**, 2787
12. Woodhead, J. S. and O'Riordan, J. L. H. (1971). Immunological properties of porcine parathyroid hormone. *J. Endocrinol.*, **49**, 79
13. O'Riordan, J. L. H., Potts, J. T., Jr. and Aurbach, G. D. (1971). Isolation of human parathyroid hormone. *Endocrinology*, **89**, 234
14. Brewer, H. B. Jr., Fairwell, T., Ronan, R., Sizemore, G. W. and Arnaud, C. D. (1972). Human parathyroid hormone, amino acid sequence of the amino terminal residues 1–34. *Proc. Nat. Acad. Sci. (U.S.A.)*, **69**, 3585
15. Jacobs, J. W., Sauer, R. T., Niall, H. D., Keutmann, H. T., O'Riordan, J. L. H., Aurbach, G. D. and Potts, J. T. Jr. (1973). High sensitivity *N*-terminal sequence analysis of human parathyroid hormone. *Fed. Proc. (Fed. Amer. Soc. Exp. Biol.)* **32**, 648 (Abstr.)

16. Potts, J. T. Jr., Tregear, G. W., Keutmann, H. T., Niall, H. D., Sauer, R., Deftos, L. J., Dawson, B. F., Hogan, M. and Aurbach, G. D. (1971). Synthesis of a biologically active N-terminal tetratriacontapeptide of parathyroid hormone. *Proc. Nat. Acad. Sci. (U.S.A.)*, **68**, 63

17. Potts, J. T. Jr., Murray, T. M., Peacock, M., Niall, H. D., Tregear, G. W., Keutmann, H. T., Powell, D. and Deftos, L. J. (1971). Parathyroid hormone: sequence, synthesis, immunoassay studies. *Amer. J. Med.*, **50**, 639

18. Hamilton, J. W., MacGregor, R. R., Chu, L. L. H. and Cohn, D. V. (1971). Isolation and partial purification of a nonparathyroid hormone calcemic fraction from bovine parathyroid glands. *Endocrinology*, **89**, 1440

19. Cohn, D. V., MacGregor, R. R., Chu, L. L. H. and Hamilton, J. W. (1972). Studies on the biosynthesis *in vitro* of parathyroid hormone and other calcemic polypeptides of the parathyroid gland. In Ref. 1, p. 173.

20. Cohn, D. V., MacGregor, R. R., Chu, L. L., Kimmel, J. R. and Hamilton, J.W. (1972). Calcemic fraction-A. Biosynthetic peptide precursor of parathyroid hormone. *Proc. Nat. Acad. Sci. (U.S.A.)*, **69**, 1521

21. Kemper, B., Habener, J. F., Potts, J. T. Jr. and Rich, A. (1972). Proparathyroid hormone. Identification of a biosynthetic precursor to parathyroid hormone. *Proc. Nat. Acad. Sci. (U.S.A.)*, **69**, 643

22. Habener, J. F., Kemper, B., Potts, J. T. Jr. and Rich, A. (1972). Proparathyroid hormone: biosynthesis by human parathyroid adenomas. *Science*, **178**, 630

23. Martin, T. J. (1973). Peptide hormone production by human tumours in cell culture. In Ref. 4

24. Segre, G. V., Singer, F. R., Habener, J. F., Benney, C. and Potts, J. T. Jr. (1972). Characterization of immunoreactive metabolites of bovine parathyroid hormone by sequence-specific radioimmunoassays. *Clin. Res.*, **20**, 883

25. Habener, J. F., Segre, G. V., Powell, D. and Potts, J. T. Jr. (1972). Characterization of the immunoreactive hormone in the circulation of man. *Nature (London)*, **238**, 152

26. Hirsch, P. F., Cooper, C. W. and Munson, P. L. (1972). Parathyroid hormone: measurement-bioassay. *Methods in investigative and diagnostic endocrinology*. Vol. 2, in the press (S. Berson, editor) (New York: American Elsevier/North Holland)

27. Dacke, C. G. and Kenny, A. D. (1972). An avian bioassay for parathyroid hormone. *Fed. Proc. (Fed. Amer. Soc. Exp. Biol.)*, **31**, 225

28. Deftos, L. J., Murray, T. M., Powell, D., Habener, J. F., Singer, F. R., Mayer, G. P. and Potts, J. T. Jr. (1972). Radioimmunoassays for parathyroid hormones and calcitonins. Ref. 1, p. 140

29. Targonovik, J. H., Rodman, J. S. and Sherwood, L. S. (1971). Regulation of parathyroid hormone secretion *in vitro:* quantitative aspects of calcium and magnesium ion control. *Endocrinology*, **88**, 1477

30. Arnaud, C. D., Tsao, H. S. and Littledike, E. T. (1971). Radioimmunoassay of human parathyroid hormone in serum. *J. Clin. Invest.*, **50**, 21

31. Cushard, W. G. Jr., Creditor, M. A., Canterbury, J. M. and Reiss, E. (1972). Physiologic hyperparathyroidism in pregnancy. *J. Clin. Endocrinol. Metab.*, **34**, 767

32. Addison, G. M., Hales, C. N., Woodhead, J. S. and O'Riordan, J. L. H. (1971). Immunoradiometric assay of parathyroid hormone. *J. Endocrinol.*, **49**, 521

33. Brand, J. S. and Raisz, L. G. (1972). Effects of thyrocalcitonin and phosphate ion on the parathyroid hormone stimulated resorption of bone. *Endocrinology*, **90**, 479

34. Raisz, L. G., Trummel, C. L. and Simmons, H. (1972). Induction of bone in tissue culture: prolonged response after brief exposure to parathyroid hormone or 25-hydroxycholecalciferol. *Endocrinology*, **90**, 744

35. Wener, J. A., Gorton, S. J. and Raisz, L. G. (1972). Escape from inhibition of resorption in cultures of fetal bone treated with calcitonin and parathyroid hormone. *Endocrinology*, **90**, 752

36. Reynolds, J. J. (1972). A sensitive *in vivo/in vitro* method for studying substances that influence the resorption of bone. Ref. 1, p. 454

37. Talmage, R. V. (1972). Further studies on the control of calcium homeostasis by parathyroid hormone. Ref. 1, p. 422

38. Neuman, W. F. (1972). The bone: blood equilibrium: a possible system for its study *in vitro*. Ref. 1, p. 389

39. Borle, A. B. (1972). Parathyroid hormone and cell calcium. Ref. 1, p. 484

40. Rasmussen, H., Kurokawa, K., Mason, J. and Goodman, D. B. P. (1972). Cyclic AMP, calcium and cell activation. Ref. 1, p. 492
41. Parsons, J. A. and Robinson, C. J. (1972). The earliest effects of parathyroid hormone and calcitonin on blood–bone calcium distribution. Ref. 1, p. 399
42. Parsons, J. A. and Robinson, C. J. (1971). Calcium shift into bone causing transient hypocalcemia after injection of parathyroid hormone. *Nature (London)*, **230**, 581
43. Parsons, J. A., Neer, R. M. and Potts, J. T. Jr. (1971). Initial fall of plasma calcium after intravenous injection of parathyroid hormone. *Endocrinology*, **89**, 735
44. Agus, Z. S., Puschett, J. B., Senesky, D. and Goldberg, M. (1971). Mode of action of parathyroid hormone and cyclic adenosine 3′,5′-monophosphate on renal tubular phosphate reabsorption in the dog. *J. Clin. Invest.*, **50**, 617
45. Goldberg, M., Agus, Z. S., Puschett, J. B. and Senesky, D. (1972). Mode of phosphaturic action of parathyroid hormone: micropuncture studies. Ref. 1, p. 273
46. Nordin, B. E. C., Peacock, M. and Wilkinson, R. (1972). The relative importance of gut, bone and kidney in the regulation of serum calcium. Ref. 1, p. 263
47. Biddulph, D. (1972). Influence of parathyroid hormone and the kidney on maintenance of blood calcium concentration in the golden hamster. *Endocrinology*, **90**, 1113
48. Olson, E. B. Jr., DeLuca, H. F. and Potts, J. T. Jr. (1972). The effect of calcitonin and parathyroid hormone on calcium transport of isolated intestine. Ref. 1, p. 240
49. Birge, S. J. and Gilbert, H. F. (1972). The influence of parathyroid hormone on intestinal Ca transport. Ref. 1, p. 247
50. Clark, I. and Rivera-Cordero, F. (1973). Effects of endogenous parathyroid hormone on calcium, magnesium and phosphate metabolism in the rat. *Endocrinology*, **92**, 62
51. Chausmer, A. B., Sherman, B. S. and Wallach, S. (1972). The effect of parathyroid hormone on hepatic cell transport of calcium. *Endocrinology*, **90**, 663
52. MacManus, J. P., Youdale, T., Whitfield, J. F. and Franks, D. J. (1972). The mediations by calcium and cyclic-AMP of the stimulatory action of parathyroid hormone on thymic lymphocyte proliferation. Ref. 1, p. 338
53. Peng, T.-C. and Munson, P. L. (1972). The thyroid gland in the prevention of nephrocalcinosis induced by parathyroid hormone in rats. *Abstr. 5th Intern. Cong. Pharmacol.*, in the press
54. Aurbach, G. D., Marcus, R., Heersche, J. N. M., Winickoff, R. N. and Marx, S. J. (1972). Cyclic nucleotides in the action of native and synthetic parathyroid and calcitonin peptides. Ref. 1, p. 502
55. Dufresne, L. R. and Gitelman, H. J. (1972). A possible role of adenyl cyclase in the regulation of parathyroid activity by calcium. Ref. 1, p. 202
56. Abe, M. and Sherwood, L. M. (1972). Regulation of secretion of parathyroid hormone by cyclic 3′,5′-AMP. *Abstr. 4th Internat. Cong. Endocrinol., Internat. Cong. Ser. 256*, 94 (Amsterdam: Excerpta Medica)
57. Reitz, R., Mayer, G. P., Deftos, L. J., and Potts, J. T., Jr. (1971). Endogenous parathyroid hormone response to thyrocalcitonin-induced hypocalcemia in the cow. *Endocrinology*, **89**, 932
58. Fischer, J. A., Oldham, S. B., Sizemore, G. W. and Arnaud, C. D. (1971). Calcitonin stimulation of parathyroid hormone secretion *in vitro*. *Horm. Metab. Res.*, **3**, 223
59. Fujita, T., Ohata, M., Orimo, H. and Yoshikawa, M. (1971). Age and parathyroid hormone inactivation by kidney tissue. *J. Geront.*, **26**, 20
60. Fang, V. S. and Tashjian, A. H. Jr. (1972). Studies on the role of the liver in the metabolism of parathyroid hormone. *Endocrinology*, **90**, 1177
61. Hirsch, P. F. and Munson, P. L. (1969). Thyrocalcitonin. *Physiol. Rev.*, **49**, 548
62. Pearse, A. G. E. and Polak, J. M. (1972). The neural crest origin of the endocrine polypeptide cells of the APUD series. Ref. 2, p. 145
63. Nunez, E. A. and Gershon, M. D. (1972). Synthesis and storage of serotonin by parafollicular (C) cells of the thyroid gland of active, prehibernating and hibernating bats. *Endocrinology*, **90**, 1008
64. Pearse, A. G. E., Polak, J. M. and Van Noorden, S. (1972). The neural crest origin of the C cells and their comparative cytochemistry and ultrastructure in the ultimobranchial gland. Ref. 1, p. 29
65. Douarin, N. and Lievre, C. (1970). Demonstration of the neural origin of the ultimobranchial body glandular cells in the avian embryo. *C. R. Acad. Sci. (Paris), Ser. D*, **270**, 2857

66. Kaplan, E. L., Hill, B. J., Sizemore, G. and Peskin, G. W. (1972). Extrathyroidal sources of calcitonin in the pig. *Clin. Res.*, **20**, 724
67. Kaplan, E. L., Sizemore, G., Hill, B. J. and Peskin, G. W. (1972). Calcitonin in non-thyroid tumors in man. *Clin. Res.*, **20**, 724
68. Voelkel, E., Tashjian, A., Davidoff, F., Cohen, R. and Perlia, C. (1972). Neuroecto-derm, calcitonin and catecholamines in man. *Abstr. 4th Internat. Cong. Endocrinol.*, *Internat. Cong. Ser.* 256, 174 (Amsterdam: Excerpta Medica)
69. Hakanson, R., Lundquist, I., Melander, A., Owman, Ch., Sjoberg, N. O. and Sundler, F. (1972). Significance of amines in polypeptide secreting endocrine cells with special regard to the C cells. Ref. 2, p. 184
70. Hakanson, R., Owman, Ch. and Sundler, F. (1971). Aromatic L-amino acid decar-boxylase in calcitonin producing cells. *Biochem. Pharmacol.*, **20**, 2187
71. Atkins, F. L., Beaven, M. A. and Keiser, H. R. (1972). High DOPA decarboxylase activity in medullary carcinoma of the thyroid. *Clin. Res,*, **20**, 884
72. Potts, J. T. Jr., Niall, H. D., Keutmann, H. T. and Lequin, R. M. (1972). Chemistry of the calcitonins: Species variation plus structure activity relations and pharmacologic implications. Ref. 1, p. 121
73. Keutmann, H. T., Lequin, R. M., Habener, J. F., Singer, F. R., Niall, H. D. and Potts, J. T. Jr. (1972). Chemistry and physiology of the calcitonins: Some recent advances. Ref. 2, p. 316
74. Pless, J., Bauer, W., Bossert, H., Zehnder, K. and Guttman, St. (1972). Synthesis of highly active analogues of salmon calcitonin. Ref. 2, p. 67
75. Orimo, H., Ohata, M., Fujita, T., Yoshikawa, M., Higashi, T., Abe, J., Watanabe, S. and Otani, K. (1972). Ultimobranchial calcitonin of Anguilla Japonica. Ref. 2, p. 49
76. Byfield, P. G. H., Clark, M. B., Turner, K., Nathanson, B. M., Foster, G. V. and MacIntyre, I. (1971). Immunochemical studies on human calcitonin-M leading to information on the shape of the molecule. *Biochem. J.*, **122**, 33
77. Brewer, H. B. Jr. (1970). Bovine thyrocalcitonin. *Calcitonin 1969*, 14 (S. Taylor, editor) (London: Heinemann)
78. Ontjes, D. A., Roberts, J. C., Hennessy, J. F., Burford, H. J. and Cooper, C. W. (1973). Biological and immunological activity of a thyrocalcitonin produced by the solid phase method of peptide synthesis. *Endocrinology*, **92**, 1780
79. Rivaille, P. and Milhaud, G. (1972). Solid phase synthesis of human thyrocalcitonin. *Helv. Chim. Acta*, **55**, 1617
80. Nieto, A. and R-Candela, J. L. (1972). Chicken calcitonin: Isolation and biological properties. Ref. 2, p. 55
81. Cooper, C. W., Hirsch, P. F. and Munson, P. L. (1972). Thyrocalcitonin: measurement-bioassay. *Methods in Investigative and Diagnostic Endocrinology*, Vol. II, in the press (S. Berson, editor) (New York: American Elsevier/North Holland)
82. Kenny, A. D. (1971). Determination of calcitonin in plasma by bioassay. *Endocrinology*, **89**, 1005
83. Kenny, A. D., Boelkins, J. N., Dacke, C. G., Fleming, W. R. and Hanson, R. C. (1972). Plasma calcitonin levels in birds and fishes. Ref. 2, p. 39
84. Gonnerman, W. A., Breitenbach, R. P., Erfling, W. F. and Anast, C. S. (1972). An analysis of ultimobranchial gland function in the chicken. *Endocrinology*, **91**, 1423
85. Raisz, L. G., Wener, J. A., Trummel, C. L., Feinblatt, J. D. and Au, W. Y. W. (1972). Induction, inhibition and escape as phenomena of bone resorption. Ref. 1, p. 446
86. Marcus, R., Heersche, J. N. M. and Aurbach, G. D. (1971). Effects of calcitonin on formation of 3′,5′-cyclic AMP in bone and kidney. *Endocrinology*, **88** (Suppl.), A-68
87. Deftos, L. J., Bury, A. E., Mayer, G. P., Habener, J. F., Singer, F. R., Powell, D., Krook, L., Watts, E. and Potts, J. T., Jr. (1972). Radioimmunoassays for calcitonins: clinical and experimental studies. Ref. 2, p. 89
88. Milhaud, G., Tharaud, D., Julbenne, A. and Moukhtar, M. S. (1972). Radioimmuno-assay of rat calcitonin. Ref. 2, p. 380
89. Buckle, R. M. (1971). Development of a radioimmunoassay for calcitonin. *J. Endo-crinol.*, **51**, 7
90. Cooper, C. W., Deftos, L. J. and Potts, J. T. Jr. (1971). Direct measurement of *in vivo* secretion of pig TCT by radioimmunoassay. *Endocrinology*, **88**, 747
91. Care, A. D., Bates, R. F. L., Swaminathan, R. and Ganguli, P. C. (1971). The role of gastrin as a calcitonin secretogogue. *J. Endocrinol.*, **51**, 735

92. Cooper, C. W., Schwesinger, W. H., Mahgoub, A. M., Ontjes, D. A., Gray, T. K. and Munson, P. L. (1972). Regulation of secretion of thyrocalcitonin. Ref. 1, p. 128
93. Tashjian, A. H. Jr., Howland, B. G., Melvin, K. E. and Hill, C. S. (1970). Immuno-assay of human calcitonin. *New Engl. J. Med.*, **283**, 890
94. Tashjian, A. H. Jr., Melvin, K. E. W., Voelkel, E. F., Howland, B. G., Zuckerman, J. E. and Minkin, C. (1972). Calcitonin in blood, urine and tissue: immunological and biological studies. Ref. 1, p. 97
95. Deftos, L. J. (1971). Immunoassay for human calcitonin. I. Method. *Metabolism*, **20**, 1122
96. Deftos, L. J., Bury, A. E., Habener, J. F., Singer, F. R., and Potts, J. T. Jr. (1971). Immunoassay for human calcitonin. II. Clinical studies. *Metabolism*, **20**, 1129
97. Deftos, L. J., Goodman, A. D., Engelman, K. and Potts, J. T. Jr. (1971). Suppression and stimulation of calcitonin secretion in medullary thyroid carcinoma. *Metabolism* **20**, 428 ,
98. Huefner, M. and Hesch, R. D. (1971). Radioimmunochemical determination of human calcitonin. *Klin. Wochenschr.*, **49**, 1149
99. Kennedy, J. W., III and Talmage, R. V. (1971). Influence of the thyroids on the rate of removal of recently deposited radiocalcium and radiophosphorus from bone. *Endocrinology*, **88**, 1203
100. Talmage, R. V., Anderson, J. J. B. and Cooper, C. W. (1972). The influence of cal-citonins on the disappearance of radiocalcium and radiophosphorus from plasma. *Endocrinology*, **90**, 1185
101. Sorensen, O. H., Hindberg, I. and Bank-Mikkelsen, O. (1971). Hydroxyproline, calcium, and magnesium content of bones in rats after long term treatment with thyrocalcitonin. *Acta Endocrinol.*, **68**, 203
102. Matrajt-Denys, H., Tun-Chot, S., Bordier, P., Hioco, D., Clark, M. B., Pennock, J., Doyle, F. H. and Foster, G. V. (1971). Effect of calcitonin on vitamin A-induced changes in bone in the rat. *Endocrinology*, **88**, 129
103. Klein, D. C. and Raizs, L. G. (1971). Role of adenosine 3′,5′-monophosphate in the hormonal regulation of bone resorption: Studies with cultured fetal bone. *Endo-crinology*, **89**, 818
104. Belanger, L. F. and Copp, D. H. (1972). Skeletal effects of prolonged calcitonin admini-stration in birds under various conditions. Ref. 1, p. 41
105. Mills, B. G., Haroutenian, A. M., Holst, P., Bordier, P. and Tun-Chot, S. (1972). Ultrastructural and cellular changes at the costochondral junction following *in vivo* treatment with calcitonin or $CaCl_2$ in the rabbit. Ref. 2, p. 79
106. Kallio, D. M., Garant, P. R. and Minkin, C. (1972). Evidence for an ultrastructural effect of calcitonin on osteoclasts in tissue culture. Ref. 1, p. 383
107. Matthews, J. L., Martin, J. H., Collins, E. J., Kennedy, J. W., III and Powell, E. L. Jr. (1972). Immediate changes in the ultrastructure of bone cells following thyro-calcitonin administration. Ref. 1, p. 375
108. Sorensen, O. H. and Hindberg, I. (1972). The acute and prolonged effect of porcine calcitonin on urine electrolyte excretion in intact and parathyroidectomized rats. *Acta Endocrinol.*, **70**, 295
109. Nielsen, S. P., Buchanan-Lee, B., Matthews, E. W., Moseley, J. M. and Williams, C. C. (1971). Acute effects of synthetic porcine calcitonins on the renal excretion of magnesium, inorganic phosphate, sodium and potassium. *J. Endocrinol.*, **51**, 455
110. Pak, C. Y. C., Ruskin, B. and Caspen, A. (1970). Renal effects of porcine thyrocal-citonin in the dog. *Endocrinology*, **87**, 262
111. Barlet, J. P. (1972). Effect of porcine, salmon and human calcitonin on urinary excretion of some electrolytes in sheep. *J. Endocrinol.*, **55**, 153
112. Haas, H. G., Dambacher, M. A., Guncaga, J. and Lauffenburger, T. (1971). Renal effects of calcitonin and parathyroid extract in man. *J. Clin. Invest.*, **50**, 2689
113. Paillard, F., Ardaillou, R., Malendin, H., Fillastre, J. P. and Prier, S. (1972). Renal effects of salmon calcitonin in man. *J. Lab. Clin. Med.*, **80**, 202
114. Bijvoet, O. L. M., van der Sluys Veer, J., deVries, H. R., and van Koppen, A. T. J. (1971). Natriuretic effect of calcitonin in man. *New Engl. J. Med.*, **284**, 681
115. Sorensen, O. H., Friis, T., Hindberg, I. and Nielsen, S. P. (1970). The effect of calci-tonin injected into hypercalcemic and normocalcemic patients. *Acta Med. Scand.*, **187**, 283

116. Sorensen, O. H., Hindberg, I. and Friis, T. (1972). The renal effect of calcitonin in hypoparathyroid patients. *Acta Med. Scand.*, **191**, 103
117. Olson, E. B., Jr., DeLuca, H. F. and Potts, J. T. Jr. (1972). Calcitonin inhibition of vitamin D-induced intestinal calcium absorption. *Endocrinology*, **90**, 151
118. Shai, F., Baker, R. K. and Wallach, S. (1971). The clinical and metabolic effects of porcine calcitonin on Paget's disease of bone. *J. Clin. Invest.*, **50**, 1927
119. Milhaud, G., Calmettes, C., Julienne, A., Tharaud, D., Block-Michel, H., Cavaillon, J. P., Colin, R. and Moukhtar, M. S. (1972). A new chapter in human pathology: calcitonin disorders and therapeutic use. Ref. 1, p. 56
120. Pak, C. Y. C., Zisman, E., Evens, R., Jowsey, J., Delea, C. S. and Bartter, F. C. (1969). The treatment of osteoporosis with calcium infusions. *Amer. J. Med.*, **47**, 7
121. Pak, C. Y. C. (1971). Parathyroid hormone and thyrocalcitonin: their mode of action and regulation. *Ann. New York Acad. Sci.*, **179**, 450
122. Gray, T. K. and Juan, D. (1973). Salmon calcitonin and the net jejunal calcium transport *in vivo*. *Clin. Res.*, **21**, 625
123. Hesch, R. D., Schmidt, M., Hufner, M., Winkler, K., Hasenjager, M., Paschen, K., Becker, H. J., Fuchs, K. and Creutzfeldt, W. (1972). Gastrointestinal effects of calcitonin in man. Ref. 2, p. 265
124. Orimo, H., Yoshida, A. and Fujita, T. (1972). Calcitonin inhibition of gastric secretion in man. *Clinical Aspects of Metabolic Bone Disease*, in the press (A. M. Parfitt and B. Frame editors) (Amsterdam: Excerpta Medica)
125. Hufner, M., Hesch, R. D., Schmidt, H., Hasenjager, M., Winkler, K., Creutzfeldt, W. and Paschen, K. (1972). Gastrointestinal effects of calcitonin. *Acta Endocrinol.*, **159** (Suppl.), 65
126. Ziegler, R., Minne, H. and Bellwinkel, S. (1972). The influences of experimentally induced hypercalcemia and hypocalcemia on gastric function in rat and man. Ref. 2, p. 307
127. Hottermuller, K. H., Go, V. L. W., Sizemore, G. W., Arnaud, C. D. and Goldsmith, R. S. (1972). Dissociation of calcitonin, parathyroid hormone, and intraluminal calcium effects on gastric secretion in man. *Clin. Res.*, **20**, 732
128. Murad, F., Brewer, H. B. and Vaughan, M. (1970). Effect of thyrocalcitonin on adenosine 3′,5′-cyclic phosphate formation by rat kidney and bone. *Proc. Nat. Acad. Sci. (U.S.A.)*, **65**, 446
129. Vaes, G. (1972). Inhibitory actions of calcitonin on resorbing bone explants in culture and on their release of lysosomal hydrolases. *J. Dent. Res.*, **51**, 362
130. Orimo, H., Ohata, M. and Fujita, T. (1971). Role of inorganic pyrophosphatase in the mechanism of action of parathyroid hormone and calcitonin. *Endocrinology*, **89**, 852
131. Feinblatt, J. D. and Raisz, L. G. (1971). Secretion of thyrocalcitonin in organ culture. *Endocrinology*, **88**, 797
132. Deftos, L. J., Watts, E. G. and Copp, D. H. (1972). Sex differences in calcitonin secretion by salmon. *Abstr. 4th Internat. Cong. Endocrinol.*, Internat. Cong. Ser. 256, 180 (Amsterdam: Excerpta Medica)
133. Cooper, C. W., Gray, T. K., Hundley, J. D. and Mahgoub, A. M. (1971). Secretion of thyrocalcitonin and its regulation. *Recent Advances in Endocrinology*, Internat. Cong. Ser. 238, 349 (E. Mattar, G. B. Mattar and V. H. T. James, editors) (Amsterdam Excerpta Medica)
134. Care, A. D. (1970). The effects of pancreozymin and secretin on calcitonin release. *Fed. Proc. (Fed. Amer. Soc. Exp. Biol.)*, **29**, 253
135. Cooper, C. W., Schwesinger, W. H., Mahgoub, A. M. and Ontjes, D. A. (1971). Thyrocalcitonin: Stimulation of secretion by pentagastrin. *Science*, **172**, 1238
136. Cooper, C. W., Schwesinger, W. H., Ontjes, D. A., Mahgoub, A. M. and Munson, P. L. (1972). Stimulation of secretion of pig thyrocalcitonin by gastrin and related hormonal peptides. *Endocrinology*, **91**, 1079
137. Care, A. D., Bates, R. F. L., Swaminathan, R. and Ganguli, P. C. (1971). The role of gastrin as a calcitonin secretagogue. *J. Endocrinol.*, **5**, 381
138. Cooper, C. W., Biggerstaff, C. R., Wiseman, C. W. and Carlone, M. F. (1972). Hypocalcemic effect of pentagastrin and related gastrointestinal hormones in the rat. *Endocrinology*, **91**, 63
139. McGuire, A., Cohen, S. and Brooks, F. P. (1972). Serum gastrin and calcium levels in man during the infusion of synthetic human gastrin. *Clin. Res.*, **20**, 734

140. Care, A. D., Bruce, J. B., Boelkins, J., Kenny, A. D., Conaway, H. and Anast, C. S. (1971). Role of pancreozymin-cholecystokinin and structurally related compounds as calcitonin secretagogues. *Endocrinology*, **89**, 262

141. Avioli, L. V., Shieber, W. M. and Kipnis, D. M. (1971). Role of glucagon and adrenergic receptors in thyrocalcitonin release in the dog. *Endocrinology*, **88**, 1337

142. Cooper, C. W., McGuigan, J. E., Ontjes, D. A., Hennessy, J. F., Schwesinger, W. H. and Gray, T. K. (1973). Control of secretion of parathyroid hormone and thyrocalcitonin. Ref. 4, in the press

143. Deftos, L. J., Habener, J. F., Krook, L. and Mayer, G. P. (1972). Multiple endocrine adenomatosis and calcitonin secretion in the bovine species. *Clin. Res.*, **20**, 544

144. Sizemore, G., Leffler, J., Fischer, J., Oldham, S., Goldsmith, R. and Arnaud, C. (1972). Physiological aspects of human calcitonin secretion. *Clin. Res.*, **20**, 441

145. Care, A. D., Bell, N. H. and Bates, R. F. L. (1971). The effects of hypermagnesemia on calcitonin secretion *in vivo*. *J. Endocrinol.*, **51**, 381

146. Bell, N. H. (1970). Effects of glucagon, dibutyryl cyclic 3′,5′-adenosine monophosphate, and theophylline on calcitonin secretion *in vitro*. *J. Clin. Invest.*, **49**, 1368

147. Care, A. D., Bates, R. F. L. and Gitelman, H. J. (1970). A possible role for the adenyl cyclase system in calcitonin release. *J. Endocrinol.*, **48**, 1

148. Powell, D. and Deftos, L. J. (1972). Secretion of calcitonin in pseudohypoparathyroidism and other hypocalcemic states. *Abstr. 4th Internat. Cong. Endocrinol.*, Internat. Cong. Ser. 256, 179 (Amsterdam: Excerpta Medica)

149. Deftos, L. J., Swenson, K. and Bode, H. (1972). Parathyroid hormone and calcitonin inter-relationships in clinical disorders of calcium metabolism. *Clin. Res.*, **20**, 424

150. Hennessy, J. F., Gray, T. K., Ontjes, D. A. and Cooper, C. W. (1973). Stimulation of thyrocalcitonin secretion by pentagastrin and calcium in two patients with medullary carcinoma of the thyroid. *J. Clin. Endocrinol. Metab.*, **36**, 200

151. Phillippo, M., Bates, R. F. L. and Lawrence, C. B. (1971). The effect of progesterone on calcitonin release in the sheep. *J. Endocrinol.*, **51**, vi

152. Copp, D. H., Byfield, P. G. H., Kerr, C. R., Newsome, F., Walker, V. and Watts, E. G. (1972). Calcitonin and ultimobranchial function in fishes and birds. Ref. 1, p. 12

153. Orimo, H., Fujita, T., Yoshikawa, M., Abe, J., Watanabe, S. and Otani, K. (1972). Ultimobranchial calcitonin in Anguilla Japonica (Japanese eel). *Abstr. 4th Internat. Cong. Endocrinol.*, Internat. Cong. Ser. 256, 181 (Amsterdam: Excerpta Medica)

154. Habener, J. F., Singer, R. F., Neer, R. M., Deftos, L. J. and Potts, J. T. Jr. (1972). Metabolism of salmon and porcine calcitonins: An explanation for the increased potency of salmon calcitonins. Ref. 1, p. 152

155. Hankers, J., Milhaud, G., Staub, J. F. and Dubert, A. (1971). Kinetics and mechanism of thryocalcitonin inactivation by different tissues. *Acta Biol. Med. Gen.*, **26**, 1157

156. Singer, F. R., Greene, E., Godin, P. and Habener, J. F. (1972). Metabolism of the calcitonins in the dog. *Abstr. 4th Internat. Cong. Endocrinol.*, Internat. Cong. Ser. 256, 180 (Amsterdam: Excerpta Medica)

157. Foster, G. V., Clark, M. B., Williams, C., Nathanson, B. M., Horton, R., Buranapong, P. and Glass, H. I. (1972). Metabolic fate of human calcitonin in dog. Ref. 2, p. 71

158. Voelkel, E. F. and Tashjian, A. H. Jr. (1970). Measurement of thyrocalcitonin-like activity in the urine of patients with medullary carcinoma. *J. Clin. Endocrinol. Metab.*, **32**, 102

159. Marx, S. J., Woodard, C. J. and Aurbach, G. D. (1972). Calcitonin receptors of kidney and bone. *Science*, **178**, 1000

160. Riggs, B. L., Arnaud, C. D., Goldsmith, R. S., Taylor, W. E., McCall, J. T. and Sessler, A. D. (1971). Plasma kinetics and acute effects of pharmacologic doses of porcine thyrocalcitonin in man. *J. Clin. Endocrinol. Metab.*, **33**, 115

161. Greenberg, P. B., Martin, T. J., Melick, R. A., Jablonski, P. and Watts, J. McK. (1972). Calcitonin clearance in the pig and in the isolated perfused pig liver. *J. Endocrinol.*, **54**, 125

162. Heaney, R. P. and Skillman, T. G. (1971). Calcium metabolism in nomal human pregnancy. *J. Clin. Endocrinol. Metab.*, **33**, 661

163. Harper, C., Kristoffersen, U. M. and Toverud, S. U. (1973). Thyrocalcitonin and parathyroid hormone in calcium homeostasis during lactation. *Abstracts, Internat. Assoc. Dental Research*, Washington, D.C., April 12–15, 1973, p. 137

164. Gray, T. K. and Munson, P. L. (1969). Thyrocalcitonin: evidence for physiological function. *Science*, **166,** 512

165. Munson, P. L. and Gray, T. K. (1970). Function of thyrocalcitonin in normal physiology. *Fed. Proc. (Fed. Amer. Soc. Exp. Biol.)*, **29,** 1206

166. Munson, P. L. (1971). Role of thyrocalcitonin in calcium metabolism. *The Action of Hormones: Genes to Populations*, 231 (P. P. Foa, editor) (Springfield: C. C. Thomas)

167. Munson, P. L., Cooper, C. W., Gray, T. K., Hundley, J. D. and Mahgoub, A. M. (1971). Physiological importance of thyrocalcitonin. *Cellular Mechanisms for Calcium Transfer and Homeostasis*, 403 (G. Nichols, Jr. and R. H. Wasserman, editors) (New York: Academic Press)

168. Munson, P. L. (1971). Thyrocalcitonin: physiological importance and significance in renal failure. *Amer. J. Med. Sci.*, **262,** 310

169. Munson, P. L., Schwesinger, W. H., Cooper, C. W., Gray, T. K. and Peng, T.-C. (1972). Physiological function of thyrocalcitonin. Ref. 2, p. 98

170. Milhaud, G., Perault-Staub, A. M. and Staub, J. F. (1972). Diurnal variation of plasma calcium and calcitonin function in the rat. *J. Physiol. (London)*, **222,** 559

171. Swaminathan, R., Bates, R. F. L. and Care, A. D. (1972). Fresh evidence for a physiologic role of calcitonin in calcium homeostasis. *J. Endocrinol.*, **54,** 525

172. Peng, T.- C., Cooper, C. W. and Munson, P. L. (1972). The hypocalcemic effect of ethyl alcohol in rats and dogs. *Endocrinology*, **91,** 586

173. Peng, T.-C., Cooper, C. W. and Munson, P. L. (1972). The hypocalcemic effect of urethane in rats. *J. Pharmacol. Exp. Therap.*, **182,** 522

174. Heath, D. A., Palmer, J. S. and Aurbach, G. D. (1972). The hypocalcemic action of colchine. *Endocrinology*, **90,** 1589

175. Charbon, G. A. and Pieper, E. E. M. (1972). Effect of calcitonin on parathyroid hormone-induced vasodilation. *Endocrinology*, **91,** 828

176. Robertson, D. R. (1972). Calcitonin in amphibians and the relationship of the paravertebral lime sacs with carbonic anhydrase. Ref. 1, p. 21

177. DeLuca, H. F. and Steenbock, H. (1972). 1,25-Dihydroxycholecalciferol: identification, regulation and mechanism of action. Ref. 2, p. 452

178. Wong, R. G., Myrtle, J. F., Tsai, H. C. and Norman, A. W. (1972). Studies on calciferol metabolism: the occurrence and biological activity of 1,25-dihydroxy-vitamin D_3 in bone. *J. Biol. Chem.*, **247,** 5728

179. Kodicek, E. (1972). The intermediary metabolism of vitamin D: 1,25-dihydroxycholecalciferol, a kidney hormone affecting calcium metabolism. Ref. 2, p. 444

180. Boyle, I. T., Gray, R. W., Omdahl, J. L. and DeLuca, H. F. (1972). Calcium control of the *in vivo* biosynthesis of 1,25-dihydroxy vitamin D_3-Nicolaysen's endogenous factor. Ref. 2, p. 468

181. Galante, L., Colston, K., MacAuley, S. and MacIntyre, I. (1972). Effect of parathyroid extract on vitamin D metabolism. *Lancet*, Vol. No. **985**

182. Garabedian, M., Holick, M. F., DeLuca, H. F. and Boyle, I. T. (1972). Control of 25-hydroxycholecalciferol metabolism by parathyroid glands. *Proc. Nat. Acad. Sci. (U.S.A.)*, **69,** 1673

183. Rasmussen, H., Wong, M., Bikle, D. and Goodman, D. B. (1972). Hormonal control of the renal conversion of 25-hydroxycholecalciferol to 1,25 dihydroxycholecalciferol. *J. Clin. Invest.*, **51,** 2502

184. Galante, L., Colston, K., MacAuley, S. J. and MacIntyre, I. (1972). Effect of calcitonin on viatmin D metabolism. *Nature (London)*, **238,** 271

9
Pineal–Anterior Pituitary Gland Relationships

R. J. REITER
The University of Texas

9.1 INTRODUCTION

Although among early anatomists the epiphysis cerebri attracted much attention, physiologists generally did not recognise the pineal as a legitimately functioning gland until recent years. Inferential evidence for the pineal gland being an endocrinologically-active structure had sporadically accumulated for a half century, but until the isolation and identification of its potential hormones the gland suffered from a vestigiality complex it had acquired through many years of disquieting experimental results. In light of more recently acquired substantive data, the evidence for an interaction between the secretory products of the pineal gland and the pituitary hormones presently seems well established. The physiological relationship imputed most frequently is with the gonadotrophins, however, the present survey will deal also with the influence of the pineal gland on the other anterior hypophyseal hormones.

Even though the most parsimonious scientists may admit that there now exists incontrovertible evidence for an endocrine function of the pineal gland, there still are numerous unsolved questions relative to the influences governing the biosynthetic and secretory activity of the pineal gland as well as the mechanisms of action of its hormonal products. Several of these unclarified facets will be considered in the initial sections of this report. After identifying these problem areas the interaction of the pineal and its constituents with specific pituitary hormones will be discussed.

9.2 FUNCTIONAL PINEAL INNERVATION: SYMPATHETIC v. PARASYMPATHETIC

Detailed anatomical studies of the mammalian pineal reveal that, unlike this organ in some submammalian species, it is totally devoid of sensory cells. With the exception of the primates, where some axons may enter the pineal directly from the epithalamus, many of the nerve fibres which terminate within the mammalian pineal gland have their perikarya within the superior cervical ganglia[1,2]. These fibres enter the pineal in conjunction with blood vessels or as two well delineated nerve bundles, the nervi conarii. The fibres are primarily disposed in the perivascular spaces but also ramify among the pinealocytes.

The endocrine activity of the pineal gland is at least partially governed by the prevailing environmental photoperiod. Usually light which enters the lateral eyes is considered to be inhibitory to pineal synthetic and secretory activity while darkness exaggerates the capabilities of this organ[3,4]. Although in this scheme it is known that the lateral eyes are required for light detection, the classic photoreceptor elements (e.g. the rods in the rat retinas) seem not to be involved[5]. Indeed, the specific retinal receptors for the photic stimuli which drive pineal activity remain in doubt. Regardless of the nature of the receptor, however, the photoperiodic information travels to the pineal through a series of pathways which includes axons located in the optic nerve, the inferior accessory optic tract, and the peripheral autonomic nervous system[1,2,6].

For more than a decade it was felt that the exclusive autonomic innervation of the pineal gland was sympathetic in nature and was derived from the superior cervical ganglia. The terminations of the postganglionic fibres within the pineal are known to contain norepinephrine (NE)[7] and, when released, the neurotransmitter acts on β receptors[8]. One action of NE on the pineal is to stimulate the conversion of serotonin to melatonin[3,9]. Surgical removal of the superior cervical ganglia obliterates the rhythms in pineal

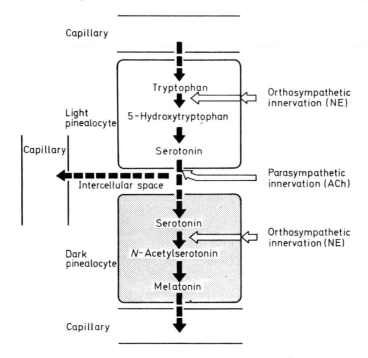

Figure 9.1 Theoretical model for the control of melatonin synthesis in the pineal gland of the rabbit. Under the influence of norepinephrine (NE), tryptophan is converted to serotonin in the light pinealocyte. Acetylcholine (ACh) causes the release of serotonin from the light cell. Serotonin is taken up by the dark pinealocytes where NE again acts to convert it to melatonin. (From Romijn[16], by courtesy of Nederlands Centraal Instituut voor Herseronderzock.)

enzymes which are normally impelled by environmental lighting conditions[3,10] and also renders the pineal incapable of modulating reproductive functions[11].

Because of such convincing results, few workers currently deny a role for the sympathetic nervous system in mediating certain pineal biochemical changes which are determined by incoming neural information. Unfortunately, the emphasis on the postganglionic adrenergic fibres in this system has overshadowed studies on the possible role of a parasympathetic control of pineal function. Until very recently, most investigators ignored (many still do) the potential importance of this neural component. In 1969, pharmacological evidence was presented which implicated cholinergic fibres in the modulation of the enzyme which forms melatonin, i.e. hydroxyindole-O-methyltransferase or HIOMT[12]. Oxotremorine oxalate, a parasympathomimetic, was found to have a facilitatory influence on pineal HIOMT activity in female rats kept in continual darkness. Presumed histochemical verification of a cholinergic component in the rat pineal was provided by Machado and Lemos[13]. Acetylcholinesterase (AChE), currently accepted as evidence for cholinergic fibres, was present in the pineals of both immature and adult rats. The AChE-positive nerve fibres disappeared after bilateral removal of the superior cervical ganglia, thus identifying the source of the axons. The pineal gland of the ferret is endowed with a distinct ganglion which is strongly positive for AChE, but the enzyme is more or less limited to the ganglion and, thus, may not contribute to the perivascular system of nerve endings[14]. Kenny[15] identified efferent preganglionic fibres going to the pineal of macaques; these fibres had their supposed origin from the greater superficial petrosal nerves. The axons entered the gland through the nervi conarii and theoretically synapsed on postganglionic parasympathetic neurones located within the pineal. There are obviously species variations in the course the parasympathetic fibres take to arrive at the pineal gland but their existence and functional importance should no longer be neglected.

Romijn[16] is the only investigator who has worked the pineal adrenergic and cholinergic innervation into a functional scheme. The model was devised after extensive ultrastructural and histochemical studies of the rabbit pineal gland. Romijn theorised that two types of cells (light and dark pinealocytes) are concerned with the formation of the pineal secretory product, melatonin. The precursor of melatonin, i.e., serotonin, is synthesised in the light pinealo-cyte and is at least under partial control of the noradrenergic sympathetic innervation (Figure 9.1). The cholinergic parasympathetic fibres control the release of the precursor (serotonin) from the light cell and thus allow it to gain access to the dark cell, where, under the influence of NE, melatonin formation and secretion is completed. At the ultrastructural level, bulbous enlargements of light cells invaginate the dark cells suggesting to Romijn the transfer mentioned above. He has reviewed the biochemical evidence supporting this hypothesis. Although it must be realised that this model is highly speculative and very provisional, researchers in the field should become aware of the potential interaction of the noradrenergic and cholinergic neurones in controlling pineal synthetic and secretory activity.

Finally, in that the pineal gland and the medial habenular nuclei share a common innervation from the superior cervical ganglia[17], it may be worth while to consider this nuclear group as a portion of the functional pineal complex. This idea remains virtually untested but the possibility bears scrutiny.

9.3 MODE OF PINEAL SECRETION: INTRAVASCULAR v. INTRAVENTRICULAR

Endocrine glands by definition release their secretory products into body fluids through which they travel to distant sites and cause their effects. Characteristically, the body fluid involved is the blood. In recent years,

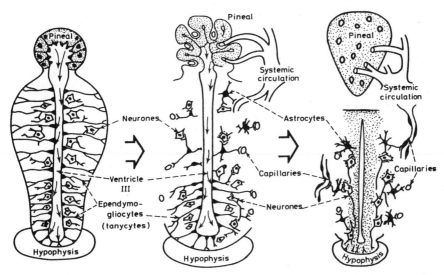

Figure 9.2 A portrayal of a proposed evolutionary derivation of the mode of secretion of pineal principles. Pineals of early vertebrates probably released their products primarily into the ventricular fluid (left) while in present day mammals the secretory route seems to be directly into the blood vascular system (right). Intermediate forms are probably represented by early tetrapods (centre). (From Quay[27], by courtesy of America Society of Zoologists.)

however, the cerebrospinal fluid (CSF) has attracted progressively more attention as a possible means for the transport of hormones between brain areas[18]. The description of ependymal tanyctes which may be capable of transmitting material between the CSF and the primary portal plexus of the median eminence makes this suggestion even more provocative[19].

For years it was tacitly assumed that the pineal released its products into the systemic circulation through which they eventually arrived at their target organs. The evolution of this notion was natural since, (1) as already noted, most classical hormones gain access to the vascular system, and (2) in many species (primarily rodents) that have been investigated the pineal gland, although lying in the subarachnoid space, was generally considered to be far removed from the ventricular system of the brain.

In 1969 a revolution in the ideas concerning the space into which the pineal extruded its products occurred. Over a short time a considerable amount of circumstantial evidence accumulated implicating the CSF as a recipient of endogenous pineal secretions[20, 21]. Although neither of these groups of workers were ready to promote unreservedly the CSF as a normal conveyer of pineal hormones, other investigators relied quite heavily on these indirect findings. After observing that intraventricularly, but not peripherally, administered melatonin blocked ovulation in mature rats, Collu and associates[22, 23] suggested that the physiological route of secretion and of transport of the pineal principles is probably through the CSF.

To date this point remains unproven and the evidence is becoming more, rather than less, tenuous. Melatonin has been shown to inhibit ovulation and the associated rise in plasma levels of luteinising hormone (LH) even when the indoleamine is given as an intraperitoneal injection[24]. This indicates that peripherally administered melatonin reaches the brain in sufficient quantity to interfere with the neural mechanisms governing LH release. Moreover, meticulous anatomical studies of the pineal gland offer little evidence to support a ventricular route of secretion. The ultrastructural features of the organ and its venous drainage are consistent with a mode of secretion into the vascular system[16, 25]. In that there is no known portal system connecting the pineal with the third ventricle, a means whereby the pineal principles would have indirect access to the ventricles seems also to be precluded. Finally, the identification of melatonin in the blood of chickens and its disappearance after pinealectomy is very strong evidence that the pineal releases at least one of its hormones into the systemic circulation[26]. The present consensus seems to be that the pineal extrudes its materials into the systemic circulation. Quay[27] has summarised the possible evolutionary changes associated with the eventual release of pineal hormones into the blood and their action on the brain. This sequence is portrayed in Figure 9.2.

9.4 PINEAL HORMONES: POLYPEPTIDES *v.* INDOLES

Researchers investigating the chemical nature of the pineal hormones have clearly aligned themselves into two camps. One group of workers claims the pineal hormones are polypeptides while the other contends the pineal is responsible for elaborating and secreting indoles. The two schools are not mutually exclusive and it seems probable that the pineal may be capable of releasing several hormones, some from each category. Although the literature on the pineal polypeptides has the longest heritage, generally more is known about the indoles. With only a few exceptions, the polypeptides have been promoted predominantly by scientists in Europe and Asia while American workers have advanced the indoles. The majority of investigators have concerned themselves with the antigonadotrophic capabilities of pineal substances but, as will be discussed later, they have inhibitory influences on other pituitary-regulated endocrine glands as well.

For a number of years, Thieblot and colleagues[28] have adamantly insisted that the pineal antigonadotrophic substance is a polypeptide. According to them, the active compound is a combination of five peptides and has a molecular weight of 1000–3000. They have used exclusively biological assays to assess the influence of their extracts on the gonadotrophin content of rat pituitaries[29]. When administered peripherally to castrated rats at the dosage of 50 μg daily it significantly reduced the gonadotrophic potency of their pituitaries. Not only has this group pushed the polypeptides to the forefront, but they have denied the gonad-inhibiting potential of melatonin, a pineal indoles with alleged antigonadotrophic properties. Accordingly, they claim that in low doses (<250 μg/day) melatonin lacks any reproductive effects while in greater amounts (>250 μg/day) it is actually progonadotrophic.

In their quest to establish the peptidic nature of the pineal antigonadotrophic material, Thieblot and associates have received substantial support from other workers as well. Milcu, Pavel and Neacsu[30, 31] have long advocated the peptidic nature of the pineal antigonadotrophin. They were convinced the compound they had isolated from bovine pineal glands was identical to arginine vasotocin. When compared with synthetic arginine vasotocin, the extracted material proved to have equivalent gonad-inhibiting activity[32, 33]. The bovine pineal compound tentatively identified as arginine vasotocin by Milcu *et al.*[30] has also been isolated recently by Cheesman and Farris[34]. Structural elucidation by amino acid analysis and mass spectrometry has shown it to be 8-arginine vasotocin.

Successful isolations of antigonadotrophic compounds from acetone-dried bovine pineal powder have also been conducted by Ebels, Moszkowska and Scémama[35-37]. After gel filtration on Sephadex G-25, two peaks from the column eluent possessed demonstrable biological activity; one of these had a stimulatory influence on the *in vitro* secretion of hypophyseal gonado-trophin[37]. The molecular weight of the partially-purified inhibitory compound was estimated to be about 700 and the data are strongly suggestive of it being a polypeptide[35, 36].

Benson *et al.*[38, 39] have isolated from bovine pineal tissue a presumptive polypeptide with a molecular weight in the range of 500–1000 which may be identical to that found by Ebels and colleagues. Benson's compound, which was labelled pineal antigonadotrophin or PAG, was judged to be 60–70 times more potent than melatonin when tested in an assay system involving the inhibition of compensatory ovarian hypertrophy in female mice. Addition-ally, PAG was shown to reduce ventral prostate and seminal vesicle weights in male mice suggesting a rather specific anti-LH effect. Whether the compound is identical to arginine vasotocin remains undetermined.

The second category of potential pineal hormones embraces those with indole properties. This group is typified by one substance in particular, namely, *N*-acetyl-5-methoxytryptamine or melatonin. As a representative of the indole category, melatonin has been widely investigated as to its endocrine capabilities. It is remarkable how many different experimental systems are influenced by this compound.

Melatonin was first isolated from bovine pineal tissue in 1958 by Lerner and colleagues[40] and, a year later, the same group definitively characterised the compound[41]. This discovery, because of its paramount importance, served as a stimulus for a foray of experiments on the biochemical and physiological properties of melatonin[3]. The enzymatic formation of the *O*-methylated indole from *S*-adenosylmethionine within the pineal was elucidated by Axelrod and Weissbach[42]. The melatonin forming enzyme was named hydroxyindole-*O*-methyltransferase (HIOMT) and it is probably localised in the soluble cytoplasmic fractions of pinealocytes. One especially interesting feature of HIOMT was that it appeared to be relegated, in mammals, exclusively to the pineal gland. This meant that the potential pineal hormone, melatonin, was produced only within this diencephalic structure. This concept has not withstood further experimentation in that HIOMT apparently exists also in mammalian retinas[43] and Harderian glands[44].

Vaginal opening time is delayed and ovarian growth is retarded in maturing rats if they are treated daily with microgram quantities of melatonin[45]. Peripherally or centrally injected melatonin blocks ovulation and the associ-ated rise in plasma LH levels in immature PMS-treated rats[24] and reduces plasma LH levels in adult female rats[46]. Implantation of melatonin depots either subcutaneously[47] or directly into the brain[23] has similar retardative effects on reproductive physiology. Although there are exceptions to the inhibitory effect of melatonin on the activity of the neuroendocrine axis, they are in the minority. It should be noted that rather large amounts of melatonin must usually be administered to elicit a discernible effect; the reasons for this may be manifold.

The intense investigation of melatonin as an endocrinologically-active substance has drastically overshadowed studies on other pineal indoles. 5-Methoxytryptophol, another product of HIOMT, seems to be at least as potent as melatonin in curtailing reproductive organ growth and the associated sexual events[48, 49]. N-Acetylserotonin and 5-hydroxytryptophol have also been implicated in the control of gonadotrophin release[49]. Finally, 5-hydroxytryptamine (serotonin), a substance which is extremely abundant within the pineal, may also be a hormonal product of the gland[50].

There is not, of necessity, any conflict between the two schools which advocate different substances as pineal hormones. Considering the large number of systems influenced by the pineal it is easy to envisage that this multipotent organ may secrete a number of hormones, some of which could be polypeptides and some of which could be indoles. Both categories of compounds may even affect reproduction, either via different mechanisms or in different ways[51]. As an example, polypeptides could control seasonal (i.e. long term) adjustments of the reproductive system to the photoperiod whereas the indoles may influence short term (daily or cyclic) fluctuations in reproductive physiology. Or for that matter, the reverse could be true. These possibilities remain untested, however.

9.5   SITE OF PINEAL ACTION: CENTRAL v. PERIPHERAL

Although the bulk of evidence favours a site of action of the pineal constituents within the brain, there are data which show that at least one pineal product can also act directly at the level of the gonads. It would generally seem inefficient to allow secretion of the pituitary trophic hormones and then prevent their action on the target organs.

Virtually all studies conducted in which the hamster was used as the experimental animal have suggested that the pineal in this species regulates reproduction by interfering with the neuroendocrine axis[11, 52]. Even though the hamster reproductive system is profoundly sensitive to the inhibitory influence of the pineal gland, the ovaries and uteri of pineal-stimulated animals respond to treatment with gonadotrophins[52]. Furthermore, male hamsters in which the sexual organs are involuted because of an activated pineal gland also have depressed levels of circulating LH[53]. These findings are consistent with an antagonistic action of the pineal at the hypothalamic or pituitary level.

In rats, melatonin also seems to be capable of interfering with the neural mechanisms governing gonadotrophin synthesis or release. The acute rise in serum levels of LH associated with ovulation in PMS-treated rats is prevented if melatonin is given at the anticipated time of LH release from the anterior pituitary[24, 54]. In the most elegant studies along this line to date, Kamberi and colleagues[46,55] infused small quantities of melatonin into the third ventricle of rats and examined peripheral levels of LH, FSH and prolactin at periodic intervals thereafter. Within 10–30 min, they observed statistically valid depressions in both serum LH and FSH levels while prolactin titres were elevated. The concentrations of all of the hormones had returned to their pre-injection levels within 2 h after melatonin administration. By comparison, when melatonin was infused directly into a cannulated hypophyseal portal vessel which drains directly into the anterior pituitary, it was ineffective in modifying circulating concentrations of the hormones. The findings are strongly suggestive of a direct effect of melatonin on the liberation of the releasing factors into vessels of the primary portal plexus. There is one point concerning studies in which intraventricular injections are used that should be remembered, however. The infusion of a variety of compounds directly into the CSF causes the release of monoamines and catecholamines into the ventricular system which, themselves, could gain access to the portal system and affect the liberation of hormones from the adenohypophysis. Until it is proved that melatonin does not release such substances into the CSF, it is impossible to determine whether the observed consequences are directly attributable to melatonin.

Fraschini and colleagues[23,56] have proposed two neural loci of action for melatonin. On the basis of results obtained from stereotaxic implantation studies, they theorised that there are specific melatonin receptors located in the median eminence (ME) and in the midbrain reticular formation(RF). In these locations, melatonin antagonised the rise in pituitary LH levels attendant upon castration. They have also speculated on the neural sites of action (in ME and RF) of 5-hydroxytryptophol and of 5-methoxytryptophol (in RF).

The proposed midbrain location of melatonin receptors conveniently happens to coincide with the concentration of the serotoninergic neuronal cell bodies. The significance of this lies in the fact that the peripherally administered melatonin reportedly elevates brain serotonin levels[57]. Thus, melatonin may exert its influence on the hypothalamo–pituitary system by altering the metabolism of serotonin-containing neurones whose cell bodies are in the midbrain and whose axons terminate in the medial basal hypothalamus. This unencumbered model is highly theoretical and requires much more extensive investigation before it can be accepted as a mechanism of action of melatonin. For example, we have been unable to confirm the facilitatory influence of melatonin on brain serotonin concentrations (W. W. Morgan and R. J. Reiter, unpublished observations).

Another approach has been employed to attempt to define precisely where in the brain the pineal acts to control the neuroendocrine axis. By cutting various neural tracts within the CNS, one could theoretically identify the necessary neural pathways which are involved. Studies to this point have been very difficult to interpret but it appears certain that the pineal hormones do not suppress reproduction by way of the gonadotrophin-inhibiting centres located in the amygdala[58]. Conversely, fibres entering the medial basal hypothalamus anteriorly must be intact for the pineal to maintain its inhibitory influence on sexual physiology while axons entering posteriorly seem to be of lesser or no importance[59]. Although the findings generally support the notion that the axons of pineal responsive neurones can be localised, the problem is complicated by the fact that neuronal processes passing from the retinas to the pineal gland also traverse the hypothalamus[6]. Interruption of these fibres could merely render the pineal non-functional and give no information about the sites of action of the pineal neurohumoral agents[60]. Indeed, cuts in the anterior hypothalamic area prevent the night time rises in pineal N-acetyltransferase and melatonin (unpublished observations). With a combination of implantation of pineal hormones and neural pathway interruption, however, specific loci of action may yet be identified.

Evidence for a testicular level of action of melatonin has been obtained primarily from *in vitro* preparations. According to Peat and Kinson[61], the addition of melatonin to testicular incubates reduced androgen production from pregnenolone while Ellis[62] reported that melatonin interfered with androgen formation by specifically acting on 17-a-hydroxypregnene-C17-C20-lyase and 17-β-hydroxysteroid dehydrogenase in the biosynthetic pathway. In the thyroid gland as well melatonin may inhibit thyroxine synthesis by negating the effects of TSH[63]. In that melatonin is now known to get into the systemic circulation (at least in chickens[26]) a peripheral site of action is feasible.

One of the most interesting findings in this regard is that of Debeljuk and colleagues[64]. Daily treatment of rats for 22 days with melatonin (750 µg/day) significantly depressed the weights of the already involuted testes and seminal vesicles of hypophysectomised rats. The authors proposed that melatonin acted primarily on the interstitial cells of the testes. This finding could be verified by assaying the serum levels of testosterone under similar experimental conditions.

Studies on the site of action of pineal polypeptides are relatively sparse. A melatonin-free, ninhydrin-positive fraction (presumptive polypeptide with a molecular weight of 500–1000) extracted from bovine pineal glands was found to block significantly the increased ovarian weight and radioactive phosphorus uptake in hypophysectomised rats treated with gonadotrophins[65]. The observations are, of course, consistent with an ovarian level of action of the pineal factor but any effect of the peptide in the neuroendocrine axis could not be assessed with the experimental design utilised.

Other peripheral and central sites of action for the pineal hormones have been proposed by various authors[27, 66, 67] but proof for any of these awaits further investigation.

9.6 PINEAL REGULATION OF ANTERIOR PITUITARY

9.6.1 Gonadotrophins

The first tenable evidence that the pineal gland was an organ of internal secretion derived from the observations that pineal tumours in humans were sometimes associated with reproductive abberations. Even these results were perplexing because enlarging pineals could cause either precocious or delayed pubescence. This wide variation in sexual responses was probably explicable in terms of the pineal cellular element (i.e. parenchymatous or non-parenchymatous) involved in the tumourous growth.

In experimental animals, the results of experiments designed to provide proof of pineal endocrine activity were equally as baffling. Under laboratory conditions earlier investigators were struck with the inconsistent findings which followed surgical removal of the pineal gland. The variations in the response were undoubtedly attributable to a host of factors[4, 54, 68] and only after the fortuitous elucidation of the role of environmental lighting in modulating pineal activity has the physiological potential of the pineal gland been unequivocally documented. In that darkness is known to exaggerate the gonad-inhibiting capability of the pineal gland, the constraining effects of this organ on reproduction can now be routinely demonstrated[4, 60, 68].

9.6.1.1 Pineal–gonadal relationships in hamsters

In no species studied to date is the pineal gland more convincingly antigonadotropic than in the hamster. Restricting the amount of light to which hamsters are exposed rapidly and dramatically leads to involution of their sexual organs[11, 54, 69]. Accompanying the gross and microscopic atrophy of the testes and adnexae is a statistically insignificant reduction in bioassayable pituitary levels of LH[58] and FSH[59] and a diminished concentration of radioimmunoassayable LH in the plasma[53]. All these changes are nullified completely by surgical removal of the pineal gland[69, 70] or by interruption of the pineal's neural input[11, 68, 70]. In the hamster, the sequence of events which culminates in pineal-induced gonadal regression seems to be as follows: the absence of long daily periods of illumination (more than 12.5 h/day[71]) activates the pineal to synthesise and release an antigonadotrophic factor. Specifically, the nature of this factor in the case of the hamster remains unknown[60]. This yet unidentified antigonadotrophic substance probably intervenes with gonadotrophin releasing factor mechanisms in the hypothalamus which results in a cessation of pituitary gonadotrophin release. In that it requires several weeks of darkness before the pineal appreciably depresses reproductive physiology[72], the system seems to be rather slow acting. Regardless of this, the resultant sexual organs are not unlike those of hypophysectomised hamsters suggesting a total suppression of all reproductively-active hormones.

As already noted, denervation of the pineal gland renders it incapable of inducing gonadal atrophy[11, 73] whereas exposure of animals to long daily photoperiods (12–16 h light/day as is used in most animal rooms) leads to a physiological or functional 'pinealectomy'[60, 70]. In fact, it has been this common usage of long photoperiods which has effectively stymied pineal research. The usual experimental design in years past was to remove surgically the pineal gland from a group of animals, and at some predetermined time thereafter, to compare the growth of the reproductive organs in these animals with those of sham-operated controls. Whereas this is a proven method for illustrating the endocrine nature of many other organs, in the case of the pineal gland there were few, if any, observable differences between the functioning of the sexual organs in the pinealectomised and non-pinealectomised animals. When maintained in long daily photoperiods, both groups of animals were essentially pinealectomised, one group having had it surgically ablated and the other group having had it rendered non-antigonadotrophic by long daily photoperiods. Thus, any potential effects of pinealectomy were minimised[74].

9.6.1.2   Pineal and seasonal reproduction

The observation that the quantity of light to which hamsters are exposed determines directly the functional status of the pineal gland and secondarily that of the gonads led to the obvious conclusion that the pineal gland may be related to seasonal changes in sexual competence[69, 74]. It appeared that as the length of the day changes during the year the antigonadotrophic activity of the pineal gland would fluctuate accordingly. In such a scheme, during the winter months when day lengths are shortest the pineal would theoretically induce sexual quiescense.

A search of the published literature revealed several fragments of information which supported this speculation[75]. Morphological evidence for a hyperfunctional pineal gland during the winter in animals maintained under natural photoperiodic conditions was obtained over a decade ago[76, 77]. Also, hamsters kept in outdoor cages were found to have atrophic testes during the month of January unless they had been pinealectomised a month earlier[78]. In their natural habitat, hamsters are believed to hibernate during the winter and to breed only during the summer months[79, 80]. During their hibernatory period the gonads of both sexes are dormant.

To test whether the photoperiodically-induced rhythm in reproductive competence was in fact a manifestation of a change in pineal function, the

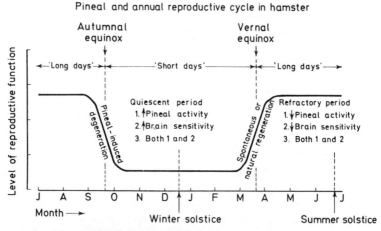

Figure 9.3   Possible relations between the pineal gland, the photoperiod and seasonal reproductive events in the hamster. During the 'short day' period (winter months) the pineal gland is maximally stimulated and the sexual organs regress. There is possibly an increased sensitivity of the brain to the pineal substances as well. In the summer ('long days') the pineal is inhibited and the gonads are reproductively capable. During the summer the reproductive system may be refractory to the influence of the pineal gland. (From Reiter[74], by courtesy of *Annual Reviews*, Inc.)

testicular morphology and serum LH levels were assessed in hamsters killed during various months of the year. Animals which had been exposed to normal daylength for the previous 8 weeks and which were killed in mid-January had remarkably involuted testes and accessory sex organs and also had depressed levels of serum LH. Conversely, control hamsters that had been pinealectomised prior to the experimental period had highly functional reproductive organs and serum LH levels comparable to those observed during the summer months[53]. The findings strongly suggest that the pineal gland is the critical determinant between seasonal reproductive fluctuations and changing photoperiodic conditions. Without this important gland, photosensitive species such as the hamster would not experience the depression in sexual competence which ensures that the young are born at an appropriate time of the year. Contrary to popular opinion, the pineal may yet be essential for survival of the species. The theoretical relationships between the environmental photoperiod, the pineal gland and gonadotrophins in the hamster are schematically depicted in Figure 9.3. During the summer months the pituitary–gonadal axis may actually be refractory to the influence of the pineal gland[74].

Herbert[14] envisaged similar relationships to be operative in the ferret. The pineal gland in this species also subserves the function of synchronising oestrous behaviour with the spring of the year. Pinealectomised ferrets kept under daylight conditions have oestrous periods which are separated by intervals greater than one year although there are no appreciable influences on the duration of the oestrous phase. The ultimate effect, then, is the same as in the hamster. In the absence of the pineal gland both hamsters and ferrets would breed during seasons which would result in parturition at a time not conducive to survival of the young. It is interesting that, despite the reliability of melatonin in moderately suppressing gonadotrophins in other species, it has proven to be inactive in the pineal-sensitive hamster and ferret[14, 60]. The effects of pineal polypeptides have not been tested in these species.

Conversely, the reproductive organs of the weasel, an animal whose heritage is closely linked to that of the ferret, appear to be acutely sensitive to melatonin[81]. Summer-captured, sexually mature weasels underwent reproductive involution after receiving weekly implants of melatonin (1 mg melatonin in 25 mg beeswax). During this time pelage colour changed from brown to white. On the other hand, reproductively dormant weasels captured in the winter experienced gonadal recrudescence when exposed to the long photoperiods of the laboratory. This light-induced regeneration was easily counteracted by subcutaneous implants of melatonin. These data certainly provide ancillary evidence supporting the concept that the pineal gland may control seasonal reproductive phenomena but do little to clarify the nature of the pineal substance which impels these rhythms in species other than the weasel.

9.6.1.3 Pineal–gonadal relationships in rats

If researchers had to depend on the rat for conclusive evidence of pineal–gonadal interactions, most investigations may still deny an endocrine function of the pineal gland. In as much as the rat is somewhat less photosensitive, changes associated with pineal manipulations are usually not so dramatic and therefore statistically less reliable. Light deprivation in rats causes only a modest delay in sexual maturation and this effect is negated by surgical removal of the pineal gland[82]. Besides stimulating an enhanced growth of the genital apparatus, pineal ablation also augments pituitary levels of both LH and FSH[83].

There are several experimental circumstances which greatly increase the sensitivity of the rat to the pineal antigonadotrophic influence. These treatments have been designated potentiating agents and they most likely modify the reactivity of the neural sites at which the pineal principles act[4, 60, 84]. The first of these to be discovered was early postnatal treatment with androgens[85, 86].

The administration of testosterone propionate (or other androgens or oestrogens) to young rats before 8 days of age severely impairs the subsequent development of the hypothalamic mechanisms which, after adulthood, are destined to govern gonadotrophin synthesis and release[87]. Female rats, having been so treated, do not ovulate spontaneously and exhibit persistent cornification of the vaginal epithelium. This constellation of signs is due to the lack of maturation of the centres which regulate cyclic LH release. For convenience, these females are usually referred to as being androgen-sterilised. Early postnatal injection of gonadal steroid hormones into male rats also affects the differentiation of the hypothalamic neuroendocrine mechanisms which regulate testes growth. After puberty, the gonads of these animals are smaller than normal and may have impaired spermatogenic activity[88].

Presumably because of the neural deficits produced by neonatal androgen treatment, the hypothalamo–pituitary–gonadal axes of these rats are more sensitive than usual to the suppressive effect of the pineal gland[85, 86]. If androgen-treated rats (either males or females) are maintained in the absence of light, the sexual apparatus either fails to mature or, more commonly, its rate of development is severely impeded. The hindrance to gonadal maturation is probably a manifestation of the inability of the gonadotropes of the anterior pituitary gland to form or secrete their trophic principles[84]. The reason these cells are not able to perform their ascribed functions is because they, or higher neural centres (releasing factor centres, for example), are being inhibited by pineal secretory products. Proof for this is provided by the observation that if androgen-sterilised rats are pinealectomised their reproductive organs mature at the usual rate even if they are deprived of light. Similarly, bilateral interruption of the nerve fibres going to the pineal gland nullifies the ability of this organ to retard sexual maturation in rats that had been exposed to steroid hormones shortly after birth.

The second obvious perturbation which exaggerates the antagonistic potential of the pineal gland is anosmia. The degree to which animals rely on olfactory stimuli for the maintenance of sexual competence varies greatly. Whereas mice seem especially sensitive to the loss of the olfactory sense[91], rats suffer little during prolonged anosmia[92]. Like androgen-sterilisation, however, anosmia renders the rats' reproductive system highly responsive to suppression by the activated pineal gland. Moreover, the mechanisms whereby these potentiating factors sensitise the neuroendocrine axis may be similar[84]. If immature female rats have their olfactory bulbs removed surgically and are also deprived of light, puberty is delayed and vaginal cyclicity and ovulation are disrupted. Near normal reproductive organ growth can be restored if the dual sensory deprived rats are pinealectomised[93]. If rats which have attained adulthood are deprived of olfactory and photic stimuli, the gonads and accessory sex glands undergo atrophy indicative of reduced stimulation by pituitary gonadotrophins. This condition is also ameliorated by extirpation of the pineal gland[70, 94].

The final potentiating factor to be considered is quantitative reduction in food intake. Restricting the amount of food male rats eat during their rapid growth phase retards only slightly development of their gonads[95]. This effect is markedly accentuated if the animals are also deprived of light by blinding. On the other hand, if blinded rats are also pinealectomised prior to the interval of underfeeding, they reach sexual maturity at the same time as control animals[96]. Other instances where nutritional changes may have increased the ability of the pineal gland to induce a lag in sexual maturation have been discussed elsewhere[84].

The results of these studies make it quite obvious that the sensitivity of the neuroendocrine axis can change under given experimental conditions. Although some of the methods employed in the investigations surely create artificial situations which animals in the field may not encounter, nevertheless, it seems likely that there also may be naturally occurring variables which render the pituitary–gonadal system less resistent to the pineal antigonadotrophic principle. In this category may be such factors as decreasing environmental temperature, decreased food availability, changes in the nutritional quality of food and different olfactory cues. In the case of opportunistic breeders even factors such as rainfall may play a paramount role in adjusting the responsiveness of the releasing factor mechanisms to inhibitory hormonal information. It may well be that many animals in their natural habitat would be continuous breeders if adverse environmental conditions did not change the ability of the pineal to induce reproductive incompetence. Hence the use of the potentiating agents may yield valuable clues relative to how exteroceptive stimuli, the pineal and seasonality in reproduction interact. Furthermore, the mechanisms of action of the pineal may be more easily elucidated in a situation which yields reproducible and dramatic pineal effects[74, 84].

In summary, it is quite apparent that the sensitivity of the neuroendocrine system to the pineal gland varies greatly from one species to another. In the hamster, the reproductive axis is sufficiently sensitive so that darkness alone, because of its stimulatory action on pineal biosynthetic and secretory processes, is sufficient to induce complete gonadal regression. On the contrary, in species such as the rat, darkness also facilitates pineal antigonadotrophic activity but the neuroendocrine axis is suppressed essentially in a subliminal manner due presumably to the resistance (insensitivity) of the system to inhibition. However, if the sensitivity of the neuroendocrine axis is increased (threshold decreased) by one of the potentiating factors (anosmia, underfeeding, or androgen sterilisation) the previously subliminal inhibition now reaches threshold and gonadotrophin output is restricted probably by a mechanism involving releasing factor inhibition. The potentiating factors do not seem capable of further increasing (in excess of that caused by darkness) the production of pineal antigonadotrophic substances[84, 94]. The final proof of this hypothesis, however, must await the identification of all pineal antigonadotrophins.

9.6.1.4 Pineal substances and reproduction

Every reasonable means of administration of pineal principles has been employed in order to illustrate the endocrine capabilities of refined and purified pineal compounds. Several decades ago the use of crude tissue extracts of the pineal gland portended the significance of this organ but the experiments in which the extracts were utilised were usually poorly designed and thus the data were widely neglected. However, after the identification of the active pineal principles and their commercial availability, researchers began to recognise the potential, if not the importance, of the pineal gland as an organ of internal secretion.

Treatment of rats with melatonin between the age of weaning (20–23 days of age) and adulthood usually causes a delay in puberty[3, 45, 47]. This phenomenon has been more widely studied in the female than in the male, simply because in the former the indices of puberty are more easily recognised. Because of the small magnitude of the changes in the sexual organs even after prolonged melatonin administration, it is not likely that the reproductive competence of the animals is jeopardised. 5-Methoxytryptophal, another pineal product, seems to be somewhat more potent than melatonin in delaying pubescence[48]. Despite this, it has never been given very serious consideration as a normal pineal envoy.

In the rat, at least, surgical removal of one ovary initiates an augmented secretion of FSH from the pituitary gland which culminates in hypertrophy of the intact gonad[97]. Whether the enlargement of the remaining ovary is exclusively a function of higher circulating levels of FSH is disputed, since an elevated concentration of LH may also be involved. The compensatory ovarian hypertrophy (COH) model has been successfully used to investigate the gonad inhibiting ability of several pineal compounds. In the rat, daily injections of melatonin were found to curtail the rise in serum FSH associated with COH[98]. Mice appear even better suited for such studies. In this species, COH is a highly uniform response which can be readily blocked by the administration of a single dose of melatonin. Depending on the strain of mouse used, the degree of enlargement of the remaining ovary within 10 days following unilateral ovariectomy ranges from 30 to 60%[99, 100]. The minimum effective dose of melatonin required to block significantly COH in the CD-1 mouse was found to be 25 μg[99]. In this experiment the melatonin was given as a single intraperitoneal dose at the time of unilateral ovariectomy. It was later determined that if a single dose of melatonin is to be given, it must be administered within the first 24 h after unilateral ovariectomy in order for it to retard significantly COH 10 days later (Figure 9.4)[101]. These data were believed to be consistent with melatonin-enhanced feed-back sensitivity to lowered oestrogen levels after removal of one ovary. In effect, then, melatonin curtailed gonadotrophin secretion.

There is no longer any doubt that melatonin can inhibit LH secretion from the anterior pituitary but there is some disagreement relative to the specificity of melatonin as an anti-LH substance. If given just prior to the predicted time of LH release in either immature PMS-treated rats or in adult rats on the day of pro-oestrous, it prevents the usual surge of LH and as a

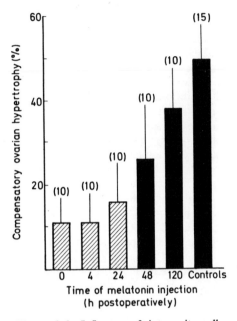

Figure 9.4 Influence of intraperitoneally injected melatonin (single 100 μg dose) administered at various time intervals after unilateral ovariectomy on compensatory ovarian hypertrophy in mice. Ovarian hypertrophy was measured 9 days after removal of the contralateral ovary. Hatched columns indicate groups in which significant ($p < 0.001$) inhibition of compensatory ovarian hypertrophy was recorded. Number of animals in parentheses. (From Vaughan *et al.*[101], by courtesy of Blackwell Scientific Publications.)

result the ova are not shed[22, 24, 102]. According to Fraschini and colleagues[23,103] melatonin specifically restricts LH synthesis and secretion but is without influence on FSH. This is in direct conflict with the data of Kamberi and co-workers[46, 55] who observed that melatonin injected intraventricularly is capable of modulating the secretion of both LH and FSH. The findings of a specific effect of melatonin on LH is also in apparent disagreement with the data of Vaughan *et al.*[100, 101] and Sorrentino[98] in which melatonin was found to block compensatory enlargement of the ovary, a response which at least partially relies on FSH secretion[97]. It would be advantageous if LH and FSH specific inhibitory pineal compounds were identified. On the basis of information presently available, however, any judgement concerning such a relationship would be wanton speculation. Besides melatonin, other natural products of the pineal which inhibit gonadotrophin metabolism include 5-methoxytryptophol, 5-hydroxytryptophol and serotonin[83].

Presumptive pineal polypeptides, although structurally unidentified, have also been implicated in the control of gonadotrophins. Moszkowska *et al.*[35, 37, 104] have summarised their findings in several recent reviews. They were able to isolate from sheep pineal glands by gel filtration on Sephadex G-25 two fractions which have opposite effects on the release of FSH by incubated pituitary glands. When added to the incubation medium, one fraction increased FSH discharge from the gonadotropes while, under similar experimental conditions, another fraction diminished FSH release. Prolonged administration of the latter compound to rats inhibited growth of the gonads and accessory sex organs. Benson and colleagues[38, 39] have had similar experiences with pineal polypeptides. Using the model of COH previously described, they estimated that on a weight basis a polypeptide with mol. wt. of 500–1000 was 60 to 70 times more potent than melatonin in inhibiting compensatory enlargement of the remaining ovary in young adult female mice. Like Moskzowska and co-workers[37], they have also isolated a compound which may have progonadotrophic properties (B. Benson, personal communication). In addition to the well known inhibitory influence of the pineal gland on reproduction, a stimulatory effect has also been proposed[105].

The present state of knowledge allows us to predict quite reliably that the pineal gland must exercise some control over seasonal reproductive rhythms but what it has to do with the daily functioning of the pituitary–gonadal axis remains enigmatic. How the pineal regulates the secretion of pituitary gonadotrophins and whether there are specific pineal antigonadotrophic hormones for LH and FSH are problems that will be solved with further experimentation. To be sure, however, endocrinologists can no longer ignore the paramount role of the pineal gland in sexual physiology.

9.6.2 Prolactin

The dominant influence of the brain on prolactin secretion from the anterior pituitary gland seems to be of an inhibitory nature. Grafting the pituitary away from its neural connections is followed by a copious secretion of prolactin while adding hypothalamic tissue to pituitary cultures restricts prolactin release and affords direct evidence for the negative control of prolactin by the brain. Relatively little attention has been focused on the pineal gland as a modulatory of prolactin synthesis or release.

According to Relkin[106], pinealectomising male rats at weaning (3 weeks of age) is followed by a transitory elevation of pituitary prolactin concentration while levels in the blood drop. The differences disappear within a week after the operation. If rats are pinealectomised at 8 weeks of age, the changes in prolactin levels (increased in the pituitary and decreased in the plasma). persist for at least a month. These results are consistent with observations by the same worker[107] showing that short term (up to 7 days) exposure to constant light resulted in higher pituitary prolactin levels and lower blood concentrations, while darkness produced the opposite findings. Thus, the effects of constant light mimicked those following pineal ablation. A shortcoming of this work is that pooled plasma and pituitary samples were used; this was unnecessary in that a sensitive radioimmunoassay was used for the prolactin analyses.

In support of this, we found that the activated pineal gland is capable of depressing the accumulation of prolactin in the pituitary[108]. In blinded anosmic rats, an experimental situation in which the neuroendocrine inhibitory effects of the pineal gland appear to be maximal[84, 94], a diminished content and concentration of pituitary prolactin was observed.

The data from the studies discussed thus far consistently fit into the following scheme. The pineal gland secretes a substance which prevents prolactin inhibiting factor (PIF) from reaching the anterior pituitary gland. In the absence of PIF, the synthesis and secretion of prolactin from the cells of the anterior pituitary proceeds unabated. The result is that the amounts of residual stored hormone in the pituitary cells are diminished. The opposite effects follow pinealectomy. In view of the findings of Kamberi et al.[55], the substance responsible for the pineal influence on prolactin may be melatonin. After the injection of this indole into the third ventricle of rats transitory rises in plasma prolactin were recorded. Presumably, the increased plasma levels were accompanied by a reduction of pituitary prolactin. These findings are consistent with the above hypothesis relative to the inhibitory effect of the pineal on PIF. Thus, although the data on pineal–prolactin relationships are scanty, they appear to be quite consistent and explicable.

9.6.3 Growth hormone

As with prolactin, the data implying a relationship between the pineal gland and somatic enlargement are comparatively new but seemingly compatible with the idea that some pineal constituent diminishes growth hormone synthesis or secretion and, as a consequence, restricts growth[109]. The lower body weights of light-deprived rats presaged this pineal function long before the actual relationships between the pineal and growth hormone (GH) were established. Removal of the eyes from rats during their rapid growth phase not uncommonly leads to lower body weight[85, 90]. This effect is exaggerated if the animals are also rendered anosmic[93, 94]. In both the singly and doubly sensory-deprived rats, the animals grew almost normally if they also had been pinealectomised. Although pinealectomy itself reportedly caused a transient acceleration of bodily growth in rats[110] this was an isolated finding and such a change cannot be considered a reliable index of pineal–growth relationships unless it is confirmed by other workers.

Judging from the tibial epiphyseal growth test, the pituitary glands of donor rats injected with bovine pineal extract contained less than the normal amount of growth promoting activity when administered to hypophysectomised recipient rats[111]. On the other hand, whereas melatonin stymied maturation of the reproductive organs in male rats it failed to curtail the growth of the animals[47]. These preliminary findings suggest that the antigrowth effect of the pineal gland may not be mediated by melatonin.

The first substantial evidence supporting a pineal–GH relationship is derived from studies in which radioimmunoassayable levels of GH were determined. As already noted, rats that have their eyes or their olfactory bulbs removed before puberty grow in a subnormal manner and their pituitaries contain less GH than those of sham-operated control rats[112]. If rats are deprived of both senses, very poor growth is observed and pituitary GH levels fall to approximately 60% of normal values. Pinealectomy in dual sensory deprived rats reversed the depressant action of blinding on the pituitary concentration of GH but did not restore the diminished GH levels which resulted from anosmia. Although plasma levels of GH in the blinded anosmic rats also tended to be lower than normal, a statistically significant depression could not be verified because of the wide variation in plasma GH levels generally. GH in adult animals is not exempt from the pineal influence since in these animals also, the combination of blinding and anosmia depresses GH metabolism unless the animals have their pineal gland ablated[113]. Presumably the changes observed are a consequence of pineal-induced decrease in GH-releasing factor synthesis or release although experiments have not yet been designed to test this. However, in that growth hormone inhibiting factor (GIF) activity has been identified in extracts of the rat hypothalamus[114], an increased production of GIF in the blinded anosmic rats cannot be precluded.

Since combined blinding and anosmia curtailed the functioning of the neuroendocrine–gonadal axis[84, 94], it was important to determine whether the reduced GH synthesis in these animals was secondary to decremental changes in gonadotrophins. Using castrated rats it was easily established that the deficient GH production and poor growth in dual sensory deprived rats was not mediated by a lack of testicular androgens[109]. Furthermore, the retarded growth also does not seem to depend on a deficiency of thyroxine.

More recently, Relkin[115] employed constant dark exposure in lieu of blinding to test the influence of the pineal gland on GH metabolism. His results are in direct support of our findings in that male rats maintained in continual darkness during their rapid growth phase (23–52 days of age) had lower pituitary and plasma GH levels, smaller body weights and shorter tail lengths. By comparison, these growth parameters in rats that had been pinealectomised prior to dark exposure were comparable to those of intact rats kept in long daily photoperiods.

9.6.4   Adrenocorticotrophin

The mammalian cortex is disposed into two functionally distinct zones. The outermost area of the cortex, the zona glomerulosa, is concerned with the elaboration and secretion of mineralocorticoids and is relatively independent of pituitary adrenocorticotrophin (ACTH). Because of this, the ostensibly direct relationships between the pineal gland and the glomerular zone were deemed beyond the scope of this review. The nexus between the pineal gland and aldosterone secretion has, however, been summarised elsewhere[4, 116].

The influence the pineal gland exerts on the inner adrenocortical area, the zonae fasciculata and reticularis, seems to be indirectly via ACTH. When pineals of mice were autografted to their enucleated adrenal glands, restoration of the zona fasciculata and zona reticularis proceeded normally whereas the zona glomerulosa hypertrophied to about twice its usual size[117, 118]. These findings were generally accepted as support for the notion that the pineal has no direct inhibitory control on the adrenocortical zones concerned with the production of glucocorticoids but that it may possess specific adrenoglomerulotrophic properties.

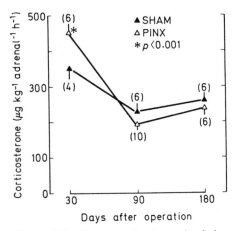

Figure 9.5 Plasma corticosterone levels in male rats at various intervals after pineal-ectomy. Animals were pinealectomised at 34–44 days of age. Blood samples were collected from cannulated left adrenal veins. (Data from Kinson *et al.*[120], by courtesy of *Gen. Comp. Endocrinol.*)

Removal of the pineal gland from adult rats reportedly leads to an elevation of plasma corticosterone levels[119, 120]. The length of time after pinealectomy at which corticosterone is measured appears to be critical, however, since the rise in this constituent in the plasma is transitory. Male rats, pinealectomised at either 34–44 or at 100 days of age, had elevated levels of plasma corticosterone one month later. At 3 and 6 months after pineal removal these differences between pinealectomised and sham-operated animals had disappeared (Figure 9.5). In these studies, the blood was collected directly from a polythene cannula inserted into the left adrenal vein. This method would likely yield more consistent results than studies dealing with peripheral blood samples and smaller changes in adrenal secretion rates could be detected since the dilution factor would be circumvented. The lighting condition employed by Kinson and colleagues[119, 120] was LD 12:12. Female, but not male, rats pinealectomised within the first 24 h after birth also had higher plasma corticosterone levels at 50 days of age[121]. The increase was quite dramatic since the levels were almost twice as high in the pinealectomised animals as compared to the unoperated controls. The blood samples in this experiment were collected by means of cardiac puncture and the lighting regimen used was not identified.

Nir *et al.*[122] tested pineal–adrenal interactions under photoperiodic conditions which are considered to be maximally inhibitory (constant light exposure) and maximally stimulatory (constant dark exposure) to pineal synthetic and secretory activity. Plasma corticosterone concentrations were found to be higher in pinealectomised than in sham-operated female rats when both groups were maintained in constant darkness for 10 days. Although

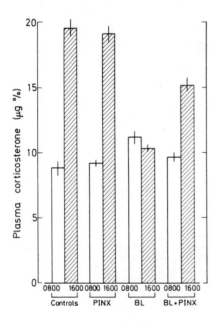

Figure 9.6 Influence of blinding (BL) and pinealectomy (PINX) on plasma corticosterone levels in rats at two times of the day. Animals were operated on at 60 days of age. Blood was collected by jugular vein puncture. Open bars = a.m. samples; hatched bars = p.m. samples. (Data from Jacobs and Kendall[126], by courtesy of Int. Congr. Endocrinology.)

pineal removal caused slight increases in corticosterone levels of rats kept in light: dark cycles of 12:12, no statistically significant differences between the plasma concentrations of this adrenal constituent in pinealectomised and intact rats were detected. Constant light exposure led to an elevation of corticosterone in the blood regardless of the status of the pineal gland. The stimulatory effects of constant light exposure and pineal removal on the pituitary–adrenal axis did not seem to be additive.

As already seen, treatments which increase the antigonadotrophic activity of the pineal gland also seem to exaggerate the adrenal inhibitory capability of the organ. Thus, blinding restricts adrenal growth in otherwise intact hamsters[123] and curtails compensatory adrenal hypertrophy in rats which have intact pineal glands[124]. In both species, pineal ablation negates the effects of blindness on adrenal growth. Likewise, the combination of blinding and anosmia, a procedure which is seriously detrimental to the functioning of the reproductive system, also greatly impairs induced growth of the remaining adrenal gland of rats that have been unilaterally adrenalectomised[125]. If the rats are additionally pinealectomised, however, compensatory adrenal hypertrophy proceeds unabated.

Plasma corticosterone levels, of course, vary according to the time of day. They are usually greatest in the late afternoon and lowest in the early morning. This rhythm is not altered in pinealectomised male rats kept in LD cycles of 12:12, but blinding reportedly obliterates the normal steroid cyclicity by depressing the afternoon peak[126]. If blinded rats also lack their pineal glands, they still exhibit a diurnal rhythm in plasma corticosterone levels but the fluctuations do not seem to be as great (Figure 9.6). This dampening of the rhythm suggests that the usual circadian periodicity is probably disturbed in the blinded pinealectomised rats although it does exist. Another explanation is that the peaks and troughs did not occur at the usual times, i.e. 0800 and 1600 h, respectively.

The consensus seems to be that all of the observed changes which follow altered environmental photoperiod or pinealectomy are due to disturbances in the secretion of pituitary ACTH. Although this may be true, pituitary and plasma ACTH levels remain to be measured in animals with reduced or exaggerated pineal function. Incubated pituitary glands of pinealectomised rats exhibit a hypersecretion of ACTH, however[127].

The use of pineal substances to clarify pineal–adrenal relationships has yielded variable results. Extracts of bovine pineal glands impede compensatory adrenal growth which follows unilateral adrenalectomy in rats[124, 128]. In the most complete study to date, in which all the pineal indoles were tested, Vaughan and colleagues[129] found that serotonin, N-acetylserotonin, melatonin, 5-hydroxytryptophol, 5-methoxytryptophol and 5-hydroxyindole acetic acid were all capable of restricting growth of the remaining adrenal gland in unilaterally adrenalectomised female mice. The indoles were administered as 100 µg doses at the time of unilateral adrenalectomy and the degree of compensatory enlargement was measured 3 days later. Conversely, there are other reports which show that crude pineal preparations stimulate ACTH secretion[130] while melatonin administered acutely or chronically does not depress either plasma corticosterone concentrations or bioassayable pituitary ACTH levels[131]. In yet other experiments, the injection of melatonin into adult male rats augmented the production of corticosterone by the adrenals[132] while the opposite finding was made by Motta et al.[133]. More recently, De Prospo and Hurley[134] injected melatonin directly into the lateral cerebral ventricles of female rats for 10 days; its administration in this manner failed to influence the neuroendocrine–adrenal axis. Only adrenal gland weights were measured, however.

Despite these inconsistencies, the present reviewer is convinced that the pineal has some regulatory control over ACTH and, thus, the secretion of adrenocorticoids. What is required to provide definite proof of this relationship is an organised effort specifically examining the adrenocortical effects of the pineal gland. Previously, many of the observations of the adrenals were merely portions of large studies dealing with other problems. That melatonin is the pineal hormone concerned with controlling ACTH secretion requires substantiation.

9.6.5 Thyrotrophin

The reliance of thyroid growth and thyroxine production on a specific hormone, i.e. thyroid stimulating hormone (TSH) or thyrotrophin, from the anterior pituitary, is well established. Experimentally, the pineal gland is ostensibly capable of modifying the function of the pituitary–thyroid axis, but the physiological significance of this interaction remains in doubt. Whereas an appreciable amount of work has been done to test pineal–thyroid interactions, the results of the studies are characterised by their inconsistencies.

The thyroid glands of mice exhibit a rather consistent, albeit rather slight, enlargement after pinealectomy[135, 136]. After similar treatment in rats the hypertrophic response of the thyroid seems to be somewhat greater but the investigators are not in agreement as to whether the thyroid glands also respond with cellular hyperplasia[137, 138]. Probably the most interesting feature is not that the weight of the thyroid gland increases after pineal removal, but that this enlargement seems to be independent of pituitary TSH. Hence, hypophysectomised rats that had also been pinealectomised were found to have larger (less atrophic) thyroid glands than rats that had only their pituitary gland removed[138, 139]. These findings support the idea that the pineal gland directly influences the growth of the thyroid.

The physiology of the thyroid gland is inconsistently altered after pinealectomy. The ability of the thyroid glands of adult rats to concentrate exogenously administered iodine is increased by about 50% after surgical removal of the pineal[137, 140]. These findings have, however, been refuted by Pazo et al.[138] who observed no significant alteration in the thyroidal radioactive iodine uptake by rats lacking their pineal gland for various lengths of time (7–49 days). Other findings include the inability of the pineal gland to alter thyroidal hormone release[141], protein bound iodine levels in the blood[121, 138], or plasma concentrations of free and bound thyroxine[142]. When the thyroid hormone secretion rate (TSR) was estimated in pinealectomised rats it was found to be elevated by roughly 12% (Figure 9.7)[143]. The TSR was measured at only one time interval (6 days) after the operation.

It was hoped that radioimmunoassays of TSH after various pineal manipulations would provide insight into the problems in this obviously perplexing area of research. Rowe and colleagues[144] estimated pituitary and plasma TSH levels in pinealectomised and intact rats kept in one of the following photoperiods (beginning when the animals were 21 days old) for 28 days: constant darkness, LD cycles of 12:12, or constant light. Under none of these conditions did the pineal gland significantly alter TSH metabolism. The experimental protocol of Rowe et al.[144] was nearly duplicated by Relkin[145] a year later but this time TSH levels were measured sooner after pinealectomy and dark exposure. Thus, male rats, 21 days old at the onset of the experiment, were pinealectomised or left intact and maintained in constant darkness for 4 or 7 days. After being without light for 4 days, both the plasma and pituitary levels of TSH of intact rats were found to be significantly depressed below those of pinealectomised animals. These differences had disappeared by the time the rats reached 28 days of age, however. Relkin[145] concluded that the pineal gland of perpuberal male rats does have an inhibitory effect on

TSH synthesis and secretion but that the effect is short-lived. TSH levels were not examined by Relkin after a longer interval of dark exposure such as was utilised by Rowe and co-workers. If Relkin's findings are, in fact, correct, such transitory changes would have been missed by Rowe *et al.*[144] In view of the short lived effect, the physiological importance of a pineal–thyroid relationship remains unclear.

As with the other pituitary trophic hormones, melatonin has been widely tested as to its potential role as a modulator of TSH secretion. Although there is one report to the contrary[146], the majority of studies indicate that subcutaneously, intraperitoneally or intraventricularly injected melatonin

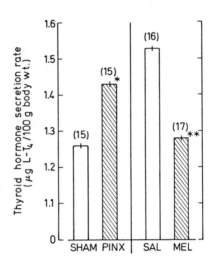

Figure 9.7 Influence of sham operation (SHAM) or pinealectomy (PINX) or treatment of rats with saline (SAL) or melatonin (MEL) on thyroid hormone secretion rate of immature rats. Melatonin was administered in the dosage of 20 μg daily for 10 days. $p < 0.05$ (*) and $p < 0.025$ (**) compared to sham-operated and saline injected groups, respectively. (Data from Ishibashi *et al.*[143], by courtesy of *Proc. Soc. Exp. Biol. Med.*)

depresses the iodine concentrating ability of the thyroid gland[147-150]. The intraventricular injections seem to rule out the possibility that melatonin acts peripherally at the level of the thyroid gland[150]. Recall that studies with hypophysectomised rats suggested a direct effect of the pineal secretions on the thyroidal follicles.

Subcutaneously administered melatonin also interferes with the TSR in young adult rats (Figure 9.7) and hamsters[151] but in older rats melatonin loses this capability[152]. On the basis of these and additional studies, Panda and Turner[63] proposed that melatonin impedes TSR by inhibiting the synthesis of iodinated hormones at the level of the thyroidal follicles, presumably by an action comparable to that of the commonly-used goitrogens. Indeed, thyroid glands of rats treated with melatonin were found to be hyperplastic and hypertrophic while bioassayable plasma TSH levels were elevated and pituitary TSH content diminished. This is characteristic of the type of reaction one would expect after goitrogen treatment. These results leave unexplained the effectiveness of intraventricularly injected melatonin on radioactive iodine uptake by the thyroid gland[150]. It would appear that melatonin may have two loci of action through which it may modulate thyroid metabolism: one at the level of the thyroid and one at the neural centre concerned with TSH-releasing factor synthesis. Alternatively, sufficient quantities of the intraventricularly injected melatonin may have gained access to the vascular system to modify thyroid activity directly.

9.7 CONCLUDING REMARKS

For many years the pineal gland was considered to be devoid of endocrine capabilities. We now find, quite to the contrary, that it may in fact secrete a heterogeneous group of substances and that these active materials may modulate the secretion of each of the adenohypophyseal hormones. It seems unlikely that the multipotent pineal depends on one hormone for its activity. Characteristically, endocrine interactions tend to be complex rather than simple. The evidence for a pineal effect on gonadotrophins is most easily defensible but it appears highly probable that it also influences the activity of other end organs which rely on trophic substances derived from the anterior pituitary gland.

Although the exact mechanisms involved remain in doubt, the most probable means by which the pineal carries out its function is by restricting hypothalamic releasing or inhibiting factor synthesis and (or) release. All of the data discussed above could be explained on this basis. The following provisional scheme of pineal action in mammals is presented. Under the influence of exteroceptive stimuli and possibly feed-back processes, the pineal produces and liberates compounds which gain access to the body fluids, i.e. either the blood or CSF but most likely the former. The pineal secretory products act on indoleamine and catecholamine containing neurones within the central nervous system. Because of the special significance of these neurones in the central control of releasing and inhibiting factor metabolism, the pineal can thus exert a regulatory influence on the secretion of hormones from the adenohypophysis. The predominant pineal effect relative to the hypothalamus is inhibitory. This is manifested at the level of the anterior pituitary as an inhibition of all of the hormones except prolactin, a hormone whose secretion is determined primarily by the amount of hypothalamic inhibiting factor which gains access to the hypothalamo–hypophyseal portal system. It will be one challenge of future endocrine research to test this theory.

References

1. Kappers, J. A. (1960). The development, topographical relations and innervation of the epiphysis cerebri in the albino rat. *Z. Zellforsch.*, **52**, 163
2. Kappers, J. A. (1965). Survey of the innervation of the epiphysis cerebri and the accessory pineal organ of vertebrates. *Prog. Brain Res.*, **10**, 87
3. Wurtman, R. J., Axelrod, J. and Kelly, D. E. (1968). *The Pineal* (New York: Academic Press)
4. Reiter, R. J. and Fraschini, F. (1969). Endocrine aspects of the mammalian pineal gland: a review. *Neuroendocrinology*, **5**, 219
5. Reiter, R. J. and Klein, D. C. (1971). Observations on the pineal gland, the Harderian glands, the retina and the reproductive organs of adult female rats exposed to continuous light. *J. Endocrinol.*, **51**, 117
6. Moore, R. Y., Heller, A., Bhatnager, R. K., Wurtman, R. J. and Axelrod, J. (1968). Central control of the pineal gland. *Arch. Neurol.*, **18**, 208
7. Owman, Ch. (1965). Localisation of neuronal and parenchymal monoamines under

normal and experimental conditions in the mammalian pineal gland. *Prog. Brain Res.*, **10**, 423

8. Strada, S. J., Klein, D. C., Weller, J. and Weiss, B. (1972). Effect of norepinephrine on the concentration of adenosine 3′, 5′-monophosphate of rat pineal gland in organ culture. *Endocrinology*, **90**, 1470

9. Klein, D. C. and Berg, G. R. (1970). Pineal gland: stimulation of melatonin production by norepinephrine involves cAMP-mediated stimulation of N-acetyltransferase. *Advan. Biochem. Physchopharmacal.*, **3**, 241

10. Klein, D. C., Weller, J. L., and Moore, R. Y. (1971). Melatonin metabolism: neural regulation of pineal serotonin: acetyl coenzyme A N-acetyltransferase activity. *Proc. Nat. Acad. Sci.*, **68**, 3107

11. Reiter, R. J. and Hester, R. J. (1966). Interrelationships of the pineal gland, the superior cervical ganglia and the photoperiod in the regulation of the endocrine systems of hamsters. *Endocrinology*, **79**, 1168

12. Wartman, S. S., Branch, B. J., George, R. and Taylor, A. N. (1969). Evidence for a cholinergic influence on pineal hydroxyindole-O-methyltransferase activity with changes in environmental lighting. *Life Sci.*, **8**, 1263

13. Machado, A. B. M. and Lemos, V. P. J. (1971). Histochemical evidence for a cholinergic sympathetic innervation of the rat pineal body. *J. Neuro-Visc. Rel.*, **32**, 104

14. Herbert, J. (1971). The role of the pineal gland in the control by light of the reproductive cycle of the ferret. *The Pineal Gland*, 303 (G. E. W. Wolstenholme and J. Knight, editors) (London: J. and A. Churchill)

15. Kenny, G. C. T. (1961). The 'nervous conarii' of the monkey. *J. Neuropath. Exp. Neurol.*, **20**, 563

16. Romijn, H. J. (1972). *Structure and innervation of the pineal gland of the rabbit, Oryctolagus cuniculus (L.), with some functional considerations* (Amsterdam: Nederlands Centraal Instituut voor Hersenonderzock)

17. Björklund, A., Owman, Ch. and West, K. A. (1972). Peripheral sympathetic innervation and serotonin cells in the habenular region of the rat brain. *Z. Zellforsch.*, **127**, 570

18. Norman, N. (1969). The cerebrospinal fluid as possible transmitter medium. *Physiology and Pathology of Adaptation Mechanisms*, 551 (E. Bajusz, editor) (New York: Pergamon Press)

19. Anand Kumar, T. C. (1968). Sexual differences in the ependyma lining the third ventricle in the area of the anterior hypothalamus of adult rhesus monkeys. *Z. Zellforsch.*, **90**, 28

20. Sheridan, M. N., Reiter, R. J. and Jacobs, J. J. (1969). An interesting anatomical relationship between the hamster pineal gland and the ventricular system of the brain. *J. Endocrinol.*, **45**, 131

21. Anton-Tay, F. and Wurtman, R. J. (1969). Regional uptake of ^{3}H-melatonin from blood or cerebrospinal fluid by rat brain. *Nature (London)*, **221**, 474

22. Collu, R., Fraschini, F. and Martini, L. (1971). Blockade of ovulation by melatonin. *Experientia*, **27**, 844

23. Fraschini, F., Collu, R. and Martini, L. (1971). Mechanisms of inhibitory action of pineal principles on gonadotropin secretion. *The Pineal Gland*, 259 (G. E. W. Wolstenholme and J. Knight, editors) (London: J. and A. Churchill)

24. Reiter, R. J. and Sorrentino, S. (1971). Inhibition of luteinizing hormone release and ovulation in PMS-treated rats by peripherally administered melatonin. *Contraception*, **4**, 385

25. Smith, A. R. (1971). The topographical relations of the rabbit pineal gland to the large intracranial veins. *Brain Res.*, **30**, 339

26. Pelham, R. W., Ralph, C. L. and Campbell, I. M. (1972). Mass spectral identification of melatonin in blood. *Biochem. Biophys. Res. Com.*, **46**, 1236

27. Quay, W. B. (1970). Endocrine effects of the mammalian pineal. *Amer. Zool.*, **10**, 237

28. Thieblot, L. and Blaise, S. (1966). Étude biochimique du principe pinéal antigonadotrope. *Prob. Act. Endocrinol. Nutr.*, **10**, 257

29. Thieblot, L. and Mersigot, M. (1971). Acquisitions récentes sur le facteur antigonadotrope de la glande pinéale. *J. Neuro-Visc. Rel.*, Suppl. X, 153

30. Milcu, S. M., Pavel, S. and Neacsu, C. (1963). Biological and chromatographic characterisation of a polypeptide with pressor and oxytocic activities isolated from bovine pineal gland. *Endocrinology*, **72**, 563

31. Pavel, S. (1963). Cercetări asupra unui nou hormon pineal cu structură peptidică. *Stud. Cercet. Endocrinol.*, **14**, 665
32. Pavel, S. and Petrescu, S. (1966). Inhibition of gonadotrophin by a highly purified pineal peptide and by synthetic arginine vasotocin. *Nature (London)*, **212**, 1054
33. Moszkowska, A. and Ebels, I. (1968). A study of the antigonadotrophic action of synthetic arginine vasotocin. *Experientia*, **24**, 610
34. Cheesman, D. W. and Fariss, B. L. (1970). Isolation and characterisation of a gonado-trophin-inhibiting substance from the bovine pineal gland. *Proc. Soc. Exp. Biol. Med.*, **133**, 1254
35. Ebels, I., Moszkowska, A. and Scémma, A. (1965). Etudé *in vitro* des extraits épiphy-saires fractionnés. Resultats préliminaires. *C. R. Soc. Biol.*, **260**, 5126
36. Ebels, I. (1967). Etudé chimique des extraits épiphysaires fractionnés. *Biol. Med.*, **56**, 305
37. Moszkowska, A. and Ebels, I. (1971). The influence of the pineal body on the gona-dotropic function of the hypophysis. *J. Neuro-Visc. Rel.*, Suppl. X, 160
38. Benson, B., Matthews, M. J. and Rodin, A. E. (1971). A melatonin-free extract of bovine pineal with antigonadotropic activity. *Life Sci.*, **10**, 607
39. Benson, B., Matthews, M. J. and Rodin, A. E. (1972). Studies on a non-melatonin pineal antigonadotrophin. *Acta Endocrinol.*, **69**, 257
40. Lerner, A. B., Case, J. D., Takahashi, Y., Lee, T. H. and Mori, W. (1958). Isolation of melatonin, the pineal gland factor that lightens melanocytes. *J. Amer. Chem. Soc.*, **80**, 2587
41. Lerner, A. B., Case, J. D. and Heinzelman, R. V. (1959). Structure of melatonin. *J. Amer. Chem. Soc.*, **81**, 6084
42. Axelrod, J. and Weissbach, H. (1960). Enzymatic 0-methylation of N-acetylserotonin to melatonin. *Science*, **131**, 1312
43. Cardinali, D. P. and Rosner, J. J. (1971). Retinal localization of the hydroxyindole-0-methyltransferase (HIOMT) in the rat. *Endocrinology*, **89**, 301
44. Vlahakes, G. and Wurtman, R. J. (1972). A Mg2+ dependent hydroxyindole-0-methyl-transferase in rat Harderian gland. *Biochim. Biophys. Acta*, **261**, 194
45. Wurtman, R. J., Axelrod, J. and Chu, E. W. (1963). Melatonin, a pineal substance: effect on rat ovary. *Science*, **141**, 277
46. Kamberi, I., Mical, R. S. and Porter, J. C. (1970). Effect of anterior pituitary perfusion and intraventricular injection of catecholamines and indoleamines on LH release. *Endocrinology*, **87**, 1
47. Sorrentino, S., Jr, Reiter, R. J. and Schalch, D. S. (1971). Hypotrophic reproductive organs and normal growth in male rats treated with melatonin. *J. Endocrinol.*, **51**, 213
48. McIsaac, W. M., Taborsky, R. G. and Farrell, G. (1964). 5-Methoxytryptophol: effect on estrus and ovarian weight. *Science*, **145**, 63
49. Vaughan, M. K., Reiter, R. J., Vaughan, G. M., Bigelow, L. and Altschule, M. D. (1972). Inhibition of compensatory ovarian hypertrophy in the mouse and vole: a comparison of Altschule's pineal extract, pineal indoles, vasopressin, and oxytocin. *Gen. Comp. Endocrinol.*, **18**, 372
50. Alberatazzi, E., Barbanti-Silva, C., Trentini, G. P. and Botticelli, A. (1966). Influence de l'epiphysectomie et du traitment avec la 5-hydroxytryptamine sur le cycle oestral de la ratte albinos. *Ann. Endocrinol.*, **27**, 93
51. Reiter, R. J. Involvement of pineal indoles and polypeptides with the neuroendocrine axis. *Progr. Brain Res.* (in press)
52. Reiter, R. J. (1967). Failure of the pineal gland to prevent gonadotrophin-induced ovarian stimulation in blinded hamsters. *J. Endocrinol.*, **38**, 199
53. Reiter, R. J. (1973). Pineal control of a seasonal reproductive rhythm in male golden hamsters exposed to natural daylight and temperature. *Endocrinology*, **92**, 423
54. Reiter, R. J. (1972). Pineal control of reproductive biology. *Biology of Reproduction: Basic and Clinical Studies*, 105. (J. T. Velardo and B. Kasprow, editors) (Mexico City: Bay Publ. Co.) (in press)
55. Kamberi, I. A., Mical, R. S. and Porter, J. C. (1971). Effects of melatonin and sero-tonin on the release of FSH and prolactin. *Endocrinology*, **88**, 1288
56. Fraschini, F., Mess, B., Piva, F. and Martini, L. (1968). Brain receptors sensitive to indole compounds: function in control of luteinizing hormone secretion. *Science*, **159**, 1104

57. Anton-Tay, F., Chou, C., Anton, S. and Wurtman, R. J. (1968). Brain serotonin concentration: elevation following intraperitoneal administration of melatonin. *Science*, **162**, 277
58. Reiter, R. J. (1973). Surgical procedures involving the pineal gland which prevent gonadal degeneration in adult male hamsters. *Ann. Endocrinol.*, **33**, 571
59. Reiter, R. J. and Sorrentino, S., Jr (1972). Prevention of pineal-mediated reproductive responses in light-deprived hamsters by partial or total isolation of the medial basal hypothalamus. *J. Neuro-Visc. Rel.*, **32**, 355
60. Reiter, R. J. (1973). Pineal regulation of the hypothalamo–pituitary axis: gonadotropins. *The Pituitary Gland and Its Control* (E. Knobil and W. H. Sawyer, editors) (Washington: American Physiological Society) (in press)
61. Peat, F. and Kinson, G. A. (1971). Testicular steroidogenesis *in vitro* in the rat in response to blinding, pinealectomy and to the addition of melatonin. *Steroids*, **17**, 251
62. Ellis, L. C. (1972). Inhibition of rat testicular androgen synthesis *in vitro* by melatonin and serotonin. *Endocrinology*, **90**, 17
63. Panda, J. N. and Turner, C. W. (1968). The role of melatonin in the regulation of thyrotrophin secretion. *Acta Endocrinol.*, **57**, 363
64. Debeljuk, L., Vilchez, J. A., Schnitman, M. A., Paulucci, O. A. and Feder, V. M. (1971). Further evidence for a peripheral action of melatonin. *Endocrinology*, **89**, 1117
65. Norris, J. T. (1971). The ovary as a potential target organ for pineal polypeptides. *Anat. Rec.*, **169**, 389
66. Bianchini, P., Osima, B., Casetta, R. and Barbanti-Silva, C. (1967). Présence dans la glanda pineale bovine de deux facteurs d'inhibition de l'oestrus. *Biochim. Biol. Sperm.*, **6**, 95
67. Quay, W. B. (1969). Evidence for a pineal contribution in the regulation of vertebrate reproductive systems. *Gen. Comp. Endocrinol.*, Suppl. 2, 101
68. Reiter, R. J. and Sorrentino, S., Jr. (1971). Reproductive effects of the mammalian pineal. *Amer. Zool.*, **10**, 247
69. Hoffman, R. A. and Reiter, R. J. (1965). Pineal gland: influence on gonads of male hamsters. *Science*, **148**, 1609
70. Reiter, R. J. (1972). The role of the pineal in reproduction. *Reproductive Biology*, 71 H. Balin and S. Glasser, editors) (Amsterdam: Excerpta Medica)
71. Gaston, S. and Menaker, M. (1967). Photoperiodic control of hamster testis. *Science*, **158**, 925
72. Reiter, R. J. (1968). Morphological studies on the reproductive organs of blinded male hamsters and the effects of pinealectomy or superior cervical ganglionectomy. *Anat. Rec.*, **160**, 13
73. Reiter, R. J. (1967). The effect of pineal grafts, pinealectomy, and denervation of the pineal gland on the reproductive organs of male hamsters. *Neuroendocrinology*, **2**, 138
74. Reiter, R. J. (1973). Comparative physiology: pineal gland. *Ann. Rev. Physiol.*, **35**, 305
75. Reiter, R. J. (1973). Evidence for a seasonal rhythm in pineal gland function. *Chronobiology* (L. E. Scheving, F. Halberg, and J. R. Pauly editors) (Tokyo: Igaku Shoin, Ltd.) (in press)
76. Quay, W. B. (1956). Volumetric and cytologic variation in the pineal body of *Peromyscus leucopus* (rodentia) with respect to sex, activity and day-length. *J. Morphol.*, **98**, 471
77. Mogler, R. K. H. (1958). Das Endokrinesystem des syrischen Goldhamster unter Berücksichtigung des Naturlichen und Experimentellen Winterschlaf. *Z. Morph. Oekol. Tiere*, **47**, 267
78. Czyba, J. C., Girod, C. and Durand, N. (1964). Sur l'antagonisme épiphyseohypophyaire et les variations saisonieres de la spermatogénése chez le hamster doré (Mesocricetus auratus). *C. R. Soc. Biol.*, **158**, 742
79. Smit-Vis, J. H. and Akkerman-Bellaart, M. A. (1967). Spermiogenesis in hibernating golden hamsters. *Experientia*, **23**, 844
80. Vendrely, E., Guerillot, C., Basseville, C. and De Lage, C. (1971). Variations saissoniéres de la spermatogenése chez le hamster doré. *Bull. Assoc. Anat.*, **152**, 778
81. Rust, C. C. and Meyer, R. K. (1969). Hair color, molt and testis size in male, short-tailed weasels treated with melatonin. *Science*, **165**, 921

82. Reiter, R. J. (1968). The pineal gland and gonadal development in male rats and hamsters. *Fertil. Steril.*, **19**, 1009
83. Fraschini, F. (1969). The pineal gland and the control of LH and FSH secretion. *The Pineal Gland*, 637 (C. Gual, editor) (Amsterdam: Excerpta Medica)
84. Reiter, R. J. and Sorrentino, S., Jr. (1971). Factors influential in determining the gonad inhibiting activity of the pineal gland. *The Pineal Gland*, 329 (G. E. W. Wolstenholme and J. Knight, editors) (London: J. and A. Churchill)
85. Reiter, R. J., Sorrentino, S. D., Hoffmann, J. C. and Rubin, P. H. (1968). Pineal, neural and photic control of reproductive organ size in early androgen-treated male rats. *Neuroendocrinology*, **3**, 246
86. Moszkowska, A. and Scemma, A. (1968). L'epiphysectomie, et la résponse photosexuelle du rat. *Arch. Anat. Histol. Embryol. Norm. Exp.*, **51**, 475
87. Gorski, R. A. (1966). Localization and sexual differentiation of the nervous structures which regulate ovulation. *J. Reprod. Fertil.*, Suppl. 1, 67
88. Swanson, H. E. and Werff ten Bosch, J. J. Van der (1963). Sex differences in growth of rats and their modification by a single injection of testosterone propionate shortly after birth. *J. Endocrinol.*, **26**, 197
89. Reiter, R. J. (1968). Pineal–gonadal relationships in male rodents. *Progress in Endocrinology*, 631 (C. Gual, editor) (Amsterdam: Excerpta Medica)
90. Reiter, R. J. (1970). Physiological effects of the pineal gland in androgen-sterilized female rats. *Acta Endocrinol.*, **63**, 667
91. Whitten, W. K. (1956). The effect of removal of the olfactory bulbs on the gonads of mice. *J. Endocrinol.*, **14**, 160
92. Aron, Cl., Roos, J. and Asch, G. (1970). Effect of removal of the olfactory bulbs on mating behaviour and ovulation in the rat. *Neuroendocrinology*, **6**, 109
93. Reiter, R. J. and Ellison, N. M. (1970). Delayed puberty in blinded anosmic female rats: role of the pineal gland. *Gen. Comp. Endocrinol.*, **2**, 216
94. Reiter, R. J., Sorrentino. S., Jr, Ralph, C. L., Lynch, H. J., Mull, D. and Jarrow, E. (1971). Some endocrine effects of blinding and anosmia in adult male rats with observations on pineal melatonin. *Endocrinology*, **88**, 895
95. Osman, P., Welshen, R. W. and Moll, J. (1972). Anti-gonadotrophic and anti-growth effects of the pineal gland in immature female rats. *Neuroendocrinology*, **10**, 121
96. Sorrentino, S., Jr, Reiter, R. J. and Schalch, D. S. (1971). Interactions of the pineal gland, blinding, and underfeeding on reproductive organ size and radioimmunoassayable growth hormone. *Neuroendocrinology*, **7**, 105
97. Benson, B., Sorrentino, S. and Evans, J. S. (1969). Increase in serum FSH following unilateral ovariectomy in the rat. *Endocrinology*, **84**, 369
98. Sorrentino. S. (1968). Antigonadotrophic effects of melatonin in intact and unilaterally ovariectomised rats. *Anat. Rec.*, **160**, 432
99. Vaughan, M. K., Benson, B., Norris, J. T. and Vaughan, G. M. (1971). Inhibition of compensatory ovarian hypertrophy in mice by melatonin, 5-hydroxytryptamine and pineal powder. *J. Endocrinol.*, **50**, 171
100. Vaughan, M. K., Benson, B. and Norris, J. T. (1970). Inhibition of compensatory ovarian hypertrophy in mice by 5-hydroxytryptamine and melatonin. *J. Endocrinol.*, **47**, 397
101. Vaughan, M. K., Reiter, R. J. and Vaughan, G. M. (1971). Effect of delaying melatonin injections on the inhibition of compensatory ovarian hypertrophy in mice. *J. Endocrinol.*, **51**, 787
102. Longenecker, D. E. and Gallo, D. G. (1971). The inhibition of PMSG-induced ovulation in immature rats by melatonin. *Proc. Soc. Exp. Biol. Med.*, **137**, 625
103. Fraschini, F. and Martini, L. (1970). Rhythmic phenomena and pineal principles. *The Hypothalamus*, 529 (L. Martini, M. Motta and F. Fraschini, editors) (New York: Academic Press)
104. Moszkowska, A., Kordon, C. and Ebels, I. (1971). Biochemical fractions and mechanisms involved in the pineal modulation of pituitary gonadotropic release. *The Pineal Gland*, 241 (G. E. W. Wolstenholme and J. Knight, editors) (London: J. and A. Churchill)
105. Hoffman, R. A. and Reiter, R. J. (1966). Responses of some endocrine organs of female hamsters to pinealectomy and light. *Life Sci.*, **5**, 1147
106. Relkin, R. (1972). Rat pituitary and plasma prolactin levels after pinealectomy. *J. Endocrinol.*, **53**, 179

107. Relkin, R. (1972). Effects of variations in environmental lighting on pituitary and plasma prolactin levels in the rat. *Neuroendocrinology*, **9**, 278

108. Donofrio, R. J. and Reiter, R. J. (1972). Depressed pituitary prolactin levels in blinded anosmic female rats: role of the pineal gland. *J. Reprod. Fertil.*, **31**, 159

109. Sorrentino, S., Jr, Schalch, D. S. and Reiter, R. J. (1972). Environmental control of growth hormone and growth. *Growth and Growth Hormone*, 330 (A. Pecile and E. Müller, editors) (Amsterdam: Excerpta Medica)

110. Malm, O. J., Skaug, O. E. and Lingjoerde, P. (1959). The effect of pinealectomy on bodily growth, survival rates and ^{32}P uptake in the rat. *Acta Endocrinol.*, **30**, 22

111. Grachev, I. I., Usanova, R. I. and Seliverstow, U. A. (1972). The influence of the pineal extract on the growth activity of the rat pituitary gland. *Sechenov Fiziol. Zh. SSSR.*, **58**, 272 (in Russian)

112. Sorrentino, S., Jr, Reiter, R. J. and Schalch, D. S. (1971). Pineal regulation of growth hormone synthesis and release in blinded and blinded-anosmic male rats. *Neuroendocrinology*, **7**, 210

113. Sorrentino, S., Jr, Reiter, R. J., Schalch, D. S. and Donofrio, R. J. (1971). Role of the pineal gland in growth restraint of adult male rats by light and smell deprivation. *Neuroendocrinology*, **8**, 116

114. Dhariwal, A. P. S., Krulich, L. and McCann, S. M. (1969). Purification of a growth hormone inhibiting factor (GIF) from sheep hypothalami. *Neuroendocrinology*, **4**, 282

115. Relkin, R. (1972). Effects of pinealectomy, constant light and darkness on growth hormone levels in the pituitary and plasma of the rat. *J. Endocrinol.*, **53**, 289

116. Quay, W. B. (1969). The role of the pineal gland in environmental adaptation. *Physiology and Pathology of Adaptation Mechanism*, 508 (E. Bajusz, editor) (New York: Pergamon Press)

117. Simionescu, N. and Scherzer, M. (1964). Un nou model experimental: simbioza pinealo-glomerulară la sobalanul alb. *Stud. Cercet. Endocrinol.*, **15**, 117

118. Simionescu, N. and Scherzer, M. (1964). Demonstrarea *in situ* a controlului hormonal al zonei glomerulare cu ajutorul 'simbiozei pinealo-glomerulare'. *Stud. Cercert. Endocrinol.*, **15**, 227

119. Kinson, G., Wahid, A. K. and Singer, B. (1967). Effect of chronic pinealectomy on adrenocortical hormone secretion rate in normal and hypertensive rats. *Gen. Comp. Endocrinol.*, **8**, 45

120. Kisnon, G. A., Singer, B. and Grant, L. (1968). Adrenocortical hormone secretion at various time intervals after pinealectomy in the rat. *Gen. Comp. Endocrinol.*, **10**, 447

121. Henzl, M. R., Spaur, C. L., Magoun, R. E. and Kincl, F. A. (1970). A note on endocrine functions of neonatally pinealectomised rats. *Endocrinol., Exp.*, **4**, 77

122. Nir, I., Schmidt, V., Hirschmann, N. and Sulman, F. G. (1971). The effect of pinealectomy on plasma corticosterone levels under various conditions of light. *Life Sci.*, **10**, 317

123. Reiter, R. J., Hoffman, R. A. and Hester, R. J. (1966). The effects of thiourea, photoperiod and the pineal gland on the thyroid, adrenal and reproductive organs of female hamsters. *J. Exp. Zool.*, **162**, 263

124. Dickson, K. L. and Hasty, D. L. (1972). Effects of the pineal gland in unilaterally adrenalectomised rats. *Acta Endocrinol.*, **70**, 438

125. Reiter, R. J. (1972). Compensatory growth of the ovaries, adrenal glands and kidneys in blinded, anosmic rats. *Experientia*, **28**, 1492

126. Jacobs, J. J. and Kendall, J. W. (1972). The effect of the pineal on rhythmic pituitary–adrenal function in the blinded rat. *Abstracts IV Int. Congr. Endocrinol.*, Washington, D.C., p. 53

127. Jouan, P. and Samperez, S. (1965). Etude de la sécretion des corticosteroides et de l'hormone adrénocorticotrope hypophysaire chez le rat epiphysectomisé. *Prog. Brain Res.*, **10**, 604

128. Anton-Tay, F., Escobar, A. and Anton, S. M. (1963). Inhibicon de la hipertrofia suprarenal compensadora por la administracion de extracto pineal. *Bol. Inst. Etud. Med. Biol.*, **20**, 281

129. Vaughan, M. K., Vaughan, G. M., Reiter, R. J. and Benson, B. (1972). Effect of melatonin and other pineal indoles on adrenal enlargement produced in male and female mice by pinealectomy, unilateral adrenalectomy, castration, and cold stress. *Neuroendocrinology*, **10**, 139

130. Nuzzi, R., De Martino, C., Pavoni, P. and Ciampalini, L. (1962). Variazioni del contento di corticotropína nella ipofisi del ratto tratto con estratti epifisari o privato di pineale. *Sperimentale*, **112**, 216
131. Barchas, J., Conner, R., Levine, S. and Vernikos-Danellis, J. (1969). Effects of chronic melatonin and saline injections on pituitary adrenal secretion. *Experientia*, **25**, 413
132. Gromova, A. E., Kraus, M. and Křeček, J. (1967). Effect of pineal substances on production of corticosterone and aldosterone by the rat adrenal gland. *Gen. Comp. Endocrinol.*, **9**, 455
133. Motta, M., Schiaffini, O., Piva, E. and Martini, L. (1971). Pineal principles and the control of adrenocorticotropin secretion. *The Pineal Gland*, 279 (G. E. W. Wolstenholme and J. Knight, editors) (London: J. and A. Churchill)
134. De Prospo, N. and Hurley, J. (1971). Effects of injecting melatonin and its precursors into the lateral cerebral ventricles on selected organs in rats. *J. Endocrinol.*, **49**, 545
135. Houssay, A. B., Pazo, J. H. and Epper, C. E. (1966). Effects of the pineal gland upon the hair cycles in mice. *J. Invest. Dermatol.*, **47**, 230
136. Lombard des Gouttes, M.-N. (1967). Epiphysectomie a la naissance chez la Souris mâle. *C. R. Acad. Sci. (Paris)*, **264**, 2141
137. Scepovic, M. (1963). Contribution á l'etude histophysiologique de la glande thyroide chez les rats epiphysectomisés. *Ann. Endocrinol.*, **24**, 371
138. Pazo, J. H., Houssay, A. B., Davison, T. A. and Chait, R. J. (1968). On the mechanism of the thyroid hypertrophy in pinealectomized rats. *Acta Physiol. Latino-Amer.*, **18**, 332
139. Houssay, A. B. and Pazo, J. H. (1968). Role of the pituitary in the thyroid hypertrophy of pinealectomized rats. *Experientia*, **24**, 813
140. Csaba, G., Kiss, J. and Bodoky, M. (1968). Uptake of radioactive iodine by the thyroid after pinealectomy. *Acta Biol. Acad. Sci. Hung.*, **19**, 35
141. Mess, B. (1968). Endocrine and neurochemical aspects of pineal function. *Int. Rev. Neurobiol.*, **11**, 171
142. Negoescu, I., Constantinescu, A., Marcean, R. P. and Dumitrescu, C. (1968). Influenta pinealaectomiei aspura tiroxinei libere se legata la sobolanul alb Wistar. *Stud. Cercet. Endocrinol.*, **19**, 125
143. Ishibashi, T., Hahn, D. W., Strivastana, L., Kumaresan, P. and Turner, C. W. (1966). Effect of pinealectomy and melatonin on feed consumption and thyroid hormone secretion rate. *Proc. Soc. Exp. Biol. Med.*, **122**, 644
144. Rowe, J. W., Richert, J. R., Klein, D. C. and Reichlin, S. (1970). Relation of the pineal gland and environmental lighting to thyroid function in the rat. *Neuroendocrinology*, **6**, 247
145. Relkin, R. (1972). Effects of pinealectomy and constant light and darkness on thyrotropin levels in the pituitary and plasma of the rat. *Neuroendocrinology*, **10**, 46
146. Naber, S. P., Goldman, M. and Peaslee, M. H. (1969). The effect of melatonin on the iodine concentrating mechanism of the thyroid gland in young adult rats. *Proc. So. Dak. Acad. Sci.*, **48**, 44
147. Baschieri, L., de Luca, F., Cramarossa, L., de Martino, C., Oliverio, A. and Negri, M. (1963). Modifications of thyroid activity by melatonin. *Experientia*, **19**, 15
148. Reiter, R. J., Hoffman, R. A. and Hester, R. J. (1965). Inhibition of ^{131}I uptake by thyroid glands of male rats treated with melatonin and pineal extract. *Amer. Zool.*, **5**, 727
149. De Prospo, N. D., Safinski, R. J., De Martino, L. J. and McGuiness, E. T. (1969). Melatonin and its precursors' effect on ^{131}I uptake by the thyroid gland under different photic conditions. *Life. Sci.*, **8**, 837
150. De Prospo, N. D. and Hurley, J. (1971). A comparison of intracerebral and intraperitoneal injections of melatonin and its precursors on ^{131}I uptake by the thyroid glands of rats. *Agents Actions*, **2**, 14
151. Singh, D. V. and Turner, C. W. (1972). Effect of melatonin upon thyroid hormone secretion rate in female hamsters and adult rats. *Acta Endocrinol.*, **69**, 35
152. Narang, G. D., Singh, D. V. and Turner, C. W. (1967). Effect of melatonin on thyroid hormone secretion rate and feed consumption of female rats. *Proc. Soc. Exp. Biol. Med.*, **125**, 184

10
Cyclic AMP as a Mediator of Hormonal Effects

S. J. STRADA and **G. A. ROBISON**

University of Texas Medical School, Houston

10.1 INTRODUCTION

Cyclic AMP (adenosine 3',5'-monophosphate) was discovered by Sutherland and Rall[1] in the course of investigating the mechanism of the hepatic glycogenolytic effects of epinephrine and glucagon. These hormones were shown to stimulate glycogenolysis in dog liver slices by increasing the activity of liver phosphorylase. This enzyme was found to exist in two forms, an active phosphorylated form and an inactive dephosphorylated form. Activation of phosphorylase involved the transfer of the terminal phosphate of ATP to the protein, under the catalytic influence of a kinase. Inactivation involved removal of this phosphate by a relatively specific phosphatase. It appeared that the hormones were acting to shift the balance between these two reactions in favour of the kinase. This was eventually demonstrated in broken cell preparations, but only if the particulate fraction containing fragments of the cell membrane was present. It was then established that the hormones were interacting with this fraction to stimulate the formation of a heat-stable factor which in turn increased the activity of phosphorylase kinase. This factor was soon identified as cyclic AMP (Figure 10.1). The activity in membrane fragments responsible for catalysing the formation of cyclic AMP from ATP was named adenyl cyclase[2], although it is more properly referred to now as adenylyl cyclase or adenylate cyclase. The reaction was shown to require magnesium ions, yielding pyrophosphate as the other product. A phosphodiesterase capable of inactivating cyclic AMP by catalysing its hydrolysis to 5'-AMP was also identified. For more detailed descriptions of the experimentation leading to the discovery of cyclic AMP, readers are referred to the introductory chapter of an earlier monograph[3] and to Professor Sutherland's Nobel Prize address[4].

Subsequently ACTH (but not glucagon or epinephrine) was to be found capable of stimulating the formation of cyclic AMP in adrenocortical slices, and the application of exogenous cyclic AMP was shown to stimulate steroidogenesis. Later a variety of other hormones was shown to stimulate adenylyl cyclase in the cells of their target organs, and these and other developments led eventually to the second messenger concept[5,6] illustrated in Figure 10.2. In

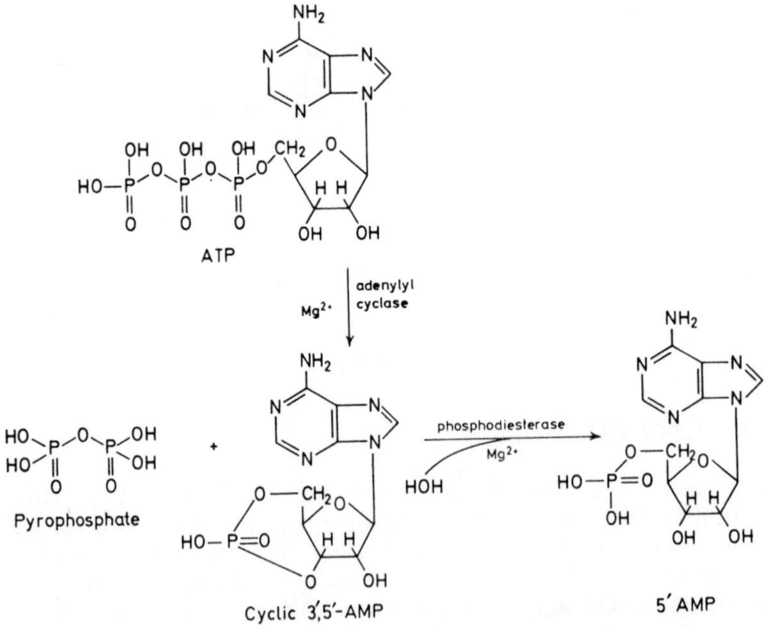

Figure 10.1   Reactions involved in the formation and metabolism of cyclic AMP

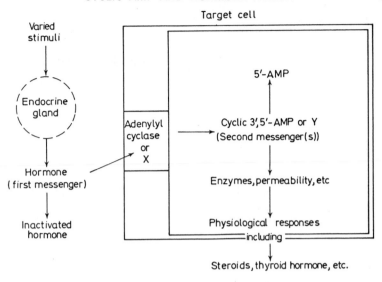

Figure 10.2   Schematic representation of the second messenger concept

brief summary, this concept states that hormones, acting as first messengers, interact with specific receptors on or near the surface of their target cells. This hormone–receptor interaction then leads, by mechanisms which are still not understood, to an increase in the catalytic activity of adenylyl cyclase and hence to a rise in the intracellular level of cyclic AMP. Acting as a second messenger, cyclic AMP then goes on to influence one or more systems inside the cell, leading ultimately to the physiological response associated with the action of the hormone.

Until recently, most research dealing with cyclic AMP was designed to elucidate the regulatory role of this nucleotide in differentiated eukaryotic cells. An involvement of cyclic AMP in lower organisms has also been established, however, and now there is evidence for an important role of cyclic AMP during growth and development. These newer developments will be discussed in this review because the role of cyclic AMP in hormone action can then be placed in better perspective. A number of other recent reviews[4, 7-13] and monographs[3, 14-16] can be consulted for more detailed discussion of certain topics and for many references to the earlier literature.

10.2   ROLE OF CYCLIC AMP IN LOWER ORGANISMS

Although we plan to emphasise the role of cyclic AMP in higher organisms in this review, it is noteworthy that cyclic AMP also plays an important role in many lower organisms. It is now apparent that these organisms possess mechanisms for survival which seem quite analogous to the 'fight or flight' system familiar to students of mammalian physiology, and that some of these mechanisms require the participation of cyclic AMP.

Data to support the role of cyclic AMP during evolution are incomplete, but there is no doubt that its role as a regulatory agent evolved at a fairly early stage. Changing requirements have caused the cyclic AMP system in higher organisms to assume a role different from that expressed in lower organisms, but many analogies can be discerned when these roles are compared.

10.2.1   Bacteria

In *E. coli* and certain other bacterial species, the cyclic AMP system is not controlled by hormones but seems rather to be controlled by the presence or absence of simple nutrients. Thus in these organisms the cyclic AMP system is invoked when their survival is threatened (e.g. following depletion of their food supply), and the effect of cyclic AMP is to enable them to utilise alternate substrates or to conserve or better utilise their stores of endogenous substrates. Mutant strains of bacteria which lack the capacity to form cyclic AMP can survive under carefully controlled experimental conditions, but are not suited for survival under the conditions of a normal environment.

The existence of cyclic AMP in *E. coli* was reported in 1965 by Makman and Sutherland, who noted that an abrupt rise in the concentration of cyclic AMP occurred in these organisms coincident with the complete utilisation of glucose. We now know, from the work of Pastan and Perlman[17] and other investigators, that cyclic AMP is required for the synthesis of a number of inducible enzymes in *E. coli* and other gram-negative organisms, and that glucose and other carbon compounds suppress the synthesis of certain enzymes (e.g. *β*-galactosidase, galactokinase, tryptophosphanase) needed in the metabolism of secondary energy sources (e.g. lactose and galactose) by reducing the concentration of cyclic AMP. Elevation of the cyclic AMP level in these bacteria leads to reversal of catabolite repression and increased enzyme synthesis. Replenishing the glucose supply leads to lower cyclic AMP levels and repression of the synthesis of secondary catabolic enzymes. The isolation of mutants of *E. coli* has provided strong evidence that cyclic AMP and a cyclic AMP receptor protein (CRP) are required for the synthesis of all inducible enzymes subject to catabolite repression.

The enzyme which has been studied in most detail from this point of view is *β*-galactosidase, the synthesis of which is controlled by the *lac* operon. The structural genes of this operon can be transcribed only when an inducer such as lactose is present, and then only in the presence of the cyclic AMP–CRP complex. Current evidence suggests that this complex binds directly to the promoter gene, thereby enabling RNA polymerase to form a pre-initiation complex with the DNA, leading to the synthesis of messenger RNA.

Mutants unable to synthesise cyclic AMP because of a deficiency in adenylyl cyclase are unable to make normal amounts of these inducible enzymes, and are therefore unable to utilise a number of carbon sources for growth. The addition of cyclic AMP to cultures of these mutants restores both enzyme synthesis and growth towards normal. Mutants lacking CRP are also unable to grow in the absence of glucose, but are unresponsive to exogenous cyclic AMP.

Another effect of cyclic AMP in these organisms is to stimulate the synthesis of flagellae, causing the cells to become motile. This is advantageous under conditions leading to cyclic AMP formation because it enables the organisms to seek a more congenial environment.

Evidence has also been presented for a role of cyclic AMP in lysogeny, the process by which certain viruses (bacteriophages) become incorporated into the bacterial DNA as silent prophages. One phage is incorporated per chromosome, and will replicate only as often as the bacteria themselves replicate. The alternative to lysogeny is that the viruses will replicate without regard to the host, leading ultimately to lysis of the bacterial cell. Hong et al.[18] showed that mutants of S. typhimurium, defective in the gene for adenylyl cyclase or in the gene for CRP, underwent lysogeny much less frequently after infection by the temperate bacteriophage P22 than did wild-type strains. Normal rates of lysogenisation could be restored to the cyclase-deficient mutants but not to the CRP-deficient ones by the addition of exogenous cyclic AMP. Similar observations have been made by others[19-21] using E. coli infected by phage λ. It would thus appear that when bacterial levels of cyclic AMP are high, as in the absence of glucose, lysogeny will be favoured over lysis. When growth conditions improve, leading to a fall in cyclic AMP, then lysis will be favoured over lysogeny. The exact point of action of the cyclic AMP–CRP complex in governing this decision has not been established, but presumably the expression of one or more of the genes necessary for lysogeny to occur must depend on cyclic AMP.

These observations are of interest because of their possible implications for mammalian physiology. Huebner and Todaro[22] have postulated that cancer results from the derepressed activity of a virus-like particle known as the oncogene. Acording to this theory, for which a substantial amount of evidence has now accumulated, the oncogene has been part of the genetic make-up of vertebrates since early in evolution. It may play an important role during early embryogenesis but is normally repressed during later life. Incorporation of the oncogene into the DNA of higher forms seems quite analogous, in principle, to the incorporation of viral DNA into the DNA of lysogenic bacteria. Factors capable of inducing lysis in lysogenic bacteria have long been known to be carcinogenic when applied to mammalian cells. By extrapolation, therefore, it might be suggested that high levels of cyclic AMP in mammalian cells would tend to repress the oncogene, whereas low levels would lead to derepression and hence to cancer. As discussed in a later section, evidence is now accumulating to implicate reduced levels of cyclic AMP in the genesis of at least some types of tumours.

Gram-positive organisms have now been studied, and it has been found that cyclic AMP occurs in some of them, such as streptococci[23], but apparently not in others, such as lactobacilli[24]. Whether some other factor assumes the role of cyclic AMP in these latter organisms remains to be determined.

10.2.2 Cellular slime moulds

At least three features characteristic of the role of cyclic AMP in higher forms were mentioned in the preceding section on bacteria. Thus, in these organisms, the intracellular level of cyclic AMP depends upon factors in the extra-cellular environment, the end result of a change in the level of cyclic AMP will depend upon factors other than cyclic AMP, and cyclic AMP does not seem to be required under all conditions. The requirement of cyclic AMP for flagella formation might suggest a fourth feature, i.e. a tendency to promote differentiation. Additional evidence for a role of cyclic AMP in differentiation has come from studies of the cellular slime mould, *Dictyostelium discoideum*.

The life cycle of this organism consists of vegetative and morphogenic phases. During the vegetative or unicellular stage, the amoebae engulf bacteria as a food source, and the accumulation of cyclic AMP does not occur. As soon as the food supply is exhausted, however, the cells cease to divide and there is a sudden increase in the extracellular level of cyclic AMP. The amoebae then begin to aggregate. Cyclic AMP functions not only as a chemotactic substance to initiate the aggregation process, but also causes the cells to become 'stickier'. After all of the amoebae have entered one or more aggregates, the cells differentiate into multicellular organisms consisting eventually of spore-forming cells supported by stalk cells. Now there is evidence that cyclic AMP functions during the morphogenic phase to trigger the differentiation of the stalk cells[25,26].

The changing levels of cyclic AMP during the life cycle of the slime mould do not appear to be regulated by rapid changes in adenylyl cyclase activity since the specific activity of the enzyme remains fairly constant throughout the cycle[27]. On the other hand, changes in phosphodiesterase activity occurring during the cycle correlate well with the known effects of cyclic AMP at various stages of growth and development, and it was known previously that the chemotactic effect of cyclic AMP during aggregation is facilitated by the extracellular release of phosphodiesterase[28]. It has been suggested that the increased phosphodiesterase activity acts to enhance the passage of chemotactic information between amoebae by maintaining a necessary concentration gradient (or signal-to-noise ratio) for cyclic AMP.

Some insights into the biochemistry of this process have come from studies showing that the activity of a membrane-bound phosphodiesterase, having a high affinity for cyclic AMP (low apparent K_m), reaches a peak during aggregation, and that the secretion of an enzyme with similar kinetic properties occurs during the stage preceding aggregation[29,30]. Because the Michaelis constants of these enzymes are in a range (*ca.* 10^{-6}M) that would provide the greatest latitude in activity at concentrations of cyclic AMP which elicit chemotactic responses (*ca.* 10^{-6}–10^{-8}M), it has been suggested that during aggregation the low K_m enzyme is the physiologically significant form. The location and release of these enzymes during development suggest that during the later stages of the cycle, when higher concentrations of cyclic AMP would be needed to trigger differentiation, the activity of this high affinity phosphodiesterase must be suppressed. Chassy[31] confirmed the presence of a low K_m form of the enzyme in slime moulds, and showed that under certain conditions it could be converted to a form having a lower affinity for cyclic AMP. Besides the possibility that an interconversion of the two forms of phosphodiesterase regulates the level of cyclic AMP, an endogenous inhibitor of phosphodiesterase, whose activity during the cell cycle is a mirror image of that for phosphodiesterase, has been found[32-34]. Some interesting differences in phosphodiesterase and inhibitor activities in non-aggregating mutants have been reported. One mutant maintained high activities of phosphodiesterase throughout the period when the wild type was derepressed by the active release of the inhibitor, and other mutants produced high amounts of inhibitor during a time when phosphodiesterase activity was increasing in the wild type.

The mechanisms by which cyclic AMP acts to produce its effects in the slime mould are completely unknown. A protein in these organisms analogous to bacterial CRP has not been reported, but may exist. A protein kinase which is inhibited by cyclic AMP has been found in the true slime mould *Physarum polycephalum*[35]. The inhibition of this enzyme by cyclic AMP was found to vary with the cell cycle with maximum inhibition occurring during the G_2 phase. A temporal relationship exists between the reversal of the cyclic AMP-inhibited protein kinase activity and the increase in DNA synthesis seen during the S phase, but the complete significance of this is unknown. Whether a similar enzyme exists in cellular slime moulds remains to be determined.

It should be noted that not all species of slime moulds are attracted by cyclic AMP, even though most of them seem capable of producing it[26]. Apparently substances other than cyclic AMP have evolved as chemotactic agents in certain species.

Some of the features of the role of cyclic AMP in these organisms seem unusual, or at least they are not commonly seen in higher forms. One is that cyclic AMP is released into the extracellular medium to affect other cells from the outside, much as hormones act in higher organisms. The release of phosphodiesterase or modulators of phosphodiesterase activity into the extracellular medium also seems unusual, although it may be more common than is realised at present.

10.2.3 Other organisms

The activity of adenylyl cyclase and the intracellular concentration of cyclic AMP in yeast cells are strongly influenced by the conditions of growth[36]. When the organisms are grown in maximally aerated-cultures with low concentrations of glucose and lactate, cyclic AMP levels are elevated twofold upon reaching the stationary phase of growth. Conversely, in cells cultured in high glucose concentrations, relatively low concentrations of cyclic AMP are maintained throughout the growth period. These findings support the notion that the growth of yeast is regulated by a positive control system which may be influenced by the level of cyclic AMP.

A protein which binds cyclic AMP with high affinity has been isolated from several strains of yeast[37]. The protein was found to be devoid of phosphokinase activity and did not inhibit yeast protein kinase. The function of this protein in yeast is unknown, but may be similar to that of CRP in bacteria.

Other primitive organisms which exhibit defined morphogenesis during each cell division and in which cyclic AMP appears to promote differentiation rather than replication are the soil amoebae *Hartmannella culbertosoni* and the eubacterium *Caulobacter crescentus*. In the former organism, taurine and magnesium ions, in the absence of other nutrients, promote the formation of cyclic AMP, causing the amoebae to be transformed into double-walled cysts[38]. In *C. crescentus*, the application of dibutyryl cyclic AMP enhanced the ability of this organism to synthesise β-galactosidase and also to grow and differentiate, although changes in endogenous cyclic AMP could not be correlated with these processes[39].

An especially intriguing series of observations from the standpoint of comparative endocrinology have been made in *Neurospora*. Glycogenolysis in this organism can apparently be increased by glucagon, and the cells were found to contain a membrane-bound adenylyl cyclase which could be activated by glucagon[40, 41]. To our knowledge, this is the most primitive organism in which a response to glucagon has been observed. Whether *Neurospora* can actually synthesise glucagon remains to be seen.

There is some evidence that cyclic AMP exists in vascular plants (see, for example, Ref. 42), but its role in these plants, if any, is at present very obscure.

10.3 ROLE OF CYCLIC AMP IN HIGHER ORGANISMS

Cyclic AMP was first recognised as a regulator of differentiated cell function, but now there is evidence that it may play an important role during growth and development, before the receptors for most hormones are even present. Since this role would be played earlier in the life of the organism than its better understood role in highly differentiated cells, we will consider it first.

10.3.1 Possible role during growth and development

Evidence that cyclic AMP regulates the expression of genetic information in certain lower organisms was summarised in preceding sections, and our purpose in this section will be to consider the evidence for a similar role in higher forms. Evidence for a role of cyclic AMP in tumorigenesis will also be considered.

Cells transformed spontaneously or by a variety of experimental procedures (e.g. infection by oncogenic viruses or exposure to carcinogenic chemicals) have certain properties which distinguish them from parent or normal cells. Thus, transformed cells lose many of the morphological features of untransformed cells; their growth is accelerated; they do not adhere to surfaces as well, although their ability to agglutinate upon exposure to certain plant lectins is increased; they fail to stop multiplying at high saturation densities (i.e., they lose the property of contact-inhibited growth); and their rate of production of specialised molecules such as acid mucopolysaccharides and glycolipids is either lost or reduced. Also, as a general rule, they tend to produce tumours when injected into a susceptible host. Several theories have been proposed as a molecular basis for transformation, and one of these, now supported by observations from a number of laboratories, suggests that reduced levels of cyclic AMP may be responsible.

One line of evidence for this is that increasing the level of cyclic AMP in transformed cells (whether by adding exogenous cyclic AMP or derivatives of cyclic AMP or through the application of agents which increase the accumulation of endogenous cyclic AMP) restores to these cells many of the properties characteristic of untransformed cells. These would include morphological properties[43, 44], reduced rates of growth[44-48] and motility[49], apparent or partial restoration of contact inhibition[50-53], biosynthetic properties[54, 55], reduced sensitivity to plant agglutinins[50], and stronger adhesion to substratum[56]. Morphological changes characteristic of a more highly

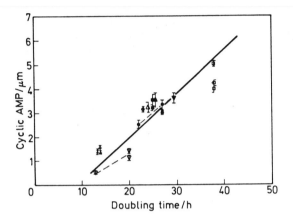

Figure 10.3 Relation of cyclic AMP levels to growth rate of fibroblasts. Each symbol represents a different cell line. Measurements were made over a 2-month period, during which cyclic AMP levels and doubling time decreased in several cell lines, as indicated by the dashed lines. (From Otten et al.[61], by courtesy of Academic Press.)

differentiated state have also been seen after exposure of untransformed cells to exogenous cyclic AMP[57-59].

Direct measurements of cyclic AMP have provided another line of evidence. Levels have generally been lower in transformed than in untransformed cells[44, 51, 53, 60] and an inverse correlation between cyclic AMP levels and growth rate has been demonstrated for a series of transformed cell lines (Figure 10.3)[61]. The relation of cyclic AMP to contact inhibition is currently in dispute. Some observations[51, 53] suggest that cell-to-cell contact may itself lead to increased accumulation of cyclic AMP, and that contact-inhibited cells stop growing *because* of the higher level of cyclic AMP. Other observations[60] indicate that the amount of cyclic AMP per cell is always higher in untransformed than in transformed cells, regardless of the cell density. This important controversy remains to be resolved. In the meantime, the undisputed point to be emphasised is that transformed cells contain less cyclic AMP than untransformed cells.

A particularly impressive demonstration of the role of cyclic AMP in transformation was provided by Pastan and his colleagues[62] using a temperature-sensitive mutant of the Rous sarcoma virus. Both it and the wild-type virus infect chick embryo fibroblasts at either 40.5 or 36°C, but the mutant is capable of producing transformation only at the lower temperature. In line with this, the wild-type virus reduced the level of cyclic AMP in the fibroblasts to *ca.* 20% of control values at either temperature, whereas the mutant was effective only at the lower temperature. The fall in cyclic AMP preceded the morphological transformation, which could be prevented by exogenous cyclic AMP. Quite apart from what it tells us about transformation, the remarkable effect on cyclic AMP of reducing the temperature from 40.5 to 36°C is noteworthy in and of itself.

It has also been found that agents which stimulate proliferation of non-transformed cells in culture, such as trypsin, insulin, or serum, produce a transient fall in the level of cyclic AMP[53, 60, 63, 64]. Addition of exogenous cyclic AMP (or agents which increase endogenous cyclic AMP) during this period prevents the proliferation which would otherwise occur[63-66].

Also of interest from the standpoint of the regulatory influence of cyclic AMP on cell growth are the studies of Voorhees and his colleagues[67, 68] who have shown that reduced levels of cyclic AMP in epidermal cells correlate well with the excessive rate of cell proliferation in psoriatic lesions. Increasing the level of cyclic AMP in these cells, either through the application of dibutyryl cyclic AMP[67] or by stimulation of adenylyl cyclase[69, 70], effectively inhibits epidermal mitosis.

The cause of the reduced levels of cyclic AMP in rapidly proliferating cells (transformed or otherwise) has not been established. Measurements of adenylyl cyclase activity in broken cell preparations have in general correlated poorly with growth rate (see, for example, Refs. 71–73), but such studies must be viewed with caution because of the danger of introducing artifacts in the course of homogenisation. The nature of this problem is well illustrated by the studies of Ney and his colleagues[74, 75] on an adrenocortical carcinoma which did not respond to ACTH with either an increase in cyclic AMP or steroidogenesis. Adenylyl cyclase in homogenates of this tumour, however, was found to be more responsive to ACTH than the cyclase from normal tissue, and was found to respond to several other hormones besides.

Changes in phosphodiesterase activity may correlate better with changing growth rates, but analysis of this relationship may be complicated by several factors. One is that numerous isozymes of phosphodiesterase have been shown to exist (see Section 10.3.4), and another is the evidence that cyclic AMP may act to induce the synthesis of phosphodiesterase[76, 77].

Regardless of the mechanisms involved, the observations that cyclic AMP is reduced in many types of transformed and rapidly-proliferating cells, together with the evidence that higher levels of cyclic AMP are associated with differentiation[55, 57-59, 78], might suggest that cyclic AMP could be involved in the control of growth and development in an interesting way. It seems possible, for example, that cyclic AMP may fall to very low levels during early embryogenesis, thereby allowing rapid cell division to occur. Subsequent increments in cyclic AMP might serve to limit the rate of cell division and to promote differentiation. Later, as hormone receptors and other mechanisms for stimulating adenylyl cyclase develop, the concentration of cyclic AMP in most cells will rise to higher levels still. At this point cyclic AMP assumes its role as a regulator of differentiated cell function, with increases above this new level leading to one effect, decreases below it to the opposite effect.

Substantial *in vivo* evidence to support this hypothesis, particularly as it relates to early embryogenesis, is not available, although it is known that embryonic levels of cyclic AMP tend to be low[80] and that pre- and post-natal levels tend to rise as hormone receptors develop[13, 81-84].

Observations which do not support this hypothesis, or at least which introduce some new considerations, are those indicating that the replication of some cells may be stimulated instead of inhibited by cyclic AMP. These would include thymic lymphocytes[85], haematopoietic stem cells[86] and salivary acinar cells[87]. Hyperplasia as well as hypertrophy of adrenal cortical cells also seems to be stimulated by cyclic AMP[12]. It should be noted that almost nothing is known about the factors determining whether a cell continues on through the cell cycle or enters the pathway leading to differentiation. There is now evidence that cyclic AMP may be capable of influencing this decision at several points in the cell cycle[65] and further research along these lines should teach us much about the factors involved.

A corollary of this hypothesis, supported especially by the studies of transformed cells *in vitro*, is that reduced levels of cyclic AMP during later life could be responsible for the production of some tumours. Recent observations that malignant hepatic nodules of ethionine-treated rats contained higher levels of cyclic AMP than uninvolved liver[88] are not necessarily at variance with this idea, since reductions in sensitivity to cyclic AMP could lead to effects essentially similar to those produced by reduced levels of the nucleotide. This general point is well illustrated by the example of bacterial mutants lacking CRP. A line of hepatoma cells[89] and an adrenocortical carcinoma[74] had previously been shown to be insensitive to cyclic AMP, and the isolation of lymphoma cell mutants resistant to the cytolytic action of cyclic AMP has just recently been reported[90]. The actual level of cyclic AMP in these cells might be quite irrelevant.

Although the rapid growth and relatively undifferentiated character of certain tumour cells could be understood in principle in terms of reduced levels of (or sensitivity to) cyclic AMP, it is not clear that the ability to metastasise could be understood in similar terms. Defects in the formation or action of cyclic AMP could be a prerequisite for malignancy, however. It is almost certain that more detailed studies of the role of cyclic AMP in growth and development will put us in a better position to understand proliferative disorders in general.

10.3.2 Regulation of differentiated cell function

As pointed out in Section 10.1, the chief established role of cyclic AMP in differentiated cells of higher organisms is to serve as a second messenger for a variety of hormones. Among the hormones which have been shown to produce at least some of their effects by this mechanism are glucagon, the catecholamines, ACTH, TSH, vasopressin, luteinising hormone, FSH and parathyroid hormone. The evidence for this has been reviewed in detail on many previous occasions[3, 11, 12, 14, 15], although the mechanism by which these hormones stimulate adenylyl cyclase is still obscure (see later).

The prostaglandins also produce some of their effects by stimulating adenylyl cyclase. The prostaglandins share with the catecholamines the distinction of being the only agents known which produce some of their effects by way of an increase in cyclic AMP and others by way of a decrease. In the case of the catecholamines, there is a relation between the type of receptor involved and the effect on cyclic AMP, with adrenergic β-receptors mediating the stimulation of adenylyl cyclase. Some[91] but apparently not all[92] α-adrenergic effects are mediated by a fall in the level of cyclic AMP. An analogous sort of relationship in the case of the prostaglandins has not been described. The mechanisms by which these and other agents (e.g. insulin) act to suppress the formation of cyclic AMP has still not been established.

It seems very probable that some of the hypothalamic-releasing hormones influence their target cells in the adenohypophysis by way of cyclic AMP. However, as discussed elsewhere[93] (see also Chapter 2 in this volume), this has been a difficult hypothesis to establish. A major problem here has been the complexity of the anterior pituitary gland, containing as it does at least six different types of hormone-producing cells, such that it has been impossible to know which cells contribute how much to observed changes in cyclic AMP.

Another hormone which may have to be added to this list is secretin, although here again the complexity of the target organ has made analysis difficult. Case and his colleagues[94] noted a bimodal response (an initial rise in cyclic AMP followed by a decline to near basal levels followed by a secondary increase) in response to secretin in the cat pancreas. The significance of this unusual response is unclear at present. A similar change has been reported to occur in the rat liver in response to partial hepatectomy[95].

The effect of a change in the level of cyclic AMP depends upon the type of cell in which the change occurs, i.e. it depends on the prior process of cellular differentiation. Some of the known effects of cyclic AMP and the tissues in which these effects have been demonstrated are listed in Table 10.1. This list is incomplete but should serve to indicate the variety of cellular processes which are subject to regulation by cyclic AMP.

The mechanisms by which most of these effects are produced are unknown, but the mechanism of the glycogenolytic effect is now understood in some detail (Figure 10.4). The first step in this sequence of events involves the binding of cyclic AMP to the regulatory (inhibitory) subunit of a protein kinase, causing the regulatory and catalytic subunits to dissociate[96]. The catalytic subunit then becomes free to catalyse the phosphorylation of phosphorylase kinase and glycogen synthetase, leading to activation in the case of phosphorylase kinase but *inactivation* in the case of glycogen synthetase. The reverse reactions are catalysed by one or more phosphatases. The same sequence occurs in muscle except that in that tissue glucose 6-phosphate is metabolised via the Embden–Meyerhof pathway to lactate and other metabolites.

Cyclic AMP-dependent protein kinases have been shown to be widely distributed throughout Nature[97] and it has been proposed that all of the biological effects of cyclic AMP in higher organisms may be mediated through the activation of these enzymes, the end result depending on the kind

Table 10.1 Some known effects of cyclic AMP

Effect	Tissue in which demonstrated
Glycogenolysis	Liver and muscle
Gluconeogenesis	Liver and kidney
Lipolysis	Adipose tissue
Steroidogenesis	Adrenal cortex and gonads
Insulin secretion	Pancreatic islets
Release of amylase	Parotid gland
Calcium mobilisation	Bone
Hyperpolarisation	Smooth muscle
Relaxation	Smooth muscle
Increased force of contraction	Cardiac muscle
Increased permeability	Many epithelial tissues
Inhibition of aggregation	Platelets
Inhibition of histamine release	Leukocytes
Inhibition of discharge frequency	Cerebellar Purkinje cells
Increased melatonin production	Pineal gland
Dispersion of melanin granules	Melanophores
Release of TSH	Anterior pituitary
Thyroid hormone release	Thyroid gland

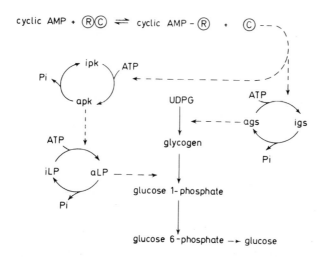

Figure 10.4 Schematic representation of the mechanism by which cyclic AMP stimulates glycogen mobilisation in the liver. R and C represent the regulatory and catalytic subunit respectively of a protein kinase. Other non-standard abbreviations are as follows: i, inactive; a, active; pk, phosphorylase kinase; LP, liver phosphorylase; gs, glycogen synthetase

of substrates phosphorylated. According to this hypothesis, each cell, and possibly each component within the cell, will have a particular substrate which is acted upon by the kinase.

Proteins which have been shown to be substrates for these enzymes, in addition to phosphorylase kinase and glycogen synthetase, include protamine, casein, certain histones[98], nuclear acidic proteins[99], adipose tissue lipase[100], a ribosomal protein[12,101], and several membrane proteins[102]. An additional intriguing possibility is that microtubular protein (tubulin) may serve as a

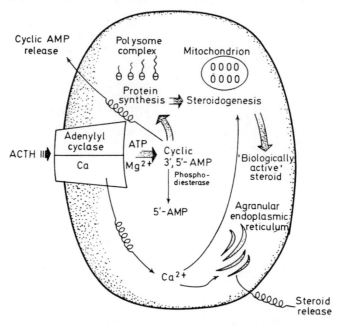

Figure 10.5 Model illustrating possible relationship between calcium and cyclic AMP in the action of ACTH on adrenocortical cells. Interaction of ACTH with its receptor leads to dissociation of Ca^{2+} from a membrane binding site, which may be necessary not only for cyclase activation but also in order for the steroidogenic effect of cyclic AMP to be expressed. (Modified from Rubin *et al.*[107], by courtesy of Macmillan.)

substrate for protein kinases under certain conditions[103] and may also be a source of the enzyme[104]. Microtubular protein is thought to play an important role in a variety of cellular functions ranging from spindle formation during mitosis through maintenance of cell morphology[59,105] to such highly specialised functions as exocytosis[103] and all of these processes are known to be influenced by cyclic AMP.

Calcium ions are involved in many cyclic AMP-mediated responses. In the process outlined in Figure 10.4, for example, calcium is required for the action of phosphorylase kinase, so that in the absence of Ca^{2+} glycogenolysis will not occur, regardless of the level of cyclic AMP. Cyclic AMP and calcium may be even more intimately involved in some hormonal responses, such as the steroidogenic response to ACTH. It was known previously that Ca^{2+}

was required for cyclase activation in response to ACTH[106]. Rubin *et al.*[107] have now presented evidence suggesting that the ACTH-receptor interaction leads to an effect on calcium translocation in addition to its effect on adenylyl cyclase, and that both effects are required in order for steroidogenesis to be stimulated. A model based on Rubin's data is shown in Figure 10.5. Similar proposals have been advanced in the cases of insect salivary gland secretion in response to serotonin[108] and the positive inotropic response to glucagon and the catecholamines[109].

The possibility that systems other than the protein kinase system might be involved in some of the actions of cyclic AMP has long seemed attractive, especially in view of the known role of CRP in bacteria. A microsomal binding protein which may play a role somewhat analogous to that of CRP has now been isolated by Donovan and Oliver[110]. This protein has high affinity for cyclic AMP and appears essential for the release of tyrosine transaminase from liver polysomes. A translational site of action for cyclic AMP in the induction of this enzyme had been postulated previously on the basis of other data[111].

Cyclic AMP may also play a role in sensory physiology, in addition to its role as a mediator of hormone action. This suggestion is based largely on the demonstration that light inactivates adenylyl cyclase in rod outer segments of the frog retina[112]. The interesting finding has also been reported that bitter but not sweet substances were capable of inhibiting phosphodiesterase activity in preparations of vertebrate taste buds[113]. It is perhaps obvious that a great deal of additional work remains to be done before the role of cyclic AMP in sensory physiology can be defined.

Unfortunately, cyclic AMP may also be a mediator of certain disease processes. The best established example of this at the present time is cholera[114].

10.3.3 Hormonal control of adenylyl cyclase activity

Earlier evidence that hormones which stimulate adenylyl cyclase do so by interacting with specific receptors on the external surface of the cell membrane has been buttressed by observations that hormones covalently linked to insoluble beads too large to possibly enter cells nevertheless retain their activity[115,116].

The mechanism by which the hormone–receptor interaction on the external surface of the membrane leads to an increase in the catalytic activity of adenylyl cyclase on the inside surface is poorly understood, although investigators are increasingly coming to grips with this problem. Some hormones, such at ACTH, seem to require Ca^{2+} in order to be effective; the calcium does not seem to be required for binding, but rather for some later step in the activation process[101]. Most hormones do not seem to have this requirement.

A requirement for GDP or GTP or related nucleoside phosphate (which may be masked in many experiments by the high concentration of ATP added as substrate) was discovered by Rodbell and his colleagues[117] for the stimulation of hepatic adenylyl cyclase by glucagon. A similar requirement has now been demonstrated for the activation of pancreatic β-cell cyclase by glucagon[118], of platelet cyclase by prostaglandin E_1 (PGE_1)[119], of toad bladder cyclase by oxytocin[120], and of thyroid cyclase by TSH or PGE_1[121]. It is beginning to appear, therefore, that this requirement may be universal. Rapid binding and dissociation of the hormone or prostaglandin appear to be essential for cyclase activation, but whether these are the most important parameters influenced by the nucleotides remains to be established.

A requirement for phospholipids has also been demonstrated, and Levey[122] has reported that different phospholipids may be required for different hormones. Levey solubilised cat heart adenylyl cyclase and found, after chromatography, that phosphatidyl serine would restore sensitivity to glucagon but not to catecholamines, whereas phosphatidyl inositol would restore sensitivity to catecholamines but not to glucagon. Current evidence suggests that phosphatidyl inositol is not required for catecholamines to bind to the β-receptor, but seems rather to be required in order for the hormone–receptor interaction to be effective in terms of cyclase activation[123]. This suggests that an earlier conclusion equating the development of sensitivity of brain slices to norepinephrine with the development of adrenergic receptors[81] may have been premature. It is equally possible that receptors develop before they become an integral part of an adenylyl cyclase system.

Numerous other factors appear to influence the hormonal sensitivity of adenylyl cyclase, and most of them are poorly understood. Studies of the pineal gland have shown that a number of physiological and pharmacological conditions increase the sensitivity of adenylyl cyclase to stimulation by catecholamines without appreciably altering basal enzymatic activity[124, 125]. An example of this enhanced stimulation by catecholamines caused by a reduction in sympathetic input is illustrated in Figure 10.6. These results might suggest that under normal conditions pineal adenylyl cyclase is resistant to excessive stimulation by catecholamines released from nerve endings because the nerves also exert an inhibitory influence on the system. Conditions which decrease sympathetic input (e.g. superior cervical ganglionectomy or continuous light exposure) remove this inhibitory influence and allow the system to respond maximally. Further studies of this system may lead to an improved understanding of the phenomenon of supersensitivity.

An interesting phenomenon observed in many tissues, including the pineal gland[124], is that cells become refractory to further stimulation after the first application of a hormone. One possible explanation of this phenomenon is that a feed-back regulator of adenylyl cyclase is released as a result of cyclase activation. There is evidence that prostaglandins[126] and other lipophilic substances[127] may function in this capacity in fat cells. Evidence of a similar role for adenosine has been presented by Fain and his colleagues[128].

An important recent finding by Schwabe and Ebert[129] has been that the accumulation of cyclic AMP in fat cells in response to hormones and other agents depends strongly on the cell density. When the cells were incubated at a concentration of 100 000 cells per ml, for example, epinephrine was found to produce only a slight effect by itself, but a substantially greater effect (of the order of five to tenfold) in the presence of theophylline. This was similar to many previous observations and could be understood simply in terms of epinephrine stimulating adenylyl cyclase and theophylline inhibiting phosphodiesterase. However, when the cells were incubated at a density of only 20 000 cells per ml, then epinephrine produced a large effect by itself,

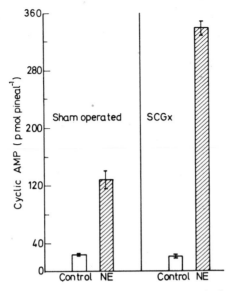

Figure 10.6 Effect of reduced sympathetic activity on the response of the pineal gland to norepinephrine. Ten weeks after bilateral superior cervical ganglionectomy (SCGx), pineal glands were incubated in the presence and absence of maximally effective concentrations of norepinephrine (50 μM). Glands were removed 10 min after the addition of norepinephrine and assayed for cyclic AMP. (From Strada and Weiss[125], by courtesy of Academic Press.)

similar to that seen at the higher density in the presence of theophylline, and theophylline did not markedly increase this, even at submaximal concentrations of epinephrine. Schwabe and Ebert interpreted these results as indicating the presence of an endogenous inhibitor of adenylyl cyclase which was diluted out at the lower cell density, and suggested that theophylline might act by antagonising the formation or action of this inhibitor. It is of interest that many of the effects of adenosine or adenosine nucleotides[130], including the ability of these agents to elevate cyclic AMP in brain tissue[131], can be antagonised effectively by theophylline. It is possible that many of the effects of the methylxanthines previously attributed to phosphodiesterase inhibition will be found instead to involve antagonism of purinergic stimulation.

The mechanism by which cholera toxin acts to stimulate adenylyl cyclase is still unknown[114, 132]. The insidious and apparently irreversible effect of this toxin is quite unlike the reversible effect produced by hormones, almost as if the toxin were acting to destroy some factor which normally maintains the cyclase in a reduced state of activity. This effect is ordinarily limited to intestinal mucosal cells, under pathological circumstances, but can be produced experimentally in many other types of cells. Cholera toxin therefore holds promise of becoming an extremely valuable tool in investigations designed to elucidate the relation of adenylyl cyclase to other membrane constituents.

10.3.4 Cyclic nucleotide phosphodiesterases

The existence of phosphodiesterase activity capable of hydrolysing cyclic AMP to 5'-AMP was established at an early date. The possible complexity of this activity, as a system, was indicated by its presence in soluble as well as particulate fractions. A puzzling feature of the early experiments was that the K_m for cyclic AMP appeared to be much higher, by several orders of magnitude, than the concentration of cyclic AMP in most cells.

It is now known[133] that most cells contain at least two forms of phosphodiesterase activity, one with a high K_m, of the order of 10^{-4} M, and the other with a lower K_m, closer to 10^{-6} M. Since the latter K_m is closer to the concentration of cyclic AMP found in most cells, it has been suggested that this form of the enzyme may be physiologically more important insofar as the metabolism of cyclic AMP is concerned. The kinetic data which led to this conclusion could also have been interpreted in terms of one enzyme showing negative co-operativity[134].

More direct evidence for the existence of multiple forms of phosphodiesterase activity has been obtained by physical separation techniques. Two fractions were separated by column chromatography, a high molecular weight fraction with a high K_m for cyclic AMP and a low molecular weight fraction with a low K_m[133, 135]. More recent experiments using gel electrophoresis have provided evidence for at least six and possibly more than six separate isozymes[136, 137], which are distributed differently in different cells and tissues.

To further complicate this picture, a number of endogenous factors have been shown to have an influence on phosphodiesterase activity. Cheung[138] described a heat-stable protein with an apparent molecular weight of *ca.* 40 000 capable of activating phosphodiesterase. Kakiuchi *et al.*[135] later showed that only one of the two peaks which they isolated chromatographically was affected by this factor, the result being that it greatly enhanced the sensitivity to stimulation by calcium ions. Similarly, it was found that only some of the isozymes obtained from rat brain by gel electrophoresis were sensitive to activation by this factor[13,137,139].

It is clear that many of the earlier experiments dealing with phosphodiesterase will have to be reconsidered, since these studies often failed to take into account the complexity of the system. The full significance of the various isozymes of phosphodiesterase and their variable distribution and sensitivities to endogenous activators and inhibitors remains to be established but already there are indications that these factors may be physiologically very important. The release of a phosphodiesterase inhibitor from certain species of cellular slime moulds was mentioned previously (Section 10.2.2). We found that the ontogenetic development of phosphodiesterase isozymes, as well as the activity of an endogenous activator, differed considerably from one part of the rat brain to another[13,83,139]. An intriguing finding by Monn *et al.*[136] was that testicular tissue contains an isozyme which is not seen until sexual maturation.

Of possible pathological significance, Amer[140] has shown that aortas from genetically hypertensive rats contain higher phosphodiesterase activity (especially the low K_m form of the enzyme) than aortas from non-hypertensive rats. This could account, at least in part, for the lower levels of cyclic AMP found in aortas from hypertensive rats. The importance of phosphodiesterase activity in the regulation of vascular tone is further supported by the correlation which has been demonstrated between the potencies of certain drugs as phosphodiesterase inhibitors and their antihypertensive activity *in vivo*[141].

It is also possible that some hormones may produce at least some of their effects by influencing phosphodiesterase activity. The mechanisms by which insulin suppresses the accumulation of cyclic AMP in liver and adipose tissue have still not been established, but evidence for an involvement of phosphodiesterase has been presented. Loten and Sneyd[142] found that exposure of fat cells to insulin raised the maximal velocity of the low K_m enzyme present in homogenates of these cells, and more recently House *et al.*[143] have reported a significant increase of low K_m activity in a sub-fraction of rat liver membranes after exposure to physiological concentrations of insulin.

An effect of pancreozymin on rabbit gall bladder phosphodiesterase has also been noted[144]. This effect was associated with a relative increase in the activity of the low K_m form of the enzyme. Such a shift might explain some of the pancreatic effects of this hormone[94] as well as its effects on smooth muscle function.

10.4 CYCLIC GMP

The biological significance of cyclic GMP (guanosine 3′,5′-monophosphate), the only 3′,5′-mononucleotide other than cyclic AMP known to occur in Nature, is still obscure. Cyclic GMP is formed from GTP under the catalytic influence of guanyl cyclase, which in many tissues appears to be a soluble rather than a membrane-bound enzyme[9, 145]. The high K_m phosphodiesterase discussed in the preceding section has generally been found to have a lower K_m for cyclic GMP. It may function *in vivo*, therefore, primarily as a cyclic GMP phosphodiesterase.

Several observations have been made during the past few years which suggest that cyclic GMP may play an important role in the regulation of biological processes. Although most of the hormones which have been shown to increase cyclic AMP levels do not seem to affect cyclic GMP, acetylcholine has been shown to increase the level of cyclic GMP in a number of tissues. In all cases studied, this has been shown to be mediated by muscarinic rather than nicotinic receptors[146, 147] and to require the presence of Ca^{2+} in the extracellular medium[148]. It seems possible, therefore, that cyclic GMP and calcium are involved in an important way in the mediation of muscarinic responses.

Hadden and Goldberg and their colleagues[149] have recently reported a remarkable increase in cyclic GMP in lymphocytes in response to phytohaemagglutinin. The preparation of phytohaemagglutinin used in these experiments possessed mitogenic activity but was free of agglutinating activity, and was found to have no effect on the level of cyclic AMP. It seems possible, therefore, that cyclic GMP may have an important role to play in regulating the immune response.

Hadden et al.[149] have suggested that cyclic AMP and cyclic GMP may act 'dualistically' as antagonists of each other, much as the sympathetic and parasympathetic divisions of the autonomic nervous system are known to oppose one another. The evidence to support this hypothesis is not overwhelming at present, but may develop. In the meantime, there are several indications that the relationship between the two cyclic nucleotides may be more complex than the simple dualistic role envisioned by Hadden and Goldberg. Although the exogenous application of cyclic GMP has been found occasionally to produce effects opposite to those produced by cyclic AMP, such as on heart rate[150] and synaptic transmission[151], in most cases exogenous cyclic GMP has been found to be inactive or to produce effects similar to those of cyclic AMP[9]. An interesting sex difference was noted in the case of the anterior pituitary gland, with cyclic GMP being more effective than cyclic AMP in stimulating growth hormone release from female pituitaries, and cyclic AMP being more effective than cyclic GMP in male pituitaries[152]. Further complexity is suggested by observations that cyclic GMP stimulates the hydrolysis of cyclic AMP in preparations of some tissues while inhibiting it in others[145].

The existence of cyclic GMP-sensitive protein kinases in some tissues suggests that cyclic GMP and cyclic AMP may at times act in a similar or complementary fashion, rather than antagonistically. Some recent observations by Greengard and his colleagues are of interest in this regard. They have studied a cyclic GMP-dependent protein kinase from lobster muscle[153]. By combining the catalytic subunit of this enzyme with the regulatory subunit of a cyclic AMP-dependent kinase from beef brain, they were able to convert the lobster enzyme to a cyclic AMP-dependent kinase.

Greengard and his colleagues[154] have also studied a heat-stable protein from lobster muscle which appears to be similar to one previously found in mammalian tissues[96]. This protein was found to inhibit the kinase-catalysed phosphorylation of most substrates, but was stimulatory in a few instances. When arginine-rich histone was used as substrate, the modulator protein was found to inhibit kinase activity in the presence of cyclic AMP but to stimulate activity in the presence of cyclic GMP. A protein with similar properties was shown to exist in several mammalian tissues. Most of the available evidence[96,155] suggests that this protein affects protein kinase activity by binding to the catalytic subunit, but how this could lead to stimulation under some conditions while inhibiting under others remains to be explained. Whether the concentration or activity of this protein ever changes in response to physiological stimuli remains to be determined.

10.5 SUMMARY

Cyclic AMP is widely distributed throughout the animal kingdom, and its role as a regulator of cell function appears to have emerged at a very early stage in the evolutionary process. In gram-negative bacteria it is required for the synthesis of inducible enzymes, and does not occur in these organism when these enzymes are not required. In certain species of cellular slime moulds its appearance serves as a signal to initiate aggregation, leading ultimately to the formation of a multicellular organism.

A series of recent observations has suggested that cyclic AMP may also play an important role during the growth and development of higher organisms. Data are insufficient at present to define this role precisely, but the bulk of experimental evidence suggests that reducing the level of cyclic AMP in most types of cells leads to rapid cell division. Conversely, increasing the level of cyclic AMP favours differentiation. Defects in the formation or action of cyclic AMP may be responsible for many proliferative disorders, including certain forms of cancer.

The chief recognised role of cyclic AMP in higher organisms is to serve as a second messenger mediating the effects of a number of hormones. These hormones act by stimulating adenylyl cyclase in the cells of their target tissues. The mechanism by which the hormone–receptor interaction on the external surface of the membrane leads to increased adenylyl cyclase activity on the other side of the membrane is still obscure. Cholera toxin, which produces an apparently irreversible increase in adenylyl cyclase activity, unlike the reversible effects produced by hormones, may become a useful tool in future studies. The hormonal sensitivity of adenylyl cyclase appears to be modulated by a variety of endogenous activators and inhibitors, although most of these factors remain to be identified.

Regulation of the metabolism of cyclic AMP appears to be much more complex than assumed originally. Phosphodiesterase activity has now been shown to be composed of a series of isozymes with different properties and sensitivities to endogenous activators and inhibitors. Some hormones, such as insulin, may produce at least some of their effects by influencing phosphodiesterase activity.

Many and perhaps most of the physiologically important effects of cyclic AMP in differentiated cells may be the result of increased protein kinase activity. Protein kinases which require cyclic AMP for activity have been shown to be widely distributed, and many proteins in addition to phosphorylase kinase and glycogen synthetase have been shown to act as substrates for these enzymes. According to one hypothesis, cyclic AMP produces different effects in different cells because the cells contain different substrates for protein kinase. It is also possible that cyclic AMP produces some of its effects by mechanisms not involving changes in protein kinase activity.

Cyclic GMP is the only 3′,5′-mononucleotide other than cyclic AMP known to occur naturally, but its biological role has yet to be established. Recent observations suggest that it may play a role in certain cholinergic responses, and a role in lymphocyte transformation during the immune response has also been suggested.

References

1. Sutherland, E. W. and Rall, T. W. (1960). The relation of adenosine 3′,5′-phosphate and phosphorylase to the actions of catecholamines and other hormones. *Pharmacol. Rev.*, **12**, 265

2. Sutherland, E. W., Rall, T. W. and Menon, T. (1962). Adenyl cyclase I. Distribution, preparation and properties. *J. Biol. Chem.*, **237**, 1220

3. Robison, G. A., Butcher, R. W. and Sutherland, E. W. (1971). *Cyclic AMP* (New York: Academic Press)

4. Sutherland, E. W. (1972). Studies on the mechanism of hormone action. *Science*, **177**, 401

5. Sutherland, E. W., Øye, I. and Butcher, R. W. (1965). The action of epinephrine and the role of the adenyl cyclase system in hormone action. *Recent Progr. Hormone Res.*, **21**, 623

6. Sutherland, E. W. and Robison, G. A. (1966). The role of cyclic AMP in responses to catecholamines and other hormones. *Pharmacol. Rev.*, **18**, 145

7. Breckenridge, B. McL. (1970). Cyclic AMP and drug action. *Ann. Rev. Pharmacol.*, **10**, 19

8. Jost, J. P. and Rickenberg, H. V. (1971). Cyclic AMP. *Ann. Review of Biochemistry*, **40**, 741

9. Hardman, J. G., Robison, G. A. and Sutherland, E. W. (1971). Cyclic nucleotides. *Ann. Rev. Physiol.*, **33**, 311

10. Cheung, W. Y. (1972). Adenosine 3′,5′-monophosphate: On its mechanism of action. *Perspect. Biol. Med.*, **15**, 221

11. Major, P. W. and Kilpatrick, R. (1972). Cyclic AMP and hormone action. *J. Endocrinol.*, **52**, 593

12. Gill, G. N. (1972). Mechanism of ACTH action. *Metabolism*, **21**, 571

13. Weiss, B. and Strada, S. J. (1973). Adenosine 3′,5′-monophosphate during fetal and postnatal development. *Fetal Pharmacology*, pp. 205–235 (L. Boreus, editor) (New York: Raven)

14. Robison, G. A., Nahas, G. G. and Triner, L. (1971). *Cyclic AMP and Cell Function* (New York: Academy of Sciences)

15. Greengard, P., Paoletti, R. and Robison, G. A. (1972). *Physiology and Pharmacology of Cyclic AMP* (New York: Raven)

16. Greengard, P., Paoletti, R. and Robison, G. A. (1972). *New Assay Methods for Cyclic Nucleotides* (New York: Raven)

17. Pastan, I. and Perlman, R. L. (1972). Regulation of gene transcription in *Escherichia coli* by cyclic AMP. *Advan. Cyclic Nucleotide Res.*, **1**, 11

18. Hong, J. S., Smith, G. R. and Ames, B. N. (1971). Adenosine 3′,5′-cyclic monophosphate concentration in the bacterial host regulates the viral decision between lysogeny and lysis. *Proc. Nat. Acad. Sci. (U.S.A.)*, **68**, 2248

19. Grodzicker, T., Arditti, R. and Eisen, H. (1972). Establishment of repression by lamboid phage in catabolite activator protein and adenylate cyclase mutants of *Escherichia coli*. *Proc. Nat. Acad. Sci. (U.S.A.)*, **69**, 366

20. Yokota, T. and Kasuga, T. (1972). Requirement for adenosine 3′,5′-cyclic phosphate for formation of the phage lambda receptor in *Escherichia coli*. *J. Bacteriol.*, **109**, 1304

21. Pearson, M. L. (1972). The role of adenosine 3′,5′-cyclic monophosphate in the growth of bacteriophage lambda. *Virology*, **49**, 605

22. Todaro, G. J. and Huebner, R. J. (1972). The viral oncogene hypothesis: new evidence. *Proc. Nat. Acad. Sci. (U.S.A.)*, **69**, 1009

23. Khandelwal, R. L. and Hamilton, I. R. (1972). Effectors of purified adenyl cyclase from *Streptococcus salivarus*. *Arch. Biochem. Biophys.*, **151**, 75

24. Sahyoun, N. and Durr, I. F. (1972). Evidence against the presence of cyclic AMP and relevant enzymes in *Lactobacillus plantarum*. *J. Bacteriol.*, **112**, 421

25. Bonner, J. T. (1971). Aggregation and differentiation in the cellular slime molds. *Ann. Rev. Microbiol.*, **25**, 75

26. Konijn, T. M. (1972). Cyclic AMP as a first messenger. *Advan. Cyclic Nucleotide Res.*, **1**, 17

27. Rossomando, E. F. and Sussman, M. (1972). Adenyl cyclase in *Dictyostelium discoideum:* A possible control element of the chemotactic system. *Biochem. Biophys. Res. Commun.*, **47**, 604

28. Goidl, E. A., Chassy, B. M., Love, L. L. and Krichevsky, M. I. (1972). Inhibition of aggregation and differentiation of *Dictyostelium discoideum* by antibodies against adenosine 3′,5′-cyclic monophosphate diesterase. *Proc. Nat. Acad. Sci. (U.S.A.)*, **69**, 1128

29. Pannbacker, R. G. and Bravord, L. J. (1972). Phosphodiesterase in *Dictyostelium discoideum* and the chemotactic response to cyclic adenosine monophosphate. *Science*, **175**, 1014
30. Malchow, D., Nagele, B., Schwartz, H. and Gerisch, G. (1972). Membrane-bound cyclic AMP phosphodiesterase in chemotactically responding cells of *Dictyostelium discoideum*. *Europ. J. Biochem.*, **28**, 136
31. Chassy, B. M. (1972). Cyclic nucleotide phosphodiesterase in *Dictyostelium discoideum*: Interconversion of two-enzyme forms. *Science*, **175**, 1016
32. Riedel, F. and Gerisch, G. (1971). Regulation of extracellular cyclic-AMP-phosphodiesterase activity during development of *Dictyostelium discoideum*. *Biochem. Biophys. Res. Commun.*, **42**, 119
33. Gerisch, G., Malchow, D., Riedel, V., Muller, E. and Every, M. (1972). Cyclic AMP phosphodiesterase and its inhibitor in slime mould development. *Nature (London)*, **234**, 90
34. Riedel, F., Malchow, D., Gerisch, G. and Nagele, B. (1972). Cyclic AMP phosphodiesterase interaction with its inhibitor of the slime mold, *Dictyostelium discoideum*. *Biochem. Biophys. Res. Commun.*, **46**, 279
35. Kuehn, G. D. (1972). Cell cycle variation in cyclic adenosine 3',5'-monophosphate-dependent inhibition of a protein kinase from *Physarum polycephalum*. *Biochem. Biophys. Res. Commun.*, **49**, 414
36. Sy, J. and Richter, D. (1972). Content of cyclic 3',5'-adenosine monophosphate and adenylyl cyclase in yeast at various growth conditions. *Biochemistry*, **11**, 2788
37. Sy, J. and Richter, D. (1972). Separation of a cyclic 3',5'-adenosine monophosphate binding protein from yeast. *Biochemistry*, **11**, 2784
38. Raizada, M. K. and Murti, C. R. K. (1972). Transformation of trophic *Hartmannella culbertsoni* into viable cysts by cyclic 3',5'-adenosine monophosphate. *J. Cell Biol.*, **52**, 743
39. Shapiro, L., Agabian-Keshishian, N., Hirsch, A. and Rosen, O. M. (1972). Effect of dibutyryl adenosine 3',5'-cyclic monophosphate on growth and differentiation in *Caulobacter crescentus*. *Proc. Nat. Acad. Sci. (U.S.A.)*, **69**, 1225
40. Flawia, M. M. and Torres, H. N. (1972). Adenylate cyclase activity in *Neurospora crassa*. I. General Properties. *J. Biol. Chem.*, **247**, 6873
41. Flawia, M. M. and Torres, H. N. (1972). Activation of membrane-bound adenylate cyclase by glucagon in *Neurospora crassa*. *Proc. Nat. Acad. Sci. (U.S.A.)*, **69**, 2870
42. Salomon, D. and Mascarenhas, J. P. (1971). Auxin-induced synthesis of cyclic AMP in *Avena coleoptiles*. *Life Sci.*, *Part II*, **10**, 879
43. Johnson, G. S., Friedman, R. M. and Pastan, I. (1971). Cyclic AMP-treated sarcoma cells acquire several morphological characteristics of normal fibroblasts. *Ann. N.Y. Acad. Sci.*, **185**, 413
44. Johnson, G. S. and Pastan, I. (1972). Role of 3',5'-adenosine monophospate in regulation of morphology and growth of transformed and normal fibroblasts. *J. Nat. Cancer Inst.*, **48**, 1377
45. Yang, T. J. and Vas, S. I. (1971). Growth inhibitory effects of adenosine 3',5'-monophosphate on mouse leukemia L-5178-YR cells in culture. *Experientia*, **27**, 442
46. Schroder, J. and Plagemann, P. G. W. (1971). Growth of Novikoff rat hepatoma cells in suspension culture in the presence of adenosine 3',5'-cyclic monophosphate. *J. Nat. Cancer Inst.*, **46**, 423
47. Paul, D. (1972). Effects of cyclic AMP on SV3T3 cells in culture. *Nature New Biol.*, **240**, 179
48. van Wijk, R., Wicks, W. D. and Clay, K. (1972). Effects of derivatives of cyclic AMP on the growth, morphology, and gene expression of hepatoma cells in culture. *Cancer Res.*, **32**, 1905
49. Johnson, G. S., Morgan, W. D. and Pastan, I. (1972). Regulation of cell motility by cyclic AMP. *Nature (London)*, **235**, 54
50. Sheppard, J. R. (1971). Restoration of contact-inhibited growth to transformed cells by dibutyryl adenosine 3',5'-cyclic monophosphate. *Proc. Nat. Acad. Sci. (U.S.A.)*, **68**, 1316
51. Heidrick, M. L. and Ryan, W. L. (1971). Adenosine 3',5'-cyclic monophosphate and contact inhibition. *Cancer Res.*, **31**, 1313

52. Smets, L. A. (1972). Contact inhibition partly restored after transformation by dibutyryl cyclic AMP. *Nature New Biol.*, **239**, 123

53. Otten, J., Johnson, G. S. and Pastan, I. (1972). Regulation of cell growth by cyclic adenosine 3'-5'-monophosphate. *J. Biol. Chem.*, **247**, 7082

54. Johnson, G. S. and Pastan, I. (1972). N^6,O^2-dibutyryl adenosine 3',5'-monophosphate induces pigment production in melanoma cells. *Nature (London)*, **237**, 267

55. Goggins, J. F., Johnson, G. S. and Pastan, I. (1972). The effect of dibutyryl cyclic adenosine monophosphate on synthesis of sulphated acid mucopolysaccharides by transformed fibroblasts. *J. Biol. Chem.*, **247**, 5759

56. Johnson, G. S. and Pastan, I. (1972). Cyclic AMP increases the adhesion of fibroblasts to substratum. *Nature (London)*, **236**, 247

57. Hsie, A. W. and Puck, T. T. (1971). Morphological transformation of chinese hamster cells by dibutyryl adenosine cyclic 3',5'-monophosphate and testosterone. *Proc. Nat. Acad. Sci. (U.S.A.)*, **68**, 358

58. Prasad, K. N. and Hsie, A. W. (1971). Morphological differentiation induced *in vitro* by dibutyryl 3',5'-cyclic monophosphate. *Nature (London)*, **233**, 141

59. Puck, T. T., Waldren, D. A. and Hsie, A. W. (1972). Membrane dynamics in the action of dibutyryl cyclic AMP and testosterone on mammalian cells. *Proc. Nat. Acad. Sci. (U.S.A.)*, **69**, 1943

60. Sheppard, J. R. (1972). Cyclic AMP: Different levels in normal and transformed cells. *Nature New Biol.*, **236**, 14

61. Otten, J., Johnson, G. S. and Pastan, I. (1971). Cyclic AMP levels in fibroblasts: Relationships to growth rate and contact inhibition of growth. *Biochem. Biophys. Res. Commun.*, **44**, 1192

62. Otten, J., Bader, J., Johnson, G. S. and Pastan, I. (1972). A mutation in a Rous sarcoma virus gene that controls cyclic AMP levels and transformation. *J. Biol. Chem.*, **247**, 1632

63. Froehlich, J. E. and Rachmeler, M. (1972). Effect of cyclic AMP on cell proliferation. *J. Cell. Biol.*, **55**, 19

64. Burger, M. M., Bombik, B. M., Breckenridge, B. McL. and Sheppard, J. R. (1972). Growth control and cyclic alterations of cyclic AMP in the cell cycle. *Nature New Biol.*, **239**, 161

65. Willingham, M. C., Johnson, G. S. and Pastan, I. (1972). Control of DNA synthesis and mitosis in 3T3 cells by cyclic AMP. *Biochem. Biophys. Res. Commun.*, **48**, 743

66. Rozengurt, E. and Pardee, A. B. (1972). Opposite effects of dibutyryl cyclic AMP and serum on growth of Chinese hamster cells. *J. Cell Physiol.*, **80**, 273

67. Voorhees, J. J., Duell, E. A. and Kelsey, W. H. (1972). Dibutyryl cyclic AMP inhibition of epidermal cell division. *Arch. Dermatol.*, **105**, 384

68. Voorhees, J. J., Duell, E. A., Bass, L. J., Powell, J. A. and Harrell, E. R. (1972). Decreased cyclic AMP in the epidermis of lesions of psoriasis. *Arch. Dermatol.*, **105**, 695

69. Bronstad, G. O., Elgjo, K. and Øye, I. (1971). Adrenaline increases cyclic 3',5'-AMP formation in hamster epidermis. *Nature New Biol.*, **233**, 78

70. Marks, F. and Grimms, W. (1972). Diurnal fluctuation and β-adrenergic elevation of cyclic AMP in mouse epidermis *in vivo*. *Nature New Biol.*, **240**, 178

71. Makman, M. H. (1971). Conditions leading to enhanced response to glucagon, epinephrine or prostaglandins by adenylate cyclase of normal and malignant cultured cells. *Proc. Nat. Acad. Sci. (U.S.A.)*, **68**, 2127

72. Allen, D. O., Munshower, J., Morris, H. P. and Weber, G. (1971). Regulation of adenyl cyclase in hepatomas of different growth rates. *Cancer Res.*, **31**, 557

73. Butcher, F. R., Scott, D. F., Potter, V. R. and Morris, H. P. (1972). Endocrine control of cyclic AMP levels in several Morris hepatomas. *Cancer Res.*, **32**, 2135

74. Ney, R. L., Hochella, N. J., Grahame-Smith, D. G., Dexter, R. N. and Butcher, R. W. (1969). Abnormal regulation of adenosine 3',5'-monophosphate and corticosterone formation in an adrenocortical carcinoma. *J. Clin. Invest.*, **48**, 1733

75. Schorr, I., Rathnain, P., Saxena, B. B. and Ney, R. L. (1971). Multiple specific hormone receptors in the adenylate cyclase of an adrenocortical carcinoma. *J. Biol. Chem.*, **246**, 5806

76. Manganiello, V. and Vaughan, M. (1972). Prostaglandin E_1 effects on cyclic AMP concentration and phosphodiesterase activity in fibroblasts. *Proc. Nat. Acad. Sci. (U.S.A.)*, **69**, 459

77. D'Armiento, M., Johnson, G. S. and Pastan, I. (1972). Regulation of adenosine 3′,5′-cyclic monophosphate phosphodiesterase activity in fibroblast by intracellular concentrations of cyclic adenosine monophosphate. *Proc. Nat. Acad. Sci. (U.S.A.)*, **69**, 459

78. Chen, S. and Tchen, T. T. (1970). Induction of melanocytogenesis in explants of *Curassus auratus*, the xanthic goldfish, by dibutyryl cyclic AMP. *Biochem. Biophys. Res. Commun.*, **41**, 964

79. Roisen, F. J., Murphy, R. A. and Braden, W. G. (1972). Neurite development *in vitro*. I. The effects of cyclic AMP. *J. Neurobiol.*, **3**, 347

80. Reporter, M. and Rosenquist, G. C. (1972). Adenosine 3′,5′-monophosphate: regional differences in chick embryos at the head process stage. *Science*, **178**, 628

81. Schmidt, M. J., Palmer, E. C., Dettbarn, W. D. and Robison, G. A. (1970). Cyclic AMP and adenyl cyclase in the developing rat brain. *Develop. Psychobiol.*, **3**, 53

82. Weiss, B. (1971). Ontogenetic development of adenyl cyclase and phosphodiesterase in rat brain. *J. Neurochem.*, **18**, 469

83. Weiss, B. and Strada, S. J. (1972). Neuroendocrine control of the cyclic AMP system of brain and pineal gland. *Advan. Cyclic Nucleotide Res.*, **1**, 357

84. Gilman, A. G. (1972). Regulation of cyclic AMP metabolism in cultured cells of the nervous system. *Advan. Cyclic Nucleotide Res.*, **1**, 389

85. MacManus, J. P. and Whitfield, J. F. (1972). Cyclic AMP binding sites on the cell surface of thymic lymphocytes. *Life Sci., Pt. II*, **11**, 837

86. Byron, J. W. (1972). Evidence for a β-adrenergic receptor initiating DNA synthesis in haemopoietic stem cells. *Exptl. Cell Res.*, **71**, 228

87. Guidotti, A., Weiss, B. and Costa, E. (1972). Adenosine 3′,5′-monophosphate concentrations and isoproterenol-induced synthesis of deoxyribonucleic acid in mouse parotid gland. *Molec. Pharmacol.*, **8**, 521

88. Chayoth, R., Epstein, S., and Field, J. B. (1972). Increased cyclic AMP levels in malignant hepatic nodules of ethionine treated rats. *Biochem. Biophys. Res. Commun.*, **49**, 1663

89. Granner, D. K. (1972). Protein kinase: altered regulation in a hepatoma cell line deficient in cyclic AMP-binding protein. *Biochem. Biophys. Res. Commun.*, **46**, 1516

90. Daniel, V., Litwack, G. and Tomkins, G. M. (1973). Induction of cytolysis of cultured lymphoma cells by cyclic AMP and the isolation of resistant mutants. *Proc. Nat. Acad. Sci. (U.S.A)*, **70**, 76

91. Robison, G. A., Langley, P. E. and Burns, T. W. (1972). Adenergic receptors in human adipocytes: divergent effects on cyclic AMP and lipolysis. *Biochem. Pharmacol.*, **21**, 589

92. Batzri, S., Selinger, Z., Schramm, M. and Robinovitch, M. R. (1973). Potassium release mediated by the epinephrine a-receptor in rat parotid slices: properties and relation to enzyme secretion. *J. Biol. Chem.*, **248**, 361

93. Zor, U., Lamprecht, S. A., Kaneko, T., Schneider, H. P. G., McCann, S. M., Field, J. B., Tsafriri, A. and Lindner, H. R. (1972). Functional relations between cyclic AMP, prostaglandins, and luteinizing hormone in rat pituitary and ovary. *Advan. Cyclic Nucleotide Res.*, **1**, 503

94. Case, R. M., Johnson, M., Scratcherd, T. and Sherratt, H. S. A. (1972). Cyclic AMP concentration in the pancreas following stimulation by secretin, cholecystokinin-pancreozymin, and acetylcholine. *J. Physiol.*, **223**, 669

95. MacManus, J. P., Franks, D. J., Youdale, T. and Braceland, B. M. (1972). Increases in rat liver cyclic AMP concentrations prior to the initiation of DNA synthesis following partial hepatectomy or hormone infusion. *Biochem. Biophys. Res. Commun.*, **49**, 1201

96. Walsh, D. A., Brostrom, C. O., Brostrom, M. A., Chen, L., Corbin, J. D., Reimann, E., Soderling, T. R. and Krebs, E. G. (1972). Cyclic AMP-dependent protein kinases from skeletal muscle and liver. *Advan. Cyclic Nucleotide Res.*, **1**, 33

97. Kuo, J. F. and Greengard, P. (1969). Widespread occurrence of cyclic AMP-dependent protein kinase in various tissues and phyla of the animal kingdom. *Proc. Nat. Acad. Sci. (U.S.A.)*, **64**, 1349

98. Langan, T. A. (1971). Cyclic AMP and histone phosphorylation. *Ann. N. Y. Acad. Sci.* **185**, 166

99. Johnson, E. M. and Allfrey, V. G. (1972). Differential effects of cyclic AMP on phosphorylation of rat liver nuclear acidic proteins. *Arch. Biochem. Biophys.*, **152**, 786

100. Corbin, J. D., Brostrom, C. O., Alexander, R. L. and Krebs, E. G. (1972). Cyclic AMP-dependent protein kinase from adipose tissue. *J. Biol. Chem.*, **247**, 3736

101. Garren, L. D., Gill, G. N. and Walton, G. M. (1971). The isolation of a receptor for cyclic AMP from the adrenal cortex: the role of the receptor in the mechanism of action of cyclic AMP. *Ann. N. Y. Acad. Sci.*, **185**, 210

102. Johnson, E. M., Tetsufumi, U., Maeno, H. and Greengard, P. (1972). Cyclic AMP-dependent phosphorylation of a specific protein in synaptic membrane fractions from rat cereberum. *J. Biol. Chem.*, **247**, 5650

103. Rasmussen, H. (1970). Cell communication, calcium ion and cyclic adenosine monophosphate. *Science*, **170**, 404

104. Soifer, D., Laszlo, A. H. and Scotto, J. M. (1972). Intrinsic protein kinase activity in lyophilized preparations of tubulin from porcine brain. *Biochim. Biophys. Acta*, **271**, 182

105. Kirkland, W. L. and Burton, P. R. (1972). Cyclic AMP-mediated stabilisation of mouse neuroblastoma cell neurite microtubules exposed to low temperature. *Nature New Biol.*, **240**, 205

106. Lefkowitz, R. J., Roth, J. and Pastan, I. (1971). ACTH-receptor interaction in the adrenal: a model for the initial step in the action of hormones that stimulate adenyl cyclase. *Ann. N.Y. Acad. Sci.*, **185**, 195

107. Rubin, R. P., Carchman, R. A. and Jaanus, S. D. (1972). Role of calcium and cyclic AMP in action of adrenocorticotrophin. *Nature New Biol.*, **240**, 150

108. Berridge, M. J. and Prince, W. T. (1972). The role of cyclic AMP in the control of fluid secretion. *Advan. Cyclic Nucleotide Res.*, **1**, 137

109. Øye, I. and Langslet, A. (1972). The role of cyclic AMP in the inotropic response to isoprenaline and glucagon. *Advan. Cyclic Nucleotide Res*, **1**, 291

110. Donovan, G. and Oliver, I. T. (1972). Purification and properties of a microsomal cyclic AMP binding protein required for the release of tyrosine aminotransferase from polysomes. *Biochemistry*, **11**, 3904

111. Wicks, W. D. (1971). Regulation of hepatic enzyme synthesis by cyclic AMP *Ann. N.Y. Acad. Sci.*, **185**, 152

112. Bitensky, M. W., Miller, W. H., Gorman, R. E., Neufeld, A. H. and Robinson, R. (1972). The role of cyclic AMP in visual excitation. *Advan. Cyclic Nucleotide Res.*, **1**, 317

113. Kurihara, K. (1972). Inhibition of cyclic nucleotide phosphodiesterase in bovine taste papillae by bitter taste stimuli. *FEBS Lett.*, **27**, 279

114. Carpenter, C. C. J (1972). Cholera and other enterotoxin-related diarrheal diseases. *J. Infect. Dis.*, **126**, 551

115. Venter, J. C., Dixon, J. E., Maroko, P. R. and Kaplan, N. O. (1972). Biologically active catecholamines covalently bound to glass beads. *Proc. Nat. Acad. Sci. (U.S.A.)*, **69**, 1141

116. Johnson, C. B., Blecher, M. and Giorgio, N. A. (1972). Activation of rat liver plasma membrane adenylyl cyclase and fat cell lipolysis by agarose-glucagon. *Biochem. Biophys. Res. Commun.*, **46**, 1035

117. Rodbell, M., Birnbaumer, L., Pohl, S. L. and Kans, H. M. J. (1971). The glucagon-sensitive adenyl cyclase system in plasma membranes of rat liver. V. An obligatory role of guanyl nucleotides in glucagon action. *J. Biol. Chem.*, **247**, 1877

118. Goldfine, I. D., Roth, J. and Birnbaumer, L. (1972). Glucagon receptors in β-cells: binding of ^{125}I-glucagon and activation of adenylate cyclase. *J. Biol. Chem.*, **247**, 1211

119. Krishna, G., Harwood, J. P., Barber, A. J. and Jamiesen, G. A. (1972). Requirement of guanosine triphosphate in the prostaglandin activation of adenylate cyclase of platelet membranes. *J. Biol. Chem.*, **247**, 2253

120. Bockaert, J., Roy, C. and Jard, S. (1972). Oxytocin-sensitive adenylate cyclase in frog bladder epithelial cells. *J. Biol. Chem.*, **247**, 7073

121. Wolff, J. and Cook, G. H. (1973). Activation of thyroid membrane adenylate cyclase by purine nucleotides. *J. Biol. Chem.*, **248**, 350

122. Levey, G. S. (1972). Phospholipids, adenylate cyclase and the heart, *J. Molec. Cell. Cardiol.*, **4**, 283

123. Lefkowitz, R. J. and Levey, G. S. (1972). Norepinephrine: dissociation of β-receptor

binding from adenylate cyclase activation in solubilized myocardium. *Life Sci., Pt. II*, **11**, 821

124. Strada, S. J., Klein, D. C., Weller, J. and Weiss, B. (1972). Effect of norepinephrine on the concentration of cyclic AMP of rat pineal gland in organ culture. *Endocrinology*, **90**, 1470

125. Strada, S. J. and Weiss, B. (1973). Supersensitivity to catecholamines of the adenylate cyclase system of rat pineal gland induced by decreased sympathetic activity. *Molec. Pharmacol.*, in the press

126. Illiano, G. and Cuatrecasas, P. (1971). Endogenous prostaglandins modulate lipolytic processes in adipose tissue. *Nature New Biol.*, **234**, 72

127. Ho, R. J. and Sutherland, E. W. (1971). Formation and release of a hormone antagonist by rat adipocytes. *J. Biol. Chem.*, **246**, 6822

128. Fain, J. N., Pointer, R. H. and Ward, W. F. (1972). Effects of adenosine nucleotides on adenylate cyclase, phosphodiesterase, cyclic AMP accumulation, and lipolysis in fat cells. *J. Biol. Chem.*, **247**, 6866

129. Schwabe, U. and Ebert, R. (1972). Different effects of lipolytic hormones and phosphodiesterase inhibitors on cyclic AMP levels in isolated fat cells. *N.-Schmied. Arch. Pharmacol.*, **274**, 287

130. Burnstock, G. (1972). Purinergic nerves. *Pharmacol. Rev.*, **24**, 509

131. Daly, J. W., Huang, M. and Shimizu, H. (1972). Regulation of cyclic AMP levels in brain tissue. *Advan. Cyclic Nucleotide Res.*, **1**, 375

132. Hynie, S. and Sharp, G. W. G. (1972). The effect of cholera toxin on intestinal adenyl cyclase. *Advan. Cyclic Nucleotide Res.*, **1**, 163

133. Thompson, W. J. and Appleman, M. M. (1971). Cyclic nucleotide phosphodiesterase and cyclic AMP *Ann. N. Y. Acad. Sci. (U.S.A.)*, **185**, 36

134. Russell, T. R., Thompson, W. J., Schneider, F. W. and Appleman, M. M. (1972). Cyclic AMP phosphodiesterase: negative cooperativity. *Proc. Nat. Acad. Sci. (U.S.A.)*, **69**, 1791

135. Kakiuchi, S., Yamazaki, R. and Teshima, Y. (1972). Regulation of brain phosphodiesterase activity: Ca^{2+} plus Mg^{2+}-dependent phosphodiesterase and its activating factor from rat brain. *Advan. Cyclic Nucleotide Res.*, **1**, 455

136. Monn, E., Desantel, M. and Christiansen, R. O. (1972). Highly specific testicular cyclic AMP phosphodiesterase associated with sexual maturation. *Endocrinology*, **91**, 716

137. Uzunov, P. and Weiss, B. (1972). Separation of multiple molecular forms of cyclic AMP phosphodiesterase in rat cerebellum by polyacrylamide gel electrophoresis. *Biochim. Biophys. Acta*, **284**, 220

138. Cheung, W. Y. (1971). Cyclic nucleotide phosphodiesterase: evidence for and properties of a protein activator. *J. Biol. Chem.*, **246**, 2859

139. Strada, S. J. and Uzunov, P. (1972). Distribution and ontogenetic development of multiple phosphodiesterase activities of rat brain. *Fed. Proc. (Fed. Amer. Soc. Exp. Biol.)*, **31**, 514 Abs

140. Amer, M. S. (1973). Cyclic adenosine monophosphate and hypertension in rats. *Science*, **179**, 807

141. Pettinger, W., Sheppard, H., Palkoski, Z. and Renyi, E. (1973). Angiotensin antagonism and antihypertensive activity of phosphodiesterase inhibiting agents. *Life Sci.*, **12**, 49

142. Loten, E. G. and Sneyd, J. G. T. (1970). An effect of insulin on adipose tissue cyclic AMP phosphodiesterase. *Biochem. J.*, **120**, 187

143. House, P. D. R., Poulis, P. and Weidemann, M. J. (1972). Isolation of a plasma membrane subfraction from rat liver containing an insulin-sensitive cyclic AMP phosphodiesterase. *Europ. J. Biochem.*, **24**, 429

144. Amer, M. S. and McKinney, G. R. (1972). Studies with cholecystokinin *in vitro*. IV. Effects of cholecystokinin and related peptides on phosphodiesterase. *J. Pharmacol. Exp. Therap.*, **183**, 535

145. Hardman, J. G., Beavo, J. A., Gray, J. P., Chrisman, T. D., Patterson, W. D. and Sutherland, E. W. (1971). The formation and metabolism of cyclic GMP. *Ann. N. Y. Acad. Sci.*, **185**, 27

146. Kuo, J. F., Lee, T. P., Reyes, P. L., Walton, K. G., Donnelly, T. E. and Greengard, P. (1972). Cyclic nucleotide-dependent protein kinases. X. An assay method for the

measurement of cyclic GMP in various biological materials and a study of agents regulating its levels in heart and brain. *J. Biol. Chem.*, **247**, 16

147. George, W. J., Wilkerson, R. D. and Kadowitz, P. J. (1973). Influence of acetylcholine on contractile force and cyclic nucleotide levels in the isolated perfused rat heart. *J. Pharmacol. Exp. Therap.*, **184**, 228

148. Schultz, G., Hardman, J. G., Schultz, K., Baird, C. E., Parks, M. A., Davis, J. W. and Sutherland, E. W. (1972). Cyclic GMP and cyclic AMP in ductus deferens and submaxillary gland of the rat. *Abstracts V Int. Congr. Pharmacol.*, p. 206

149. Hadden, J. W., Hadden, E. M., Haddox, M. K. and Goldberg, N. D. (1972). Guanosine 3′,5′-cyclic monophosphate: a possible intracellular mediator of mitogenic influences in lymphocytes. *Proc. Nat. Acad. Sci. (U.S.A.)*, **69**, 3024

150. Krause, E.-G., Halle, W. and Wollenberger, A. (1972). Effect of dibutyryl cyclic GMP on cultured beating rat heart cells. *Advan. Cyclic Nucleotide Res.*, **1**, 301

151. McAfee, D. A. and Greengard, P. (1972). Adenosine 3′,5′-monophosphate: electrophysiological evidence for a role in synaptic transmission. *Science*, **178**, 310

152. Cehovic, G. D., Robison, G. A. and Bass, A. D. (1972). Sex-dependent response in the release of growth hormone *in vitro* with different cyclic nucleotides. *Abstracts 3 Int. Congr. Endocrinol.*, p. 83

153. Miyamoto, E., Petzold, G. L., Kuo, J. F. and Greengard, P. (1973). Dissociation and activation of cyclic AMP-dependent and cyclic GMP-dependent protein kinases by cyclic nucleotides and by substrate proteins. *J. Biol. Chem.*, **248**, 179

154. Donnelly, T. E., Kuo, J. F., Reyes, P. L., Liu, Y.-P. and Greengard, P. (1973). Protein kinase modulator from lobster tail muscle. I. Stimulatory and inhibitory effects of the modulator on the phosphorylation of substrate proteins by cyclic GMP-dependent and cyclic AMP-dependent protein kinases. *J. Biol. Chem.*, **248**, 190

155. Donnelly, T. E., Kuo, J. F., Miyamoto, E. and Greengard, P. (1973). Protein kinase modulator from lobster tail muscle. II. Effects of the modulator on holoenzyme and catalytic subunit of cyclic GMP-dependent and cyclic AMP-dependent protein kinases. *J. Biol. Chem.*, **248**, 199

Index